CLASSICS
IN OBSTETRICS AND GYNECOLOGY

CLASSICS
IN OBSTETRICS AND GYNECOLOGY

INNOVATIVE PAPERS THAT HAVE CONTRIBUTED
TO CURRENT CLINICAL PRACTICE

EDITED BY T.K.A.B. ESKES AND L.D. LONGO

The Parthenon Publishing Group
International Publishers in Medicine, Science & Technology

Casterton Hall, Carnforth,
Lancs LA6 2LA, UK

One Blue Hill Plaza, Pearl River,
New York 10965, USA

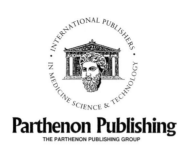

Parthenon Publishing
THE PARTHENON PUBLISHING GROUP

Published in the UK by
The Parthenon Publishing Group Limited
Casterton Hall, Carnforth, Lancs, LA6 2LA, UK

Published in the USA by
The Parthenon Publishing Group Inc.
One Blue Hill Plaza, PO Box 1564, Pearl River, New York 10965, USA

Library of Congress Cataloging-in-Publication Data
Classics in obstetrics and gynecology : innovative papers that have
   contributed to current clinical practice / edited by T.K.A.B. Eskes and
   L.D. Longo
       p. cm.
   Selection of previously published articles, accompanied by commentaries.
   Includes bibliographical references.
   ISBN 1-85070-520-8
   1. Gynecology. 2. Obstetrics. I. Eskes. T.K.A.B. (Tom Kees Anton Bonifacius)
   II. Longo, Lawrence D., 1926-
   [DNLM: 1. Obstetrics–collected works. 2. Gynecology–collected works.
WQ 100 C614 1993]
RG101.C655 1993
618–dc20
DNLM/DLC   93-32241
for Library of Congress   CIP

British Library Cataloguing in Publication Data
Classics in Obstetrics and Gynecology:
Innovative Papers That Have Contributed to Current Clinical Practice
   I. Eskes, Tom K.A.B. II. Longo, L.D.
   618
   ISBN 1-85070-520-8

Designed and Typeset by Gus Hunnybun Associates Limited, Macclesfield
Reproduction by Ryburn Publishing Services, Keele University
Printed and bound in Great Britain by Butler & Tanner Ltd., Frome and London

CONTENTS

ACKNOWLEDGEMENTS

The Editors and Publishers would like to acknowledge with thanks the following permissions that have kindly been granted for the use of material in this publication.

Classic Papers

Williams and Wilkins of Baltimore and the International Anesthesia Research Society for the paper by Apgar; Blackwell Scientific Publications Ltd. for the paper by Barcroft; The Royal Society of Medicine, London for the paper by Braxton Hicks; The Biomedical Society and Portland Press for the paper by Dale; *The Lancet* for the paper by Bevis; Georg Thieme Verlag of Stuttgart for the paper by Hegar; Mosby Year Book Inc. of St. Louis for the papers by Dieckmann, Stein and Leventhal, and Sampson; Medical Science Publishing International, Inc., Port Washington for the paper by Treloar; Organo de la Asociacion Latinoamericana de Ciencelas Fisiologicas, Buenos Aires for the paper by Pincus; and Springer Verlag of Heidelberg for the paper by Fraenkel.

Illustrations

(in addition to acknowledgements shown in the text)
The National Library of Medicine for the photographs of Barcroft, Braxton Hicks and Sampson; Springer Verlag of Berlin and Heidelberg for the photographs of Hegar, Meyer and Fraenkel; The Macmillan Company for the photographs of Aschheim, Zondek and Stein; the Elizabeth Wilcox Photographic Collection, Augustus C. Long Health Sciences Library, Columbia University for the photograph of Apgar; the Armour Pharmaceutical Company for the photograph of Dale; The Department of Obstetrics and Gynecology, University of Chicago for the photograph of Dieckmann; and Drs D.C.A. Bevis and A.E. Treloar who very kindly provided their photographs.

Cover illustrations courtesy of L.D. Longo

THE EDITORS

Professor T.K.A.B. Eskes is Chairman of the Department of Obstetrics and Gynecology, University Hospital, Nijmegen, The Netherlands. He is also the Editor-in-Chief of the European Journal of Obstetrics, Gynecology and Reproductive Biology. He has a special interest in the history of obstetrics and gynecology and one of his regular contributions to the European Journal has been a feature on 'classic illustrations' that have contributed in some special way to the development of knowledge in this field.

Professor Lawrence D. Longo is Head of the Perinatal Biology Center, and Professor of Obstetrics and Gynecology, Physiology, and Pediatrics at Loma Linda University School of Medicine in California. Professor Longo has a special interest in the history of obstetrics and gynecology. He has authored (or edited) five books in this field, as well as contributing more than 50 articles and 60 book chapters to the subject. For almost a decade he prepared the 'Classic Papers in Obstetrics and Gynecology' that were a regular feature in the *American Journal of Obstetrics and Gynecology*.

*This book is dedicated to my wife, Ada,
and my secretary, Gerda: essential ingredients.*

T.K.A.B.E.

*This work is dedicated to my wife,
Betty Jeanne.*

L.D.L.

FOREWORD

Obstetrics and gynecology, like all medical disciplines, have experienced enormous progress throughout this century. This progress has been marked by an equally vast collection of publications, some of which are now regarded as 'classics'.

For 70 years Organon has been dedicated to innovation in medical care, contributing especially to progress in endocrinology. And throughout its history, the company has always co-operated with scientists and universities all over the world. This co-operation is highly valued, and today considered an indispensable requirement of further innovative progress.

That is why we are delighted to be associated with the publication of *Classics in Obstetrics and Gynecology*, a book which commemorates some of the pioneering landmarks in the field – it is based on a concept originally developed by Organon – and illustrates yet again the spirit of co-operation between Organon and science.

The two editors of *Classics in Obstetrics and Gynecology* are eminently suited to their task. Professor T.K.A.B. Eskes from the University of Nijmegen in The Netherlands, Editor-in-chief of the *European Journal of Obstetrics and Gynecology*, has regularly contributed 'Classic illustrations' to that journal. Professor Lawrence D. Longo of Loma Linda University School of Medicine, California, prepared his series of 'Classic papers' for the *American Journal of Obstetrics and Gynecology* for ten years (1970–80). Both editors have a passionate and scholarly interest in the history of obstetrics and gynecology.

We are certain that records and commentaries presented here not only highlight achievements of the past, but also point forward to current practice and to future 'classics'. Organon is proud to be associated with this book.

Professor Hans Vemer
Medical Director
Organon International

EDITORS' PREFACE

The practice of medicine today is the result of the dedicated patient care, observation, research and experimentation undertaken by many previous generations of physicians. The building blocks of progress have been assembled over past decades and centuries by scientists whose primary objective has been to push forward the frontiers of knowledge in order to offer more effective methods of combating disease and promoting health. And fortunately that process continues today.

Amongst the many scientific developments that have led to the modern practice of obstetrics and gynecology, a relatively small number of original insights, discoveries and clinical observations stand out as having had a unique importance and seminal influence. This volume is an attempt to document some of those key developments that have acted as the signposts for clinical progress in our speciality.

Of course, there have been many important papers published in obstetrics and gynecology – and it would be impossible to reproduce all of them within the covers of a single volume. Nor do we wish to claim that the papers we have selected for inclusion in this volume are necessarily the most important ones – any assessment of significance is bound to be subjective to some extent and, in any case, is bound to vary depending on the assessment criteria used. However, what we do believe this book provides is a record of outstanding papers that have contributed notably to modern medicine and which certainly have a place of major importance in the history of obstetrics and gynecology. In addition to the 12 main papers that have been selected for publication in full, we have quoted from over 400 other papers that are relevant and important in the current context – and had space allowed we could certainly have quoted others. No doubt there will be many alternative views about other research and advances that also deserve inclusion and we should welcome readers' views on this – we hope it may be possible to consider some of the other contributions to our field for inclusion in a later volume.

In the meantime we hope that those who read this book will find that it throws some new light on past achievements and provides some valuable perspectives on present practice.

T.K.A.B. Eskes
L.D. Longo
October 1993

HISTORICAL INTRODUCTION

Some significant early contributions to obstetrics and gynecology

1. Graham, H. (1950). *Eternal Eve.* (London: Wm. Heinemann)

As must be self-evident, the history of obstetrics and gynecology goes back to the very beginning of mankind. For, as Harvey Graham noted in 1950[1],

> Everyone is a miracle in miniature with a personal history linked with the history of men and women who lived, loved, and gave birth to others since ever there were men and women.

This miracle of successful reproduction, with the delivery of sentient, thinking, feeling, working human beings, has been recorded in books since the beginning of their making. Thus it is that the history of obstetrics and gynecology comprises one of the richest records of any aspect of medicine. To reflect upon this heritage, doubly precious in that it consists of an account of the beginnings of life, as well as the record of evolution of the specialty, is the purpose of this volume. In this chapter we present illustrations from a few of the classic pre-twentieth century works which contributed in a major way to the development of the specialty. The selection is rather arbitrary, and not all are texts in obstetrics and gynecology *per se*. Nonetheless, they are among the most important volumes in the early evolution of ideas in the reproductive sciences.

Eucharius Rösslin

2. Rösslin, E. (1513). *Der Schwangern Frawen und hebammen Roszgarten.* (Strasborg: M. Flach Jr.)

With the exception of Ortolff von Bayerland's *Frauenbuchlein*, a small volume of 13 pages published about 1495, Eucharius Rösslin's [Röslin, Roesslin] (d.1526), *Der Schwangern Frauwen und hebammen Roszgarten (The Rosegarden of the Pregnant Woman's Nurse)*[2], published in both Hagenau and Strassburg in 1513, was the first printed book dealing exclusively with the subject of obstetrics apart from medicine and surgery. This illustrated obstetrical manual for the use of midwives has a lovely dedicatory woodcut which shows the author presenting the book to Countess Katherine, Duchess of Brunswick and Luneburg, Saxony, to whom he dedicated the volume. An accompanying woodcut (see figure below) shows a midwife about to deliver a woman seated on a birth stool.

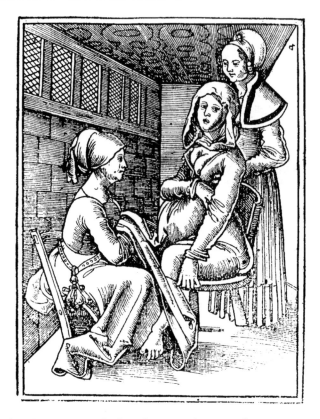

*Midwife with parturient on birth stool. From Eucharius Rösslin's Roszgarten, 1513.
The legend reads 'Come to my aide in the time of a difficult agonizing birth which is
marked by great anxieties, worries, and distress. As this has been reported in chapter
after chapter, so it must be acknowledged so here it is written.'*

The work contains little that is original. Rather, Rösslin compiled writings of the medical authors of antiquity, including Hippocrates, Galen, Soranus of Ephesus, as recorded in Moschion (Muscio or Mustion, fl circa 500), and Rhazes and Avicenna. Rösslin began his work with a preface in verse inveighing against contemporary obstetrical practice, and the ignorance, carelessness, and superstition of midwives, who had a hand in the unnecessary deaths of numberless newborns. Infant mortality, Rösslin labelled murder, for which the guilty ones deserved to be buried alive, or 'broken on the wheel' instead of receiving an honorarium for their services. The instructions in the work are simple and direct. Rösslin described and illustrated for the first time, with twenty woodcuts derived from Moschion's illustrations in manuscripts, normal and abnormal fetal positions, and twins, including Siamese twins. He also referred to podalic version and difficult deliveries. In addition, he described positions for delivery, methods of assisting at delivery, and use of the birth stool. Rösslin included instructions on the care of the child from birth until weaning and the diseases of infancy.

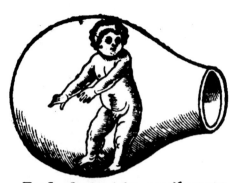

Rurfum fi partus in latus procideret, ope ram dare obftetricem decet, quo in priftinum locum atq; habitum illum reducat, ac deinde ad legitimam conuerfionem, exitumq; promoueat.

Aut fi contingat ut pedibus diuffis ana diftortis, quale eft quod in præfenti figura depingitur, partus progrediatur, cura dum itidem eft, ut pedes in unum reuocentur atq; coniungantur, ac deinde partus ad exitum, cautione tamen ubiq; circa manus illa quam diximus, obferuata, deducatur.

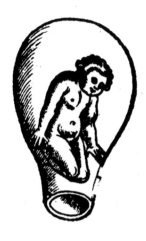

C iiij

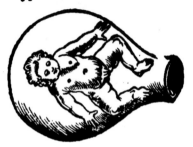

Figures of the fetus in utero, from the first Latin edition of Rösslin's Rozgarten, 1532

Numerous editions followed, including the first Latin edition 'De partu hominis ...'[3] published by Rösslin's son (also named Eucharius) in 1532 (see figure above). It was from this Latin edition that most other translations were made, rather than from the original German. The first English edition 'The Byrth of Mankynde, otherwise named The woman's book'[4] was published in London in 1540. Rösslin's work was popular, and went through over 100 editions including translations. For nearly two centuries it served as the authoritative treatise on obstetrics throughout Europe. Probably no medical book in history has been so widely translated and distributed.

Eucharius Rösslin became apothecary of Freiburg in 1493. In 1506 he was elected physician to the City of Frankfurt am Main and in 1508 he entered service at the court of Katherine. When he published this book he was working as the town physician and supervisor of midwives in Worms. In 1517 he returned to Frankfurt in the same capacity, serving in that post until his death in 1526. His son Eucharius succeeded him as town physician of Frankfurt am Main.

3. Rösslin, E. (1532). *De partu hominis, et quae circa ipsum accidunt. Medici*, Franc. Chri. Egen. Francofurti. xix., Octobris

4. Rösslin, E. (1540). *The Byrth of Mankynde* by Thomas Raynalde. T.R., London

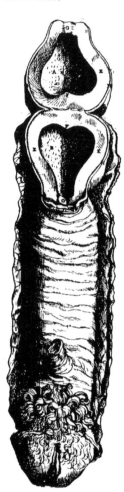

Female organs of reproduction from Andreas Vesalius' Fabrica of 1543. The specimen illustrated, as bifid and split longitudinally, was from a parous woman who had been hanged. The legends may be translated: "A,A,B,B - Sinuses of the fundus uteri. C,D - A line, somewhat like a suture, projecting slightly into the fundus uteri. E,E - The thickness of the inner and proper tunic of the fundus uteri. F,F - A portion of the inner fundus uteri; projecting downward, from its surface. G,G - Orifice of the fundus uteri. H,H - Second and external covering of the fundus uteri reflected from the peritoneum. I,I et cetera - By this we indicate the membranes on both sides which are reflected from the peritoneum and contain the uterus. K - The substance of the cervix uteri, L - A part of the neck of the bladder." (The urethra is incorrectly shown opening into the vagina)

Andreas Vesalius

The epic work which revolutionized the understanding of human anatomy was Andreas Vesalius' (1514–1564) *De humani corporis fabrica libri septum* published in Basel in 1543[5]. The *Fabrica* was a milestone in that in its seven books, one for each major system (bones, muscles, arteries, spinal cord and nerves, abdomen, thorax, head and brain), Vesalius gave a more complete and accurate depiction of human anatomy than any of his predecessors. The woodcut plates are the most famous anatomical illustrations of all time. Vesalius explained the dissections, and insisted that examination of the body must be performed by the physician himself. By undermining the religious-like reverence for authority in science, Vesalius prepared the way for independent observations in anatomy and clinical medicine. Thus, the *Fabrica* is one of the greatest works in medicine.

In Book 1, Vesalius accurately described the human pelvis for the first time. He also demonstrated that it was impossible for the pelvic bones to separate during labor, as was commonly believed at that time. In Book V he first carefully described the uterus, and confirmed Berengario's observation that it contained a single chamber (see figure above). Vesalius also described the insertion of the tubes, the ligaments, and the vasculature.

A native of Brussels, Vesalius studied medicine at Paris, Louvain, and Padua, becoming public prosector of anatomy at the latter institution. He was 29 years old when he published the *Fabrica*. The illustrations have been attributed to Titian's pupil Jan Stephan Kalkar. Following a second, and more complete, edition in 1555, he became court physician to Emperor Charles V and later to Philip II. On the return journey from a pilgrimage to Jerusalem, 1563–1564, he died on the Greek island of Zante.

5. Vesalius, A. (1543). *De humani corporis fabrica libri septem*. (Basel: Ioannis Oporini)

Jacob Rueff

Jacob Rueff (1500–1558), who was responsible for the instruction and examination of midwives in Zurich, improved upon Rosslin's manual. His book for midwives and pregnant women, *De conceptu et generatione hominis* (Zurich, 1554)[6] (see figure below), stressed the importance of knowledge of the anatomy of the female pelvis. The illustrations, derived from Rosslin and Vesalius, were the first in an obstetric book to be based on anatomic reality, rather than showing diagrammatic figures in a bottle or balloon. He described forceps for extraction of the dead fetus. Rueff also discussed cephalic version by combined external and internal version, and manual delivery of the placenta. Rueff portrayed the birth stool with drapery rather than boards on the lower portion, 'So that the child will not be injured and so that ... women assisting the midwife can insert their hands.' Although Rueff believed strongly in astrologic influences on pregnancy, particularly in the development of monsters, his book, with

6. Rueff, J. (1554). *De conceptu et generatione hominis*. (Zurich: C. Froschoverus)

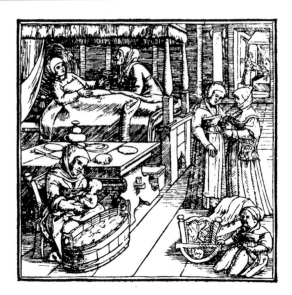

*Frontispiece from Jacob Rueff's De conceptu et generatione..., 1554,
showing scene in lying-in chamber[6]*

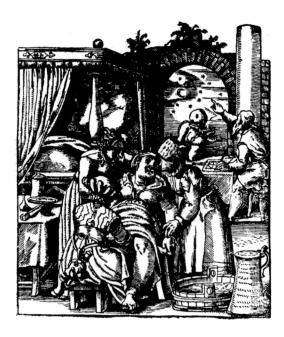

7. Rueff, J. (1580). *De conceptu et generatione
hominis: de matrice et eius
partibus ....* (Frankfurt am
Main: Sigismund
Feyerabend)

*Illustration by Amman for the second edition of Rueff's De conceptu ..., 1580[7].
Shown is the bedchamber of a pregnant noblewoman with a midwife in atten-
dance. An astrologer notes the alignment of the heavenly bodies at the moment
of birth to fortell the infant's future*

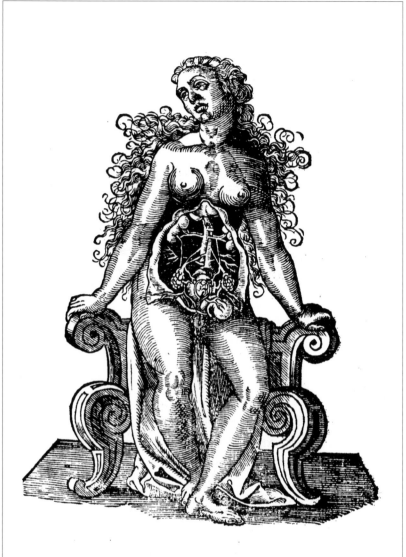

Figure of a pregnant woman from the first English edition of Jacob Rueff's The Expert Midwife, 1637[9]. This figure appeared in Rueff's original edition of 1554

8. Rueff, J. (1554). *Ein schon lustig Trostbuchle von den Empfengknussen und Geburten der Menschen ...*, Tiguri, Apud Frosch [overum]

9. Rueff, J. (1637). *The Expert Midwife, or an Excellent and most necessary Treatise of the generation and birth of Man ....* London, Printed by E. Griffin for S. Burton

Rösslin's, had a great influence on improving obstetric care. An edition in the German vernacular appeared the same year, and was titled Trostbuchle[8] or *"... a comforting booklet of encouragement concerning the conception and birth of man, and its frequent accidents and hindrances, et cetera.* The second edition, with dramatic illustrations by the Swiss artist Jost Amman, was published in 1580[7] (see previous figure). An English translation, *The Expert Midwife*[9], appeared in 1637 (see figure above).

Girolamo Fabrici

10. Fabrizio, G. (1604).
De formato foetu.
Venetiis, per F. Bolzettam,
1600. (Colophon:
Laurentius Pasquatus)

In his magnificently illustrated embryological atlas, *De formato foetu*[10] (Venice, 1604), Girolamo Fabrici (Hieronymus Fabricius ab Aquapendente) (1533–1619) presented more accurately than anyone before, and for long after, the relation of the fetus to the umbilical vessels, the fetal membranes, the placenta, the urachus, and the uterus. Fabricius also described the fetal right and left atria, foramen ovale, ductus arteriosus, vena cava, and pulmonary vein.

The work contains 34 plates which illustrate, in some instances for the first time, various aspects of the anatomy of the uterus and fetus in humans (see figure below), and in other species including sheep, cows, and

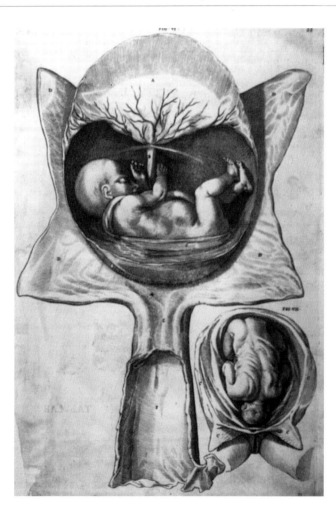

Fetus in utero with placenta and umbilical cord from Fabricius ab Aquapendente's De formato foetu, 1604[10]

horses. Fabricius was the first to study and to illustrate the decidua of the human uterus, and the uterine crypts in animals (interpreted as the open ends of uterine vessels).

An outstanding anatomist, Fabricius published many other works including *De venarum ostiolis* in 1603[11] and *De formatione ovi et pulli* in 1621[12]. The former work played a key role in his student William Harvey's development of the idea of the circulation of the blood.

Adriaan van der Spieghel

During the seventeenth century, anatomic dissection reached a high state of competence and its illustration marked a new epoch when the use of copper plate engravings replaced wood blocks. One of the most exquisite of the anatomic atlases published in that time was that attributed to Adriaan van der Spieghel (1578–1625). Spigelius succeeded Giulio Casserio (1561–1616), an outstanding anatomist, to the Chair of Anatomy at the University of Padua. Casserius had supervised the execution of superb Carreggio-like plates by an unknown artist for a work he planned to publish, the *Theatrum anatomicum*. Spigelius had written a treatise on the pregnant uterus, placenta, and infant. After the deaths of both Casserius and Spigelius, the German physician Daniel Rindfleisch (Bucreitus) carried out his promise to Spigelius to publish his unillustrated treatise on anatomy, enlisting the help of Spigelius' son-in-law Liberalis Crema, who had acquired a number of Casserius' plates from the latter's grandson. Thus, Crema, at his own expense, published with Bucreitus the *De formato foetu...*[13] (Padua, 1626), which consisted of Spigelius' text and Casserius' plates.

The nine plates deal with the pregnant uterus, placenta, and the child, and are among Casserius' most beautiful engravings. Four depict full-length female figures, showing the *foetus in utero* (see figure below), two are of the pregnant uterus and placenta, and three are infants showing their internal organs. Regarding these 'eviscerated beauties', Oliver Wendell Holmes[14] observed 'The figures ... will always attract attention, for the grace and beauty of the females who display their viscera as if they were jewels and laces. These are not likely to be overlooked by the lovers of undisguised nature and naked truth.'

Spigelius was the first in obstetrics to begin by describing the external female genitals (previously all such works had begun with the description of the uterus). He first observed the occurrence of milk in female breasts at birth, denied the presence of nerves in the umbilical cord, and argued against the idea that meconium in its intestines implied that the fetus ate *in utero*. Spigelius believed that maternal blood flows directly from the uterine vessels into the ends of the umbilical vein (rejecting Aranzio's view), to be carried to the fetal liver. However, he correctly stated that the umbilical arteries terminate in the placenta and do not communicate with the uterine arteries.

11. Fabrici, G. (1603). *De venarum ostiolis,* Patavii, ex typ. L. Pasquati

12. Fabrici, G. (1621). *De formatione ovi et pulli,* Patavii, ex off. A. Bencÿ

13. Spigelius, A. (1626). *De formato foetu liber singulairs, aeneis figuris exornatus...* Pataurii, Apud Io. Bap. de Martinis, & Liuiu Pasquatu

14. Holmes, O.W. (1889). *Boston Med. Surg. J.,* **120**, 129

Spigelius, a native of Brussels, studied medicine at Louvain and Padua. After a short period of travelling and work in Belgium, Germany, and Moravia, he succeeded the recently deceased Casserius to the Chair of Anatomy and Surgery at the University of Padua. He improved upon anatomical terminology, and his name is eponymized in the Spigelian lobe (caudate lobe) of the liver and van der Spieghel's line (*the linea semilunaris*).

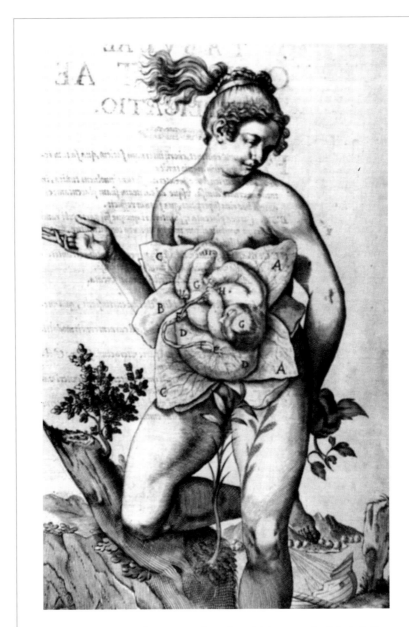

Pregnant woman with near-term fetus, from Adriaan van der Spieghel's De formato foetu, 1626[13]

François Mauriceau

The most outstanding textbook of the mid-seventeenth century, François Mauriceau's (1637–1709) *Des maladies des femmes grosses et accouchées* ...[15], published in Paris in 1668, established obstetrics as a separate specialty and science, and was the dominant force in seventeenth century obstetrical practice. The text includes 30 copper plate engravings of birth figures and obstetric instruments.

Perhaps the first obstetric text in the modern sense, it treats the subject with logical order, clarity, and erudition. Its lengthy subtitle recommends it as useful for surgeons and necessary for midwives. Much of the work was a synthesis of prior teachings. In the preface, Mauriceau advised the reader: 'The doctrine of books, which is one of the most wholesome effectual remedies we have to chase away ignorance, is wholly useless to men's wits, when not disposed to receive it.' Although he recommended the reading of other 'learned' authors, he cautioned that '... the most part of them, having never practiced the art they undertake to teach, resemble ... those geographers, who give us the description of many countries which they never saw.'

Following the introduction which describes anatomic landmarks (see figure), the work is divided into three sections which deal with diseases and abnormalities from conception to the end of pregnancy, normal childbirth, and the care of the mother and newborn infant, including the choice of a suitable wet nurse. The expectant mother was admonished to help shorten the duration of labor by walking about the chamber so that the weight of the child would help dilate the cervix. Furthermore, her pains would be stronger and more frequent. If the midwife perceived that the child was not presenting properly, Mauriceau cautioned her to ' .. send speedily for an expert and dextrous surgeon in the practice, and not delay, as too many of them very often do, till it be reduced to extremity', and admonished her to reassure the patients.

Among the important new features included in Mauriceau's work were the delivery of women in bed rather than in the obstetric chair, treatment of the various gestational periods, and discussion of many difficult cases. He also presented an analysis of the mechanism of labor, and maintained that during labor the uterus is the active agent with the fetus playing a passive role. He gave the earliest account of the prevention of congenital syphilis by antisyphilitic treatment during pregnancy. He was also the first to refer to tubal pregnancy, complications of prolapse of the umbilical cord, and epidemic puerperal fever. Mauriceau practiced podalic version, but condemned both cephalic version and Caesarean section. He gave rules for the management of placenta previa, and advanced the concept of primary repair of perineal lacerations. Mauriceau discredited the observation of Pare and others that the pubic bones separated during childbirth. He also denied that the uterus contains two cavities, and that the amniotic fluid is

15. Mauriceau, F. (1668). *Des maladies des femmes grosses et accouchées.* Paris, chez l'Auteur

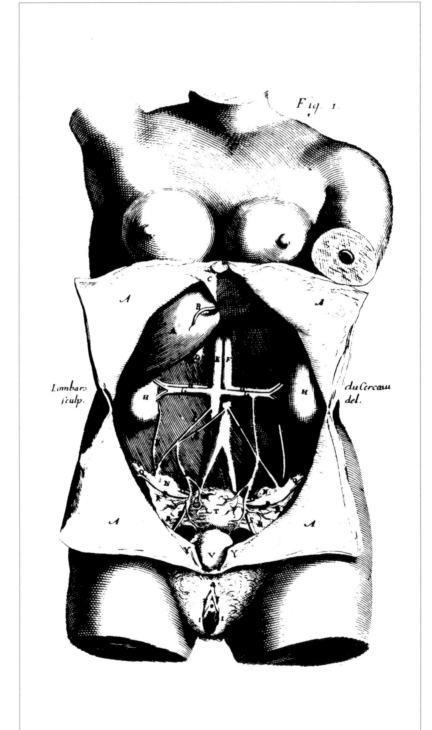

Female pelvic organs, from François Mauriceau's Des maladies des femmes ..., 1668[15]

an accumulation of menstrual blood or milk. He argued against the common misconceptions that a child born at seven months' gestation had a greater chance of survival than one born at eight months, and that a woman can give birth to only two children at a time because of the presence of two breasts. In the third edition (1681), he first described management of the aftercoming head in breech delivery with the aid of an index finger in the infant's mouth, now called the 'Mauriceau-Smellie-Viet' maneuver.

Mauriceau was born in Paris, and practiced in the maternity wards of the Hôtel Dieu, where he gained considerable experience and established a brilliant reputation for himself, becoming accoucheur-in-chief. Although not a graduate in medicine, he was a sworn mastersurgeon of Saint-Come. The book also records the author's adventure with the celebrated Hugh Chamberlen, of the Huguenot family, who succeeded in keeping their invention of an obstetrical forceps a family secret for almost 200 years. Chamberlen translated the present work into English in 1673. From the third edition of 1681, Mauriceau published a Latin edition. To the fourth edition of 1694, Mauriceau appended a collection of 283 aphorisms concerning pregnancy, delivery, and the diseases of women. German (1680), Dutch (1683), and Italian (1684) translations also appeared, and the work was widely regarded for several generations.

Regnier De Graaf

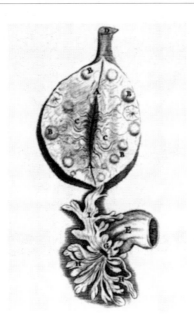

A bisected human ovary with follicles and the fimbriated end of the Fallopian tube. In Regnier De Graaf's De mullierum organis ..., 1672[16]

16. De Graaf, R. (1672). *De mulierum organis generationi inservientibus tractatus novus ... Lugduni Batavorum, ex off., Hackiana*

17. De Graaf, R. (1664). *De succi pancreatici natura ex usu exercitatio anatomico-medica.* Lugduni Batavorum, ex off. Hackiana

18. De Graaf, R. (1668). *De vivorum organis generationi inservientibus, declysteribus et de usu siphonis in anatomia.* Lugduni Batavorum, ex off. Hackiana

During the latter part of the seventeenth century, the idea gained credence that the female testes, as the ovary of birds, was the site of egg formation – as opposed to the Aristotelian doctrine of the egg being formed in the uterus as a result of activation of the menstrual blood by the male semen. Jan Swammerdam (1637–1680) and Johannes Van Horne (1621–1670), both of Leiden, and Niels Stensen (1638–1686) of Copenhagen, independently developed this hypothesis, but their works were never published.

Regnier De Graaf (1641–1673), in his *De mulierum organis generationi ...*[16] (Leiden, 1672) (in which he credits Van Horne), contains the first thorough description of the mammalian female gonad and establishes that this organ produces the ovum (see figure above). He incorrectly assumed the entire follicle was the ovum, an understandable error in the premicroscopic era. Besides describing the follicle, which several authors had noted previously, he described the corpus luteum for the first time. De Graaf concluded, 'Thus, the general function of the female testicles is to generate the ova, to nourish them, and to bring them to maturity, so that they serve the same purpose in the woman as the ovaries of birds. Hence, they should rather be called ovaries than testes ..., many have considered these bodies useless, but this is incorrect, because they are indispensable for reproduction.'

De Graaf, a practicing physician in Delft, also published important studies on the pancreatic secretions (*De succi pancreatici ...*, 1664)[17] and the male reproductive system (*De virorum organis ...*, 1668)[18].

Godfried Bidloo

19. Bidloo, G. (1685). *Anatomia humani corporus, centum et quinque tabulis, per artificiosiss ...* Amstelodami, vid J. a Someren

20. Cowper, W. (1698). *The Anatomy of Human Bodies, with figures drawn after the life by some of the best masters of Europe.* (Oxford: Som. Smith)

One of the outstanding anatomical works of the seventeenth century was that of Godfried Bidloo (1649–1713), Professor of Anatomy at The Hague and at Leiden. In his *Anatomia humani corporis*[19] (Amsterdam, 1685), Bidloo presented with 105 illustrations one of the finest anatomical atlases of the Baroque period. The plates of the reproductive system were exceptionally well done. For instance, Bidloo illustrated the female reproductive tract, including the clitoris, labia, vagina, the opened cervix and endometrial cavity, the Fallopian tubes, ovaries, and broad ligaments. Bidloo also included several plates of the fetus *in utero* and its anatomy (see figure below). He erroneously claimed to have discovered glands in the umbilical cord responsible for the elaboration of amniotic fluid.

In one of the most notorious cases of plagiarism in scientific publication, in 1698 the English anatomist William Cowper (1666–1709) published Bidloo's work under the title '*The Anatomy of Human Bodies ...*'[20] as his own, only adding nine perfunctory plates and translating the text into English. When William of Orange visited England in 1688, Bidloo accompanied him as his personal physician.

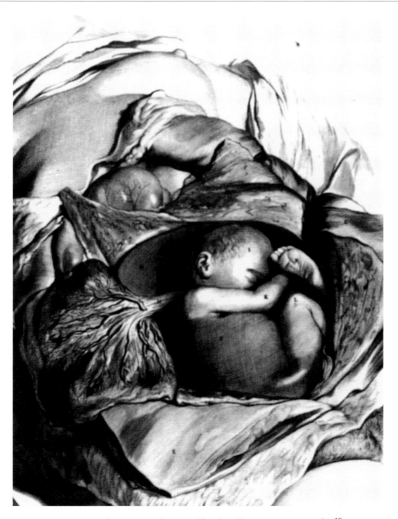

Near-term fetus in situ from Godfried Bidloo's Anatomia, 1685[19]

Hendrik van Deventer

In his *Manuale operatien, 1. deel zijnde een nieuw ligt voor vroed-meesters en vroed-vrouen* (new light for midwives) (The Hague, 1701)[21], van Deventer (1651–1724) gave the first accurate description of the female pelvis (see figure below), which he included in a textbook for midwives. He also described pelvic deformities and stressed their role in complicating labor. Deventer emphasized the need of midwives' knowledge of pelvic anatomy, '... for without a clear knowledge of that matter they proceed uncertainly, and make use of their hands, like those that are blind.' He was also the first to use the term 'placenta previa' and to advise version after piercing the placenta.

21. Deventer, H. van. (1701). *Manuale operatien, 1. deel zijnde een nieuw ligt voor vroed-meesters en vroed-vrouen.* The Hague, The author

Deventer played a key role in founding modern obstetrics. As a practitioner in his native city of den Hague, he directed his greatest efforts to pregnancy and to the study of its many unsolved problems. He was also interested in orthopedics and spent a great deal of time studying the bones of the pelvis and spinal deformity. A Latin translation of his work was published in Leiden the same year, and an English translation appeared in 1724. His work remained authoritative for one and a half centuries.

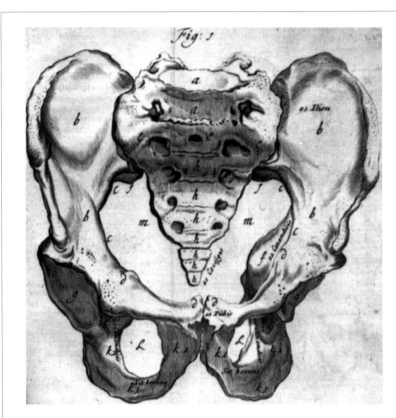

The first accurate depiction of the female pelvis by Hendrik van Deventer (1701)[21], showing the rigid structure through which the fetal head has to pass

William Smellie

22. Smellie, W. (1754). *A Sett of Anatomical Tables, with Explanations, and an Abridgment of the Practice of Midwifery ... London*

23. Smellie, W. (1752). *A Treatise on the Theory and Practice of Midwifery.* (London: D. Wilson)

William Smellie's (1697–1763) *Sett of Anatomical Tables ...*[22] (London, 1754) was intended as a supplement to his text *Treatise on the Theory and Practice of Midwifery*[23] (London, 1752), to illustrate as accurately as possible the female pelvis and fetus. Smellie, the foremost obstetrician of the eighteenth century, described more accurately than any previous writer the mechanical relation of the fetal head to that of the mother's pelvis during parturition, i.e. the mechanism of labor. He also was the first to measure the internal, or diagonal, conjugate of the pelvis, and to illustrate a rachitic pelvis. He introduced the English lock on the obstetrical forceps,

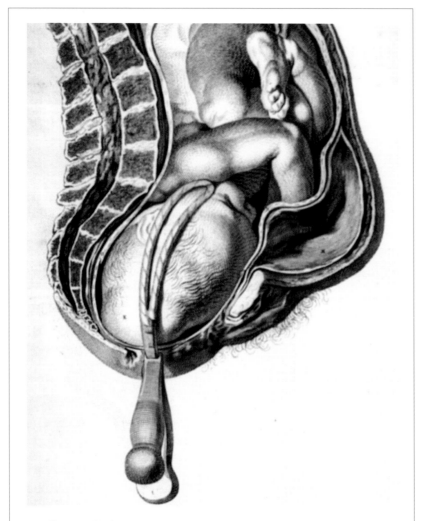

William Smellie first applied forceps with consideration of the position of the fetal head and performed a forceps rotation. He independently described the pelvic curve, which had been reported several years earlier by Levret, and probably designed the 'English lock' used today

and, coincidentally with Levret of Paris, added the pelvic curve (see figure above). He was the first to rotate the fetal head with forceps and to use them on the aftercoming head of a breech delivery. He also invented several important obstetric instruments.

The *Atlas*, a classic of illustrated obstetrics, is alleged to have been printed in only 100 copies. The anatomic plates are far superior to any which had hitherto appeared; they give everywhere a masterly representation, true to nature, of the relations of the parts of the mother and child, and have perhaps achieved more in the spread of correct ideas of labor than all the books which had previously been written on the subject. Of the 39 plates,

24. Smellie, W. (1754). *A Collection of Cases and Observations in Midwifery ...* (London: D. Wilson & T. Durham)

25. Smellie, W. (1764). *A Collection of Preternatural Cases and Observations in Midwifery.* (London: D. Wilson & T. Durham)

26 are by the Dutch comparative anatomist Jan van Rymsdyck, who later made the drawings for Hunter's *Gravid Uterus* (see below).

The first volume of the *Treatise*, based on 1150 deliveries, is a general discussion of normal obstetrics, as well as pathological problems. Smellie was the first to lay down rules regarding the safe use of the forceps, which remain valid today. The second and third volumes, published in 1754[24] and 1764[25], respectively, were largely case histories (531) collected from Smellie's extensive practice. Smellie began compiling volume three in his retirement in Lanark, and following his death it was completed by his friend, the novelist Tobias Smollett, who also practiced midwifery. The three-volume *Treatise*, as well as the anatomical atlas, went through several editions.

Smellie was born in Lanarkshire, Scotland. Following an apprenticeship with a local apothecary-physician, naval service, and general practice, he moved to London where he taught obstetrics in his own home. Smellie used a mannequin fabricated from pelvic and fetal bones covered with leather to teach obstetrics from a scientific basis. Practicing among the poor, Smellie became a popular teacher, giving over 280 courses of midwifery to more than 900 pupils, among whom was the celebrated William Hunter.

William Hunter

26. Hunter, W. (1774). *Anatomia uteri humani gravidi tabulis illustrata ....* (Birmingham: John Baskerville)

One of the most magnificent obstetric atlases ever published, William Hunter's (1718–1783) *Anatomia uteri humani gravidi tabulis illustrata ...*[26], *The Anatomy of the Human Gravid Uterus Explained by Figures* (Birmingham, 1774) is anatomically exact and artistically perfect. Hunter began the work in 1751, when it was expected to contain ten plates. The number later rose to 36 (two plates of which were discarded, leaving the present 34), and it required nearly 25 years to complete. Hunter spared no expense in having one of the leading artists of the time, Jan van Rymsdyck, draw the plates. The work was printed by John Baskerville, and is one of only two medical books to have received the attention of the finest printer of that period. The life-size line engravings achieve effects of depth and contrast, and present a wide range of normal and pathologic conditions of the womb and fetus (see figure below). Each page of text is printed in two columns, one in Latin and the other in English.

Hunter first described retroversion of the uterus. With his brother John he also described the separate maternal and fetal circulations of the placenta. The brothers later quarreled over who should receive recognition for this work, and separated professionally several years before William's death.

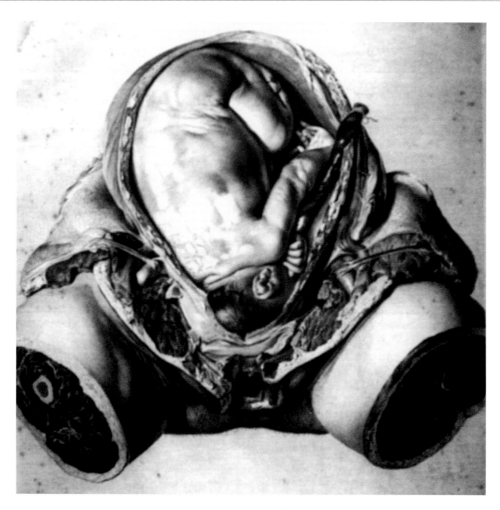

William Hunter's atlas, one of the finest ever produced (1774)[26], greatly influenced the development of obstetrics. The plates were drawn to natural size. Hunter stated, regarding the dissection shown, 'Every part is represented just as it was found; not so much as one joint of a finger having been moved to show any part more distinctly, or to give it a more picturesque effect'

William Hunter was born in Scotland, and studied at the University of Glasgow for a career in the ministry. Soon, however, he discovered his love for medicine. After an apprenticeship with William Cullen and a year in Edinburgh with Alexander Munro, he moved to London to study under William Smellie. Beginning in 1746, he offered a course in anatomy from his home. From Hunter's Great Windmill Street Anatomical School came many of the leading anatomists and surgeons of the day. In 1762 Hunter attended Queen Charlotte during her first confinement, in which she was delivered of the Duke of Cornwall. In 1767 he was elected to fellowship in the Royal Society, and the following year George III appointed Hunter Professor of Anatomy at the Royal Academy. Outside the field of obstetrics, he is remembered for the first description of arteriovenous aneurysm, and for clarifying the anatomy and physiology of the lymphatics. Following his death, Hunter's magnificent collection of books and manuscripts went to the University of Glasgow.

Ephraim McDowell

27. McDowell, E. (1817). Three cases of extirpation of diseased ovaria. *Eclect. Rep. Analyt. Rev.,* **7**, 242

Ephraim McDowell (1771–1830) of Danville, Kentucky reported the first successful removal of an ovarian tumor in *Three Cases of Extirpation of Diseased Ovaria.* (*Eclectic Repertory and Analytical Review* ..., 1817)[27]. Following a medical apprenticeship in Virginia, McDowell studied at Edinburgh, part of this time under John Bell, who taught the feasibility of ovariotomy, but apparently never performed it. However, McDowell left the university without his medical degree to return to the Ohio River Valley. After practicing there for 14 years, on Christmas morning in 1809, in 25 minutes in his home he performed the first successful ovariotomy in recorded history. McDowell used a 'long' ligature tied around the pedicle of the Fallopian tube and ovarian ligament, the free ends brought out through the incision and serving as a drain. The operation was particularly remarkable when one considers that he operated without the aid of anesthesia, without knowledge of antisepsis, and without trained assistants. McDowell performed a similar 'experiment' in 1813 and another in 1816, in which both patients survived. Despite this notable achievement, he waited for 8 years to publish his account in one of the two American medical journals published at that time (see figure below).

28. McDowell, E. (1819). *Eclect. Rep. Analy. Rev.,* **9**, 546

The report is remarkable for its brevity, naively portraying one of the greatest incidents in the annals of surgery. His paper so directly opposed the accepted teaching of the era, e.g. that exposure of the peritoneum and intestines would invariably lead to inflammation and prove fatal, that it was met initially with disbelief, derision, and sarcasm. McDowell's only other publication appeared 2 years later[28] in which he described two further cases, in the last of which the patient died.

29. Smith, N. (1822). Case of ovarian dropsy, successfully removed by a surgical operation. *Am. Med. Recorder,* **5**, 124

McDowell is believed to have performed a total of 13 ovariotomies with eight recoveries. Apparently, neither of his reports was read widely, and the operative procedure received slow acceptance by the medical profession. Nathan Smith of New Hampshire reported a similar operation in 1822[29], apparently unaware of McDowell's earlier achievements.

McDowell became well known as a surgeon in the Ohio Valley and, in fact, performed a lithotomy on James K. Polk, who in 1845 became President of the United States. In 1825 McDowell received an honorary doctor of medicine degree from the University of Maryland. His first ovariotomy patient, Jane Todd Crawford, a cousin of Mary Todd, wife of Abraham Lincoln, outlived by 11 years the great ovariotomist, who died in 1830.

242

ORIGINAL PAPERS.

——

Three Cases of Extirpation of diseased Ovaria.

By EPHRAIM M'DOWELL, M. D. of Danville, Kentucky.

In December 1809, I was called to see a Mrs. Crawford, who had for several months thought herself pregnant. She was affected with pains similar to labour pains, from which she could find no relief. So strong was the presumption of her being in the last stage of pregnancy, that two physicians, who were consulted on her case, requested my aid in delivering her. The abdomen was considerably enlarged, and had the appearance of pregnancy, though the inclination of the tumor was to one side, admitting of an easy removal to the other. Upon examination, per vaginam, I found nothing in the uterus; which induced the conclusion that it must be an enlarged ovarium. Having never seen so large a substance extracted, nor heard of an attempt, or success attending any operation, such as this required, I gave to the unhappy woman information of her dangerous situation. She appeared willing to undergo an experiment, which I promised to perform if she would come to Danville, (the town where I live) a distance of sixty miles from her place of residence. This appeared almost impracticable by any, even the most favourable conveyance, though she performed the journey in a few days on horseback. With the assistance of my nephew and colleague, James M'Dowell, M.D., I commenced the operation, which was concluded as follows: Having placed her on a table of the ordinary height, on her back, and removed all her dressing which might in any way impede the operation, I made an incision about three inches from the musculus rectus abdominis, on the left side, continuing the same nine inches in length, parallel with the fibres of the above named muscle, extending

Ephraim McDowell's 1817 report of the first successful removal of an ovarian tumor[27]

The underlying principles of the operation, as described by McDowell, obtain today, namely, adequate exposure, ligation of the blood supply to the tumor, division at its point of attachment, and closure of the abdomen.

Thus, it was that a modest and relatively unknown physician of the American frontier proved the feasibility of abdominal surgery. McDowell's operation launched the beginning of not only pelvic surgery, but abdominal surgery, in general. He demonstrated that an operation within the abdomen was not necessarily fatal. From this report, and with the introduction of anesthesia and Lister's antisepsis, the modern era of intra-abdominal surgery became possible.

Robert Lee

30. Lee, R. (1842). *On the Ganglia and Other Nervous Structures of the Uterus.* (London: Richard and John E. Taylor)

Until the mid-nineteenth century, there was no agreement as to whether the uterus possessed nerves. Although William Hunter[26], in his monograph of the anatomy of the human gravid uterus described such nerves, also noting their increase in size during pregnancy, many anatomists denied their existence. Robert Lee (1793–1877) gave the first careful and accurate description of these nerves and the cervical ganglion[30]. He recorded the background of the serendipitous discovery:

> On the 8th of April, 1838, while dissecting a gravid uterus of seven months, I accidentally observed the trunk of a large nerve proceeding upward from the cervix to the body of the uterus along with the right uterine vein, and sending off branches in its course to the posterior surface of the uterus, some of which accompanied the ramifications of the vein, and others were inserted into the peritoneum. A broad band, resembling a plexus of nerves, was seen extending across the posterior surface of the uterus, and covering the nerve midway between the fundus and the cervix. On the left side the same appearances were seen, and several branches of the great plexus crossing the body of the uterus.

Lee carefully described these nerves and their ramifications, and concluded,

31. Beck, T.S. (1846). *Phil. Trans. R. Soc. Lond.,* Part II, 213

32. Lee, R. (1848). *Engravings of the Ganglia and Nerves of the Uterus and Heart....* (London: Churchill)

> These dissections prove that the human uterus possesses a great system of nerves, which enlarges with the coats, blood-vessels and absorbents during pregnancy, and which returns after parturition to its original condition before conception takes place. It is chiefly by the influence of these nerves, that the uterus performs the varied functions of menstruation, conception, and parturition, and it is solely by their means, that the whole fabric of the nervous system sympathises with the different morbid affections of the uterus.

These papers were also published separately as *On the Ganglia and Other Nervous Structures of the Uterus*[30] (London, R. and J.E. Taylor, 1842) (see figure below). Sadly, Lee's findings were misrepresented by his former student, Thomas Snow Beck[31] and only after a prolonged battle were Lee's claims recognized. Lee then extended his findings in his 1848 publication *Engravings of the Ganglia and Nerves of the Uterus and Heart ...*[32] Twenty-five years later Ferdinand Frankenhaeuser[33] redescribed these structures in somewhat greater detail.

33. Frankenhaeuser, F. (1867). *Die Nerven der Gebaermutter und ihre Endigung in den Glatten Muskelfasern.* (Jena: F. Mauke)

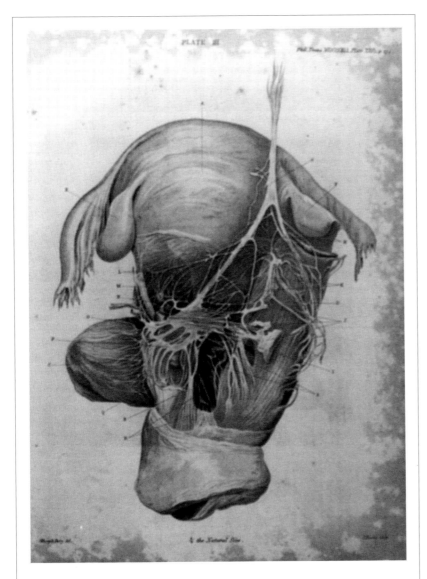

Robert Lee's 1842 depiction of the nerves of the uterus at 4 months' gestation from the posterior lateral aspect, showing the utero-cervical ganglion and its connections to the uterus, vagina, rectum, and bladder. Lee was particularly impressed with the increase in size of these structures during gestation[30]

Lee, a native of Scotland and an Edinburgh graduate, was physician to the British Lying-In Hospital, and lecturer on midwifery at St. George's Hospital, London. Although he ardently opposed ovariotomy, Lee made numerous contributions to the specialty. He apparently first used the term 'cervicitis'. From dissections on cadavers he demonstrated that leukorrhea orginates from the uterus rather than from the tubes or vagina. Lee also noted the similarity of pathologic findings in cases of puerperal fever and erysipelas, and wrote on the discovery of the obstetrical forceps by the Chamberlens.

Oliver Wendell Holmes

34. Holmes, O.W. (1842/1843). The contagiousness of puerperal fever. *N. Engl. Q. J. Med. Surg.*, **1**, 503

In one of the greatest American contributions to medicine, Oliver Wendell Holmes' (1809–1894) report 'The contagiousness of puerperal fever'[34], published in Boston in 1843, established that puerperal fever was contagious, and was carried by the unwashed hands of the physician from bed to bed. Holmes amassed considerable evidence for his thesis, and wrote with clear argument. His advice to accouchers to wash their hands in calcium chloride, and to change their clothes after treating cases of puerperal fever or performing post-mortems, aroused the scorn and animosity of his fellow physicians. *The New England Quarterly Journal of Medicine and Surgery* ran for only one year, producing this single and now scarce volume. Holmes concluded his essay:

> The woman about to become a mother, or with her new-born infant upon her bosom, should be the object of trembling care and sympathy wherever she bears her tender burden, or stretches her aching limbs. The very outcast of the streets has pity upon her sister in degradation when the seal of promised maternity is impressed upon her. The remorseless vengeance of the law, brought down upon its victim by a machinery as sure as destiny, is arrested in its fall at a word which reveals her transient claim for mercy. The solemn prayer of the liturgy singles out her sorrows from the multiplied trials of life, to plead for her in the hour of peril. God forbid that any member of the profession to which she trusts her life, doubly precious at that eventful period, should hazard it negligently, unadvisedly, or selfishly! (See figure below).

35. Holmes, O.W. (1855). *Puerperal Fever as a Private Pestilence*. (Boston: Ticknor and Fields)

Following publication of this work, Holmes regretfully recognized that his original thesis had never received adequate attention by his fellow physicians. Certainly, it had not received the wide circulation given to the views of his out-spoken opponents. To remedy the situation, in 1855 Holmes reprinted his essay[35], together with a 21-page introduction answering his opposition and mentioning the steps already taken by Semmelweis. He added a two-page list of additional references and cases at the end.

Sir William Osler called Holmes 'The most successful combination which the world has ever seen of the physician and a man of letters.' He was Professor of Anatomy at Dartmouth College and Harvard Medical School, and Dean of Harvard Medical School from 1847 to 1853. His other medical essays of note include: 'Homeopathy', and 'Intermittant Fever in New England.' Near the end of his productive life, Holmes presented his library of about 1000 rare books to the Boston Medical Library.

Contagiousness of Puerperal Fever. 529

sister in degradation when the seal of promised maternity is impressed upon her. The remorseless vengeance of the law, brought down upon its victim by a machinery as sure as destiny, is arrested in its fall at a word which reveals her transient claim for mercy. The solemn prayer of the liturgy singles out her sorrows from the multiplied trials of life, to plead for her in the hour of peril. God forbid that any member of the profession to which she trusts her life, doubly precious at that eventful period, should hazard it negligently, unadvisedly, or selfishly !

There may be some among those whom I address, who are disposed to ask the question, What course are we to follow in relation to this matter? The facts are before them, and the answer must be left to their own judgment and conscience. If any should care to know my own conclusions, they are the following; and in taking the liberty to state them very freely and broadly, I would ask the inquirer to examine them as freely in the light of the evidence which has been laid before him.

1. A physician holding himself in readiness to attend cases of midwifery, should never take any active part in the post-mortem examination of cases of puerperal fever.

2. If a physician is present at such autopsies, he should use thorough ablution, change every article of dress, and allow twenty-four hours or more to elapse before attending to any case of midwifery. It may be well to extend the same caution to cases of simple peritonitis.

3. Similar precautions should be taken after the autopsy or surgical treatment of cases of erysipelas, if the physician is obliged to unite such offices with his obstetrical duties, which is in the highest degree inexpedient.

4. On the occurrence of a single case of puerperal fever in his practice, the physician is bound to consider the next female he attends in labor, unless some weeks, at least, have elapsed, as in danger of being infected by him, and it is his duty to take every precaution to diminish her risk of disease and death.

5. If within a short period two cases of puerperal fever happen close to each other, in the practice of the same physician, the disease not existing or prevailing in the neighborhood, he would do wisely to relinquish his obstetrical practice for at least one month, and endeavor to free himself by every available means from any noxious influence he may carry about with him.

Oliver Wendell Holmes' essay on Puerperal Sepsis (1842/43)[34].
See text for details

Ignaz Phillip Semmelweis

One of the epoch-making works in the history of medicine, Ignaz Phillip Semmelweis' (1818–1865) discovery of the etiology and prevention of childbed fever was of the greatest importance in saving the lives and preventing suffering of women in childbirth[36].

36. Semmelweis, I.P. (1861). *Die Aetiologie, der Bergriff und die Prophylaxis des Kindbettfiebers.* (Pest, Wien & Leipzig: C.A. Hartleben)

In 1844 Semmelweis, a native of Hungary, was appointed assistant lecturer in the First Obstetrical Clinic of the Allgemeines Krankenhaus, Vienna under Johann Klein. At the time, particularly in maternity hospitals, the mortality from puerperal sepsis was almost unbelievable. In Klein's clinic the rate rarely was under 5% and between 1841 and 1843, of 5139 parturient women, 829 died, a mortality rate of 16%. Semmelweis was impressed that this rate prevailed only in the wards attended by students and not in the wards managed by the midwives, in which the death rate averaged about 2%. Semmelweis later observed, 'All was uncertain, all was doubtful, all was inexplicable, only the enormous number of deaths was an indubitable fact.' He later wrote that it was the death of his friend Kolletschka from a dissecting wound that 'revealed to my mind an identity' with the fatal puerperal cases. It was from this tragic event that the beginning of the knowledge of the pathology of septicemia was made. Semmelweis reasoned correctly that students carried infective material directly from the autopsy dissecting rooms to the delivery room. In 1847 he instituted the cleansing of the hands with chlorinated lime water in the maternity divi-

56

1 8 4 7.

	Geburten	Todesfälle	Percente
Juni	268	6	2.38
Juli	250	3	1.20
August	264	5	1.89
September	262	12	5.23
October	278	11	3.95
November	246	11	4.47
December	273	8	2.95
	1841	56	3.04

Es starben mithin von den innerhalb sieben Monaten verpflegten 1841 Wöchnerinnen 56, 3.04. Im Jahre 1846, in welchem die Chlorwaschungen noch nicht im Gebrauche waren, starben von 4010 an der ersten Gebärklinik verpflegten Wöchnerinnen 459, d. i. 11.4 Percent. An der zweiten Abtheilung starben im Jahre 1846 von 3754 Wöchnerinnen 105, d. i. 2., Percent. Im Jahre 1847, wo gegen Mitte Mai die Chlorwaschungen eingeführt wurden, starben an der ersten Abtheilung von 3490 verpflegten Wöchnerinnen 176, d. i. 5.0 Percent. An der zweiten Abtheilung starben von 3306 Entbundenen 32, d. i. 0., Percent. Im Jahre 1848, wo das ganze Jahr hindurch die Chlorwaschungen emsig geübt wurden, starben von 3556 Wöchnerinnen 45, 1.27 Percent. An der zweiten Abtheilung starben im Jahre 1848 von 3219 Entbundenen 43, d. i. 1.33 Percent.

Die einzelnen Monate des Jahres 1848 verhielten sich an der ersten Abtheilung wie folgende Tabelle zeigt:

Ignaz Phillip Semmelweis showed that cleansing of the operators' hands with chloride of lime, with other antiseptic measures, lowered the maternal mortality rate from 12.4% to 2.4%, a rate that continued that year at 3%[36]

sion. Within one month the mortality from puerperal fever plummeted from 12.4 to 2.4%, a rate that continued that year at about 3% (see figure above). The following year, the rate fell further to 1.3%, even surpassing the rate of the midwives. His superior Klein, however, largely through vanity and jealousy, remained unconvinced and finally succeeded in driving Semmelweis from Vienna in 1849.

Semmelweis returned to Pest where he later was appointed obstetric physician in the maternity department of St. Rochus Hospital. In 6 years he reduced the mortality there to 0.85%. The controversy in medical circles which Semmelweis' Lehre, or doctrine, inaugurated was exceptionally bitter. As a tragic end to the conflict, in 1865 Semmelweis was committed to an asylum, suffering from extreme mental disturbance, where he died within a few weeks.

James Marion Sims

James Marion Sims (1813–1883) first described the successful surgical cure of vesico-vaginal fistula. After repeated, fruitless attempts (about 40 in number) to cure several wretched creatures who were victims of fistulas, Sims ultimately succeeded with the aid of silver sutures, the improved exposure provided by the knee-chest position, and a vaginal speculum now named for him (see figure below). Sims' technique, reported in 1852 'On the treatment of vesico-vaginal fistula'[37], initiated a new era in the history of gynecology, which offered hope to women suffering from this scourge. In 1858, in his anniversary discourse before the New York Academy of Medicine 'Silver Sutures in Surgery'[38], he reviewed the trials and tribulations which led to his eventual success. In addition, he presented his experience with the use of silver sutures for other operative procedures.

Sims also wrote *Clinical Notes on Uterine Surgery*[39] (London, 1866), while he was in Europe during the Civil War. It includes the description of Sims' duck-bill speculum and controversial research on artificial and instrumental impregnation. Sims' method of uterine investigation made it possible to determine pathologic conditions with unprecedented ease and precision. His examination of cervical mucus soon after intercourse led to important insights into the role of the cervix in infertility. Nonetheless, it also led to bitter criticism from his more conservative colleagues.

Sims, a native of South Carolina and Alabama, moved to New York City in 1853 for health reasons. Two years later he founded the Women's Hospital in New York which opened 4 May 1855. The first American institution devoted exclusively to the treatment of gynecologic disorders, it was the forerunner of the present Memorial Sloan Kettering Cancer Center. Here Sims and his colleagues achieved a brilliant record for their fistula repairs and vaginal plastic operations, and established modern gynecologic surgery in the United States. Sims attained international renown as one of the world's foremost gynecologists.

37. Sims, J. M. (1852). On the treatment of vesico-vaginal fistula. *Am. J. Med. Sci.* n.s. **23**, 59

38. Sims, J.M. (1858). *Silver Sutures in Surgery.* (New York: Samuel, S. and Wood, W.)

39. Sims, J. M. (1866). *Clinical Notes on Uterine Surgery, with Reference to the Management of the Sterile Condition.* (London: R. Hardwicke)

proximal ends of the wires, and to push it along them into the vagina, till it occupies a position in front of the fistula, corresponding exactly with the one behind it.

Fig. 15 shows the two clamps, one on each side of the fistula, and every-

Fig. 15.

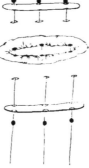

Fig. 16.

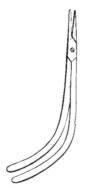

thing ready for closing it. The proximal clamp is pushed up by the crescent-shaped fork, while the wires are held firmly. This brings the denuded edges of the fistula into such close contact that it would be difficult to enter a common sized probe between them. The force necessary for tightening the clamps will depend upon the judgment of the operator; not enough will allow the parts to gape, while too much, which is the most frequent fault, will produce the bad effects formerly alluded to.

A simple and perfect contrivance now serves to hold the clamps in their proper places. A small bird shot, perforated, is passed along each wire close against the prox-imal clamp; when, the wires being held se-curely, they are gently but firmly compressed by means of a long strong pair of forceps (Fig. 16), whereby they are made to perform the office of a knot in preventing the clamp from slipping off the wire. The wires are cut off about a fourth or eighth of an inch from the shot, and then bent over, which effectually prevents their slipping off.

Fig. 17.

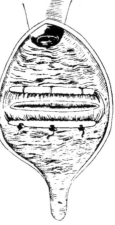

Fig. 17 shows the appearance of the fistula and suture apparatus after the

James Marion Sims in 1852 first successfully closed a persistent vesico-vaginal fistula by the use of silver sutures[37]

Summary of references

1. Graham, H. (1950). *Eternal Eve*. (London: Wm. Heinemann)

2. Rösslin, E. *Der Schwangern Frawen und hebammen Roszgarten*. (Strasborg: M. Flach Jr)

3. Rösslin, E. (1532). *De partu hominis, et quae circa ipsum accidunt. Medici,* Franc. Chri, Egen, Francofurti. xix., Octobris

4. Rösslin, E. (1540). *The Byrth of Mankynde* by Thomas Raynalde. T.R., London

5. Vesalius, A. (1543). *De humani corporis fabrica libri septem*. (Basel: Ioannis Oporini)

6. Rueff, J. (1554). *De conceptu et generatione hominis*. (Zurich: C. Froschoverum)

7. Rueff, J. (1580). *De conceptu et generatione hominis: de matrice et eius partibus ....* (Frankfurt am Main: Sigismund Feyerabend)

8. Rueff, J. (1554). *Ein schon lustig Trostbuchle von den Empfengknussen und Geburten der Menschen ...,* Tiguri, Apud Frosch [overum]

9. Rueff, J. (1637). *The Expert Midwife, or an Excellent and most necessary Treatise of the generation and birth of Man....* London, Printed by E. Griffin for S. Burton

10. Fabrizio, G. (1604). *De formato foetu*. Venetiis, per F. Bolzettam, 1600. (Colophon: Laurentius Pasquatus)

11. Fabrici, G. (1603). *De venarum ostiolis*, Patavii, ex typ. L. Pasquati

12. Fabrici, G. (1621). *De formatione ovi et pulli*, Patavii, ex off. A. Bencÿ

13. Spigelius, A. (1626). *De formato foetu liber singulairs, aeneis figuris exornatus...* Pataurii, Apud Io. Bap. de Martinis, & Liuiu Pasquatu

14. Holmes, O.W. (1889). *Boston Med. Surg. J.,* **120**, 129

15. Mauriceau, F. (1668). *Des maladies des femmes grosses et accouchées*. Paris, chez l'Auteur

16. De Graaf, R. (1672). *De mulierum organis generationi inservien tibus tractatus novus ....* Lugduni Batavorum, ex off., Hackiana

17. De Graaf, R. (1664). *De succi pancreatici natura ex usu exercitatio anatomico-medica*. Lugduni Batavorum, ex off. Hackiana

18. De Graaf, R. (1668). *De vivorum organis generationi inservientibus, declysteribus et de usu siphonis in anatomia*. Lugduni Batavorum, ex off. Hackiana

19. Bidloo, G. (1685). *Anatomia humani corporus, centum et quinque tabulis, per artificiosiss ....* Amstelodami, vid J. a Someren

20. Cowper, W. (1698). *The Anatomy of Human Bodies*, with figures drawn after the life by some of the best masters of Europe. (Oxford: Som. Smith)

21. Deventer, H. van. (1701). *Manuale operatien, 1. deel zijnde een nieuw ligt voor vroed-meesters en vroed-vrouen*. The Hague, The author

22. Smellie, W. (1754). *A Sett of Anatomical Tables, with Explanations, and an Abridgment of the Practice of Midwifery* .... London

23. Smellie, W. (1752). *A Treatise on the Theory and Practice of Midwifery.* (London: D. Wilson)

24. Smellie, W. (1754). *A Collection of Cases and Observations in Midwifery* ... (London: D. Wilson & T. Durham)

25. Smellie, W. (1764). *A Collection of Preternatural Cases and Observations in Midwifery.* (London: D. Wilson & T. Durham)

26. Hunter, W. (1774). *Anatomia uteri humani gravidi tabulis illustrata....* (Birmingham: John Baskerville)

27. McDowell, E. (1817). Three cases of extirpation of diseased ovaria. *Eclect. Rep. Analyt. Rev.,* **7**, 242

28. McDowell, E. (1819). *Eclect. Rep. Analy. Rev.,* **9**, 546

29. Smith, N. (1822). Case of ovarian dropsy, successfully removed by a surgical operation. *Am. Med. Recorder,* **5**, 124

30. Lee, R. (1842). *On the Ganglia and Other Nervous Structures of the Uterus.* (London: Richard and John E. Taylor)

31. Beck, T.S. (1846). *Phil. Trans. R. Soc. Lond.,* Part II, 213

32. Lee, R. (1848). *Engravings of the ganglia and nerves of the uterus and heart....* (London: Churchill)

33. Frankenhaeuser, F. (1867). *Die Nerven der Gebaermutter und ihre Endigung in den Glatten Muskelfasern.* (Jena: F. Mauke)

34. Holmes, O.W. (1842/1843). The contagiousness of puerperal fever. *N. Engl. Q. J. Med. Surg.,* **1**, 503

35. Holmes, O.W. (1855). *Puerperal Fever as a Private Pestilence.* (Boston: Ticknor and Fields)

36. Semmelweis, I.P. (1861). *Die Aetiologie, der Bergriff und die Prophylaxis des Kindbettfiebers.* (Pest, Wien & Leipzig: C.A. Hartleben)

37. Sims, J.M. (1852). On the treatment of vesico-vaginal fistula. *Am. J. Med. Sci. n.s.* **23**, 59

38. Sims, J.M. (1858). *Silver Sutures in Surgery.* (New York: Samuel, S. and Wood, W.)

39. Sims, J.M. (1866). *Clinical Notes on Uterine Surgery, with Reference to the Management of the Sterile Condition.* (London: R. Hardwicke)

THE APGAR SCORE

Classic
Paper
No.1

A proposal for a new method of evaluation of the newborn infant

VIRGINIA APGAR, M.D., NEW YORK, N.Y.

*Department of Anesthesiology, Columbia University,
College of Physicians and Surgeons and the Anesthesia Service,
The Presbyterian Hospital*

1. Apgar, V. (1953).
A proposal for a new
method of evaluation
of the newborn infant.
*Curr. Res. Anesth.
Analg.*, **32**, 260

The first paper chosen for inclusion in this book was published in 1953 and it is undoubtedly a 'classic' of its kind. Virginia Apgar recognized that there were 'no precise data . . . concerned with infant resuscitation' and in her paper she set out to establish a semiquantitative scoring system for the neonate, emphasizing the most important vital signs. The paper made an immediate impact, and today the Apgar score is a standard measurement tool that all obstetricians utilize. More recently, through the development and refinement of ultrasonography, it can now also be applied to the fetus as well as to the neonate.

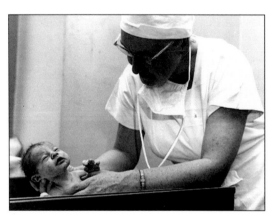

Virginia Apgar assessing an Apgar score

A Proposal for a New Method of Evaluation of the Newborn Infant.*

Virginia Apgar, M.D., New York, N. Y.

Department of Anesthesiology, Columbia University, College of Physicians and Surgeons and the Anesthesia Service, The Presbyterian Hospital

RESUSCITATION OF INFANTS at birth has been the subject of many articles. Seldom have there been such imaginative ideas, such enthusiasms, and dislikes, and such unscientific observations and study about one clinical picture. There are outstanding exceptions to these statements, but the poor quality and lack of precise data of the majority of papers concerned with infant resuscitation are interesting.

There are several excellent review articles[1] [2] but the main emphasis in the past has been on treatment of the asphyxiated or apneic newborn infant. The purpose of this paper is the reestablishment of simple, clear classification or "grading" of newborn infants which can be used as a basis for discussion and comparison of the results of obstetric practices, types of maternal pain relief and the effects of resuscitation.

The principle of giving a "score" to a patient as a sum total of several objective findings is not new and has been used recently in judging the treatment of drug addiction.[3] The endpoints which have been used previously in the field of resuscitation are "breathing time" defined as the time from delivery of the head to the first respiration, and "crying time" the time until the establishment of a satisfactory cry.[4] Other workers have used the terms mild, moderate and severe depression[5] to signify the state of the infant. There are valid objections to these systems. When mothers receive an excessive amount of depressant drugs in the antepartum period, it is a common occurence that the infants breathe once, then become apneic for many minutes. Evaluation of the breathing time is difficult. A satisfactory cry is sometimes not established even when the infant leaves the delivery room, and in some patients with cerebral injury, the baby dies without ever having uttered a satisfactory cry. Mild, moderate and severe depression of the infant leaves a fair margin for individual interpretation.

A list was made of all the objective signs which pertained in any way to the condition of the infant at birth. Of these, five signs which could be determined easily and without interfering with the care of the infant were considered useful. A rating of zero, one or two, was given to each sign depending on whether it was absent or present. A score of ten indicated a baby in the best possible condition. The time for judging the five objective signs was varied until the most practi-

*Presented before the Twenty-Seventh Annual Congress of Anesthetists, Joint Meeting of the International Anesthesia Research Society and the International College of Anesthetists, Virginia Beach, Va., September 22-25, 1952.

cable and useful time was found. This is sixty seconds after the complete birth of the baby. Insofar as possible, the rating was done by two observers only, but as the series progressed, the score as determined by the anesthesia resident present at the delivery was found to be sufficiently accurate. These ratings have been included in the present series.

The signs used are as follows:

(1) Heart Rate.—This was found to be the most important diagnostic and prognostic of the five signs. A heart rate of 100-140 was considered good and given a score of two, a rate of under 100 received a score of one, and if no heart beat could be seen, felt or heard the score was zero. If one attends the baby alone, it is easy to learn to look briefly at the epigastrium or precordium for visible heart beat, while palpation of the cord about two inches from the umbilicus is the most satisfactory method for determining the heart rate quickly, and avoids the area of clamping or tying of the cord. It is of great assistance to the person caring for the baby to have an assistant demonstrate by motion of a finger of one hand the heart rate as palpated by the other hand. In only three cases was a heart rate of over 140 detected, accompanied by arrhythmia in two of these infants. I was puzzled as to the proper way to rate this in these patients, but they were given a full score of two points. The tachycardia and arrhythmias were apparently related to an overdosage of a vasopressor drug during spinal anesthesia for cesarean section.

(2) Respiratory Effort.—An infant who was apneic at 60 seconds after birth received a score of zero, while one who breathed and cried lustily received a two rating. All other types of respiratory effort, such as irregular, shallow ventilation were scored one. An infant who had gasped once at thirty or forty-five seconds after birth, and who then became apneic, received a zero score, since he was apneic at the time decided upon for evaluation.

(3) Reflex Irritability.—This term refers to response to some form of stimulation. The usual testing method was suctioning the oropharynx and nares with a soft rubber catheter which called forth a response of facial grimaces, sneezing or coughing. Although spontaneous micturition and defecation are not a response to an applied stimulus, they were considered to be favorable signs if they occurred.

(4) Muscle Tone.—This was an easy sign to judge, for a completely flaccid infant received a zero score, and one with good tone, and spontaneously flexed arms and legs which resisted extension were rated two points. We are unable to agree with Flagg's description of spasticity[6] as a sign of asphyxiation of the infant. The use of analeptics in the baby did not influence this score because of the standardized early time of observation and rating.

(5) Color.—This is by far the most unsatisfactory sign and caused the most discussion among the observers. All infants are obviously cyanotic at birth because of their high capacity for carrying oxygen and their relatively low oxygen content and saturation.[7] The disappearance of cyanosis depends directly on two signs previously

considered—respiratory effort and heart rate. Comparatively few infants were given a full score of two for this sign, and many received zero in spite of their excellent score for other signs. The foreign material so often covering the skin of the infant at birth interfered with interpreting this sign, as did the inherited pigmentation of the skin of colored children, and an occasional congenital defect. Many children for reasons still mysterious to us, persist in having cyanotic hands and feet for several minutes in spite of excellent ventilation, and added oxygen. A score of two was given only when the entire child was pink. Several hundred children were rated at three or five minutes as well as at sixty seconds and in almost all cases a score of two could be given for color at these later times. This finding agrees well with the heel blood oxygen studies in 402 infants, conducted at Sloane Hospital during 1947-48.[8] In an occasional instance the color was worse at five minutes than at sixty seconds, and these cases were therefore missed with our usual method of evaluation.

It has been most gratifying to note the enthusiastic interest and competitive spirit displayed by the obstetric house staff who took great pride in a baby with a high score. The same trend of interest has been noted in another hospital which has undertaken the ratings of babies in this manner.[9]

Material

DURING THE PERIOD of this report (seven and one-half months) 2096 infants were born in the Sloane Hospital for Women. Eighty four per cent of the anesthesia records of these births are on file. The missing 16 per cent are chiefly those with pudendal blocks or "natural childbirth" patients. The omission of these cases is regrettable for they form the best control group for any study on infant resuscitation. Little attempt will be made to analyze these figures statistically for the groups are still too small for such treatment.

Seventeen hundred and sixty charts were available for study. Twenty-seven infants were stillbirths, or a rate of 1.5 per cent. One thousand and twenty-one of the infants born alive were rated by the method just described and comprise the data for this report. Seven hundred and twelve infants were not rated.

Type of Delivery and Score	No. Infants	Average Score
Low forceps or spontaneous	843	8.4
Cesarean section	141	6.8
Midforceps delivery	17	6.9
Breech delivery	16	6.7
Version and breech extraction	4	6.3

The infants in the best condition one minute after birth are those born vaginally with the occiput the presenting part. The incidence of the use of low forceps in this clinic is 34 per cent and after a two year daily observation of routine deliveries it did not seem to be of value to separate the spontaneous deliveries from those in which low forceps were used. Delivery by any other means produced no difference in the infants. The score for all these was slightly less favorable than those born spontaneously or with low forceps.

Cesarean Sections.—The cesarean section rate at Sloane Hospital is 10.5 per cent during this period. The anesthesia methods for the 141 rated infants born by cesarean section are listed:

	Infants	Average Score
Spinal anesthesia	83	8.0
General anesthesia	54	5.0
Epidural or caudal	4	6.3

The method used for spinal anesthesia was a single dose of nupercaine 0.25 per cent made hyperbaric with dextrose, in doses ranging from 6 to 7.5 mg., or pontocaine® 0.3 per cent, hyperbaric, from 7 to 9 mg. A 22 gauge needle was used. No supplementary anesthesia was given to these patients until after the birth of the infant. General anesthesia in all cases was accomplished with cyclopropane and oxygen. In 20 cases to be discussed later a relaxant was used with cyclopropane. Fractional epidural or caudal anesthesia (0.75 per cent xylocaine®) was continued in 4 cases for cesarean section after a trial of labor.

The indications for general anesthesia in cesarean section are thought to be a history of syphilis, septicemia, severe hemorrhage, or a history of traumatic experience with spinal anesthesia. Although this method does not take into account maternal risk or antepartum fetal problems, it is apparent that the mothers of the potentially poor risk infants received spinal anesthesia. In spite of this and the frequent maternal hypotension, the condition of the infants after spinal anesthesia was definitely better than after general anesthesia. The average time for delivery of the infant after induction of general ansthesia was fourteen minutes and twenty-four minutes after the administration of spinal anesthesia.

There is questionable support of the theory[10] that infants who have been subjected to a trial of labor are in better condition than those in whom cesarean section was chosen electively, as indicated below.

	Infants	Average Score
Patients in labor	57	7.1
Patients not in labor	84	6.7

These small groups have been analyzed statistically[11] and are not statistically significant.

In obstetric circles there has been the subtle impression that the lower the cesarean section rate in a clinic, the better was the practice of obstetrics. There is a slight trend away from this idea, and that at times even cesarean section is a conservative form of therapy.[12]

263

We have felt that with individual attention to selection of anesthetic agents and their administration by competent anesthesiologists, that infant survival after elective cesarean section might be made as successful as after an uncomplicated vaginal delivery. That we have not yet reached this point is illustrated in the next table. The group of cesarean section patients who had no antepartum problems and in whom labor was not present (secondary and tertiary sections) was compared with a similar group of vaginal deliveries in whom no problems of any kind were apparent. All received spinal anesthesia. The condition of the infants delivered vaginally was better than those delivered by cesarean section.

	Infants	Average Score
Normal, elective sections	38	7.7
Normal, low forceps or spont.	38	9.0

The most obvious difference between the two groups is the presence of labor in those delivered vaginally and the absence of labor in the section group. We do not know whether this implies some beneficial effect of labor on respiration, circulation and general well-being of the infant.

The experimental reports on the lack of placental transfer of d-tubocurarine, flaxedil,® decamethonium[13] [14] [15] [16] are intriguing. Several clinical reports seem to bear out this somewhat surprising finding. Other papers are in disagreement.[17] In an effort to test this possibility clinically, 20 patients received a relaxant intravenously as a means of keeping the patient from moving, accompanied by as light a plane of cyclopropane as would produce unconsciousness. Seventeen received d-tubocurarine, and 1 patient each received flaxedil,® succinylcholine and decamethonium bromide. Thirteen infants were rated.

	Infants	Average Score
Sections: Cyclopropane without relaxant	41	5.0
Sections: Cyclopropane with relaxant	13	5.0

In addition to the fact that there was no difference in the infant's condition with or without the use as a relaxant, 70 per cent of the infants with relaxant needed oxygen administration in some form, while the number needing oxygen after cyclopropane anesthesia alone was likewise 70 per cent. The infants are not in better condition with relaxants and nothing is to be gained by the use of curare or similar drugs for cesarean section anesthesia. The occasional maternal respiratory depression necessitating assisted respiration is a distinct disadvantage to the technique.

Breech Deliveries.—There were 16 cases of breech deliveries excluding twins and version and breech extraction. All but one who precipitated without anesthesia were anesthetized with general anesthesia in a plane as light as compatible with the obstetric maneuvers. Nitrous oxide, ethylene or cyclopropane were used for this purpose. The average score was 6.7, essentially the same as for cesarean section infants. Regional methods were not used in this small group.

Twins.—Nine pairs of twins were delivered by a variety of methods. The average score of the 18 babies was remarkably good, 8.6, and probably reflects the use of minimal medication during the first stage of labor. The use of regional anesthesia, however, again produced better results than general anesthesia in this small series.

	Infants	Average Score
Twins—general anesthesia	14	8.2
Twins—regional anesthesia	4	9.8

The condition of the first twin was somewhat better than the second.

	Infants	Average Score
Twin A	9	8.9
Twin B	9	8.2

Midforceps Delivery.—The condition of the infants following midforceps delivery was the same as by section or by breech delivery. There was no difference relating to the anesthetic method.

	Infants	Average Score
Midforceps, general anesthesia	11	6.8
Midforceps, regional anesthesia	6	7.0

Low Forceps and Spontaneous Deliveries.—This large group showed some improvement in the infant's condition following the use of regional anesthesia.

	Infants	Average Score
General anesthesia	692	8.2
Spinal anesthesia	25	8.9
Epidural, caudal anesthesia	102	9.1
Pudendal or no anesthesia	24	9.2

Prematurity

THERE WERE 70 infants in this series whose birth weights were between 500 and 2500 grams. The nonviable premature infants, under 500 grams, were excluded and considered to be abortions. The youngest child who has survived in the Premature Nursery of the Babies Hospital weighed 580 grams. Regional anesthesia again was associated with a better score for the child.

	Infants	Average Score
Premature, general anes.	44	8.0
Premature, regional anes.	24	9.2
Premature, no anes. ppt.	2	2.0

Resuscitation

OXYGEN, SUCTION, some method of positive pressure, endotracheal tubes and an infant laryngoscope are present in every delivery room. Oxygen was used freely if the infant's condition was not good. The three types of administration used are:

(1) Face oxygen, in which method oxygen is added to inspired air, but without increase in pressure at the face.

(2) Positive pressure mask, in which a small mask is held snugly on the infant's face, and some degree of positive pressure is applied

to the pharynx.

(3) Endotracheal oxygen, in which direct laryngoscopy is performed, additional suction used if necessary, and intubation accomplished. Positive pressure usually with added oxygen is implied in this method.

The details of these methods and indications for their use as well as discussion of other resuscitative measures will be the subject of other communications.

Three hundred thirty six or 19.4 per cent of the 1733 living infants received oxygen by some method. Of this group

156 or 46 per cent received face oxygen.
111 or 33 per cent received positive pressure mask.
13 or 4 per cent received endotracheal oxygen.
56 or 17 per cent received an unspecified method.

The survival rate following the use of endotracheal oxygen in this clinic over a 3 year period is between 60 and 70 per cent of the cases in which it has been employed.

The incidence of the use of oxygen for the infant following the various routes of deliveries is as follows:

Cesarean section	54 per cent
Midforceps	8 per cent
Breech delivery	37 per cent
Low forceps and spont.	15 per cent

In 217 of 336 infants who received oxygen, ratings were obtained and the method of administration was recorded.

	Cases	Average Score
Face oxygen	117	6.7
Positive pressure mask	90	3.9
Endotracheal oxygen	10	2.1

In 14 of the group of 117 cases receiving face oxygen, a score of 9 or 10 was given, and these infants undoubtedly did not need the oxygen so administered.

Neonatal Deaths

THERE WERE 25 neonatal deaths in the entire group of 2096 deliveries, or a rate of 1.2 per cent. If the 38 stillbirths over 500 grams are included, the total fetal loss was 64 infants, or a rate of 3.0 per cent of total infants born. The distribution by type of delivery is as follows:

Type	Cases	Neonatal Deaths	Per Cent of type
Cesarean section	220	2	0.9 per cent
Breech deliveries	54	5	9.3 per cent
Low, midforceps and spont.	1822	18	1.0 per cent

Fourteen of the infants who died were under 2500 Gm. birth weight, representing a mortality of 7.8 per cent of the total number of premature infants born alive. Of the 11 mature infants who died, all had obstetric or medical reasons for their deaths. In this series anesthesia complications apparently did not contribute to the death of any case. Twelve of the infants who later died were rated at birth and averaged 2.3 points.

In order to check the approximate accuracy of the various scores, the fate of the infants in poor, fair and good condition was examined. After this initial experience, it seems to us that groups 8, 9, and 10 indicate infants in good condition, 0, 1, and 2, poor condition, and the remaining scores, fair condition.

Infants receiving 0, 1 or 2 scores	65
Deaths in this group 9 or 14 per cent	
Infants receiving 3, 4, 5, 6, 7 scores	182
Deaths in this group 2 or 1.1 per cent	
Infants receiving 8, 9, 10 scores	774
Deaths in this group 1 or 0.13 per cent	

Thus, the prognosis of an infant is excellent if he receives one of the upper three scores, and poor if one of the lowest 3 scores. From this we may also conclude that color as a sign is relatively unimportant when observed one minute after birth.

Summary

$\mathcal{A}$ PRACTICAL METHOD of evaluation of the condition of the newborn infant one minute after birth has been described. A rating of ten points described the best possible condition with two points each given for respiratory effort, reflex irritability, muscle tone, heart rate and color. Various applications of this method are presented.

The author wishes to acknowledge gratefully the assistance and encouragement of H. C. Taylor, Jr., M. D. The data were collected with the technical assistance of Rita Ruane, R.N.

Bibliography

1. Little, D. M., Jr., and Tovell, R. M.: Collective Review: A Physiological Basis for Resuscitation of the Newborn, *Internat. Abstr. Surg.* 86:417-428 (May) 1948.

2. Smith, C. A.: Effects of Birth Processes and Obstetric Procedure upon the Newborn Infant. Advances in Pediatrics. Interscience Publishers. New York. 1948, vol. 3, chan. 1 pp. 1-54.

3. Kolb, L., and Himmelsbach, C. K.: Clinical Studies of Drug Addiction III, Washington, Public Health Reports. U. S. Treas. Dept., 1938, Supplement 128, pp. 23-31.

4. Hapke, F. B., and Barnes, A. C.: The Obstetric Use and Effect on Fetal Respiration of Nisentil,® *Am. J. Obst. & Gynec.* 58:799-801 (Oct.) 1949.

5. Eckenhoff, J. E.; Hoffman, G. L.; and Dripps, R. D.: N-allyl Normorphine, an Antagonist to the Opiates, *Anesthesiology* 13:242-251, (May) 1952.

6. Flagg, P.: The Art of Rescuscitation, New York, Reinhold Publishing Co., 1944, p. 124.

7. Eastman, N. J.: Foetal Blood Studies. I. The Oxygen Relationships of the Umbilical Cord at Birth, *Bull. Johns Hopkins Hosp.* 47:221-230, 1930.

8. Apgar, V.: Oxygen as Supportive Therapy in Fetal Anoxia, *Bull. N. Y. Acad. Med.* 26:2nd series, 474:478 (July) 1950.

9. Fleming: Personal communications.

10. Bloxsom, A.: The Difficulty in Beginning Respiration Seen in Infants Delivered by Cesarean Section, *J. Pediat.* 20:215-222 (Feb.) 1942.

11. Frumin, J.: Personal communication.

12. Harris, J. M., et al.: The Case of Reevaluation of Indications for Cesarean Section, *West. J. Surg.* 59:327-356, 1951.

13. Harroun, P., and Fisher, C. W.: The Physiological Effects of Curare, *Surg., Gynec. & Obst.* 89:73-75, 1949.

14. Young, I. M.: Abdominal Relaxation with Decamethonium Iodide During Cesarean Section, *Lancet* 1:1052-1053, 1949.

15. McMann, W.: Curare with General Anesthesia for Vaginal Deliveries, *Am. J. Obst. & Gynec.* 60:1366-1368 (Dec.) 1950.

16. Scurr, C.: A Comparative Review of the Relaxants, *Br. J. Anaesth.* 23:103-116 (Apr.) 1951.

17. Davenport, H. T.: D-Tubocurarine Chloride for Cesarean Sections: Report of 210 Cases *Br. J. Anaesth.* 23:66-80 (Apr.) 1951.

This paper has been reproduced by kind permission of the International Anesthesia Research Society and Williams & Wilkins, Baltimore.

Commentary on Classic Paper No. 1

In this manuscript, Virginia Apgar[1], Anesthesiologist at Columbia University, encouraged clinicians to observe all newborns during the first minutes after delivery and to score their condition.

The proposed scoring system covered five 'signs' to be observed in the neonate – heart rate, respiratory effort, reflex irritability, muscle tone, and color. Each sign was allocated a rating of 0, 1 or 2, a total score of 10 indicating the best possible condition.

The intended functions of the Apgar score were twofold: first, to quantify the neonatal condition; and second, to compare the results of obstetric practices and the effects of resuscitation.

Virginia Apgar had already noticed that the individual components of the score were not alike. She found, for example, that the color of the infant was the most unsatisfactory sign because all infants are cyanotic at birth. She thus recognized the fact that circulation and respiration were most important and that the scale was non-parametric.

The choice of 1 min postdelivery as the time of assessment of the condition of the newborn infant was undoubtedly an arbitrary one, which led subsequently to assessment at 5 and/or 10 min.

Emphasis on asphyxia

As an anesthesiologist, Virginia Apgar was particularly interested in the asphyxiated baby, the necessity of prompt resuscitation and a scoring system to observe the progress in vital functions. In this regard, animal studies in sheep, monkeys and guinea pigs, as reported by Geoffrey Dawes[2] in the United Kingdom and William Windle[3] and Ronald Myers[4] in the United States, are of special importance.

The sequence of events in cases of acute asphyxia were elegantly described by Dawes[2] in 1968 when he wrote:

> 'When a normal foetal rhesus monkey is delivered without general anaesthesia near term, the umbilical cord is tied and the head is covered with a small bag of warm saline, a characteristic series of changes ensues. Within about half a minute of tying the cord a short series of respiratory efforts begin, often of a rhythmic character. These are interrupted by a convulsion of series of clonic movements accompanied by an abrupt and profound fall in heart rate after which the animal lies inert with no muscular tone. The skin is by this time cyanosed and during the next five minutes

1. Apgar, V. (1953). A proposal for a new method of evaluation of the newborn infant. *Curr. Res. Anesth. Analg.*, **32**, 260

2. Dawes, G.S. (1968). *Fetal and Neonatal Physiology*. p.149. (Chicago: Year Book Medical Publishers)

3. Windle W. F. and Becker R. F. (1943). Asphyxia neonatorum. An experimental study in the guinea pig. *Am. J. Obstet. Gynecol.*, **45**, 183

4. Myers, R. E. (1972). Two patterns of perinatal brain damage and their conditions of occurrence. *Am. J. Obstet. Gynecol.*, **112**, 246

becomes blotchy and finally white as vasoconstriction spreads to produce asphyxia pallida. The initial period of apnoea (primary apnoea) lasts for 0.5–1.0 minutes. The monkey then begins to gasp, and 4–5 minutes after the onset of asphyxia the rate of gasping increases somewhat. Thereafter, there is little change in rate, the gasps merely becoming weaker terminally. There then follows secondary or terminal apnoea and, if resuscitation is not begun within a few minutes, death. If the arterial pH is low on delivery, as a result of placenta praevia, maternal hypotension or other causes (say 7.0–7.1) there are no rhythmic respiratory efforts preceding primary apnoea. If the initial pH is lower still (< 6.8) there may be no gasps at all. The pH on delivery is the most powerful determinant of the time to the last gasp (when body temperature is maintained).'

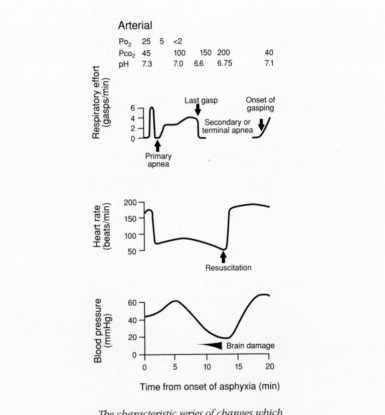

The characteristic series of changes which ensue when a normal fetal rhesus monkey is delivered without general anesthesia near term, the umbilicus tied, and the head covered with a small bag of warm saline. Adapted from Dawes (1968)[2] with permission

5. Niswander, K., Gordon, M. and Berendes, H. (1972). *The Women and Their Pregnancies.* (Philadelphia: W.B. Saunders Company)

Based on the observations made between 1930 and 1935, and the clinical fact that the fetus could only be observed as a neonate in those days, a large multicenter prospective study was launched by the National Institutes of Health (NIH) comprising 54000 women and their pregnancies[5].

The prospective study of the National Institutes of Health

This collaborative study in which 15 large obstetric units participated was performed in North America and linked obstetric data with the sequelae of the neonate, concentrating on neonatal mortality and morbidity. Perinatal morbidity was especially centered around cerebral palsy, mental retardation and other neurological and sensory disorders of infancy and childhood.

Each infant in the study received a neurological examination at 1 year of age. The children were examined by neurologists or pediatricians who had received relevant instruction and who had no previous knowledge of the prenatal history or findings. The neurological diagnosis was recorded as 'normal', 'suspect' or 'abnormal', and the collected data were forwarded to the National Institute of Neurological Diseases and Blindness for review, coding and final computer analysis.

From the prospective NIH study, two important conclusions could be drawn.

Prognostic value of the Apgar score is limited

Review of the data showed that there was a strong association between low Apgar scores and neonatal mortality, and that this mortality occurred during the first 2 days of extrauterine life, as documented by Drage and colleagues in 1965[6]. In 1966, Drage and co-workers[7] also reported that the 5-min scores were strongly associated with neonatal morbidity and that low birth weight was associated with low scores. In 1969, Drage and Berendes[8] indicated that investigation of infants at 1 year of age showed that 1.9% of 14 115 were neurologically abnormal. Within the 1-min score groups, 3.6% of the infants had scores between 7 and 10, and within the low 5-min score group, 7.4% were abnormal compared with 1.7% of the high-score group. Neurological abnormality within birth-weight groups showed more than a sixfold difference between infants weighing 1001–2000 g at birth and those weighing 2501 g and over.

Both low birth weight and low 5-min scores were associated with an increased percentage of abnormality. When controlled for birth weight, a threefold difference remained.

The same study also indicated that 95% of full-term neonates with low Apgar scores were not neurologically abnormal at 1 year of age.

Drage and Berendes also suggested that 'the low Apgar score, the neonatal mortality and the infant morbidity may each be a manifestation in sequence of some underlying pathologic state'; this thought led to further

6. Drage, J.S., Kennedy, C. and Schwartz, B.K. (1965). The Apgar score as an index for neonatal mortality. *Obstet. Gynecol.*, **24**, 222

7. Drage, J.S., Kennedy, C. and Schwartz, B.K. (1966). The Apgar score as an index for neonatal morbidity. *Dev. Med. Child. Neurol.*, **8**, 141

8. Drage, J.S. and Berendes, H. (1969). Low Apgar scores and outcome of the newborn. *Pediatr. Clin. N. Am.*, **13**, 635

9. Little, W.J. (1862). On the influence of abnormal parturition, difficult labours, premature birth, and asphyxia neonatorum, on the mental and physical condition of the child, especially in relation to deformities. *Trans. Obstet. Soc. London*, **3**, 293

10. Nelson, K.B. and Ellenberg, J.H. (1986). Antecedents of cerebral palsy: multivariate analysis of risk. *N. Engl. J. Med.*, **315**, 81

11. Nelson, K.B. and Ellenberg, J.H. (1988). Antecedents of cerebral palsy. Multivariate analysis of risk. In Kubli, F., Patel, N., Schmidt, W. and Linderkamp, O. (eds.) *Perinatal Events and Brain Damage in Surviving Children.* (Berlin, Heidelberg, New York, London, Paris, Tokyo: Springer Verlag)

12. Hagberg, B. and Hagberg, G. (1989). The changing panorama of infantile hydrocephalus and cerebral palsy over forty years. A Swedish survey. *Brain Dev.*, **11**, 368

13. Rosen, M.G. and Dickinson, J.C. (1992). The incidence of cerebral palsy. *Am. J. Obstet. Gynecol.*, **167**, 417

detailed investigations to determine antecedents of morbidity with a concentration on cerebral palsy already described in 1862 by Little[9].

Cerebral palsy is not always due to hypoxia during labor

From data gathered in the NIH study, Nelson and Ellenberg[10], in 1986, reported that, on multivariate analysis of 189 children with cerebral palsy studied up to the age of 7 years, the leading predictors of the disease were maternal mental retardation, birth weight below 2001g, fetal malformations and breech presentation.

In a later report published in 1988, also by Nelson and Ellenberg[11], data were presented in the form of pie diagrams (see figure below), which indicated that, when considering the 5% of the population at highest predicted risk, prepregnancy factors contributed 13% of the cases of cerebral palsy.

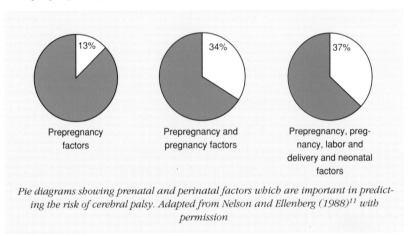

Pie diagrams showing prenatal and perinatal factors which are important in predicting the risk of cerebral palsy. Adapted from Nelson and Ellenberg (1988)[11] with permission

Taking into account congenital malformations, gestational age and birth weight, and breech presentation among characteristics determined by the moment before labor began, prepregnancy and pregnancy stage factors contributed 34% of the cases of cerebral palsy. The addition of information from labor, delivery, and the neonatal period led to a negligible increase in predictive ability (a further 3%). Of the 189 children with cerebral palsy, only 40 had symptoms of clinical asphyxia during labor such as bradycardia or a low Apgar score at 5 min.

The clinical and technological improvements have not led to a decrease in the incidence of cerebral palsy[12].

More recent studies of Rosen and Dickinson[13] in 1992, concluded that 70% of cerebral palsy cases were of antepartum or unknown origin, the incidence of risk for the term infant being one in 2000 births.

In 1979, Ronald S. Illingworth, a pediatrician from the Children's Hospital, Sheffield, in the UK, joined the research front on perinatal mortality and morbidity, and published a paper in the *British Medical Journal* – Why blame the obstetrician? A review[14]. He searched the literature thoroughly on the subject of causes of submental status and cerebral palsy, and, in addition, he drew on his own extensive clinical experience. In his review, evidence is given for underlying causes acquired during pregnancy which lead to difficulties during labor, rather than the reverse. For example, as reported by Hagberg and colleagues in 1976[15], maternal bleeding during pregnancy occurs three times more frequently among pregnancies result-ing in cerebral palsy than in controls.

Another significant study on the effect of the birth process on subnormal mental performance was carried out by Penrose in 1949[16]. He found that, of 1280 mentally defective patients, in only 11 did the clinical history war-rant a diagnosis of birth injury as a cause. Cerebral palsy undoubtedly is linked to hypoxia/anoxia. In 1969, Towbin[17] demonstrated through mor-phological studies that the brain of the developing fetus could be 'marked' at the time that hypoxia occurred.

Much more frequent causes of cerebral palsy and mental retardation than hypoxia during labor are placenta previa or abruption, chronic toxemia, placental insufficiency with fetal growth retardation and multiple gesta-tions. Furthermore, fetal brain death has been documented[18].

To date, these findings are in line with those of Illingworth[14]. However, the conclusion of this paper must not be used to deliver babies with poor Apgar scores. Medical litigation is an increasing phenomenon in industrial-ized countries and both the law courts and the people still assume that any infant who develops neonatal or infant neurological morbidity must have been damaged by intrapartum mismanagement. The fact, that much can happen during the 9 months of pregnancy and that parturition can make things worse, calls for accurate documentation of events and new tech-niques for the early detection of fetal hypoxia and acidosis leading to dis-tress.

Refined semiquantitative methods of neonatal neurology

Although cerebral palsy is a rather strictly defined syndrome in terms of neurological symptoms, a more 'refined' and 'unbiased' neurology which could be applied to the neonate was most definitely welcomed.

In 1964, Heinz Prechtl and D. Beintema[19], of the Department of Developmental Neurology, University of Groningen, The Netherlands, pre-sented a manual for clinical use, entitled *The Neurological Examination of the Full-term Newborn Infant*, which described a standard neurological examination technique for the full-term newborn infant in the 2nd week after birth. A further edition of the book, edited by H. Prechtl, was pub-

14. Illingworth, R.S. (1979). Why blame the obstetrician? A review. *Br. Med. J.*, **1**, 797

15. Hagberg, G., Hagberg, B. and Olow, I. (1976). The changing panorama of cerebral palsy in Sweden 1954–1970. *Acta Paediatr. Scand.*, **65**, 403

16. Penrose, L.S. (1949). Birth injury as a cause of mental defect: the statisti-cal problem. *J. Ment. Sci.*, **95**, 373

17. Towbin, A. (1969). Cerebral hypoxic damage in fetus and newborn. Basic patterns and their clinical significance. *Arch. Neurol.*, **20**, 35

18. Nijhuis, J. G., Kruijt, N. and Van Wijck, J.A.M. (1988). Fetal brain death. Two case reports. *Br. J. Obstet. Gynaecol.*, **95**, 197

19. Prechtl, H.F.R. and Beintema, D. (1964). *The Neurological Examination of the Full-term Newborn Infant,* 1st edn. (London: W. Heinemann)

20. Prechtl, H.F.R. (1977). *The Neurological Examination of the Full-term Newborn Infant,* 2nd edn. (London: W. Heinemann)

21. Prechtl, H.F.R. (1967). Neurological sequelae of prenatal and perinatal complications. *Br. Med. J.,* **4**, 763

22. Brazelton, T.B. (1973). *Neonatal Behavioral Assessment Scale.* (Philadelphia: J.B. Lippincott)

23. Manning, F.A., Platt, L.D. and Sipos, L. (1980). Antepartum fetal evaluation: development of a fetal biophysical profile. *Am. J. Obstet. Gynecol.,* **136**, 787

24. Vintzileos, A.M., Campbell, W.A., Ingardia, C. J. and Nochimson, D. J. (1983). The fetal biophysical profile and its predictive value. *Obstet. Gynecol.,* **62**, 271

lished in 1977[20]. The examination takes into account the behavioral state of the neonate as well as the development and possibilities of the central nervous system at that particular age. A protocol of semiquantitative reflex testing has to be performed in a specific sequence. The total neurological score of 42 variables in earlier studies or of 60 variables in later studies completes the examination.

The number of optimal neurological responses correlated negatively with the number of non-optimal obstetric conditions. In 1967, Prechtl[21] reported that quantitation of non-optimal conditions could identify babies at risk for neurological damage. Prechtl's methodology was used for the study of obstetrical –neonatal neurological relationships, especially in the Netherlands. Prechtl's concept of neonatal behavioral states also lead to the description of those states in the fetus (see Paper 2). In 1973, Brazelton[22] expanded the concept of Prechtl in clinical tests for the capacity of the infant to control its environment, and a variety of perinatal influences (particularly maternal medication) was investigated.

'The Apgar score *in utero*'

As a consequence of the development of ultrasound imaging techniques, in 1980, F.A. Manning and co-workers[23] were able to carry out an important study on the assessment of fetal biophysical variables. Antepartum fetal evaluation is particularly important where perinatal mortality is the outcome and even more so in cases of intrauterine fetal death.

In this paper, five biophysical variables were introduced – fetal breathing movements, fetal body movements, fetal tone, amniotic fluid volume, and fetal heart rate reactivity.

Analogous with the Apgar score, 0–2 points were allocated to each variable, a total of 10 being the maximum possible for 'fetal condition' and the combination of variables was considered to be far more accurate in antepartum fetal evaluation than any single test. As with the Apgar score, the variables are, however, not independent of each other.

In the Apgar score, respiration is the dominant factor and should have had more than 2 points. The same physiological reasoning applies to the 'Manning' score. For example, fetal respiratory movements are necessary for lung development and extrauterine survival and not for fetal oxygenation and deserve less than 2 points. In contrast, the volume of amniotic fluid is a sign of a good or bad chronic balance of compartmental exchanges and probably warrants allocation of more than 2 points. In cases of acute distress, cardiac reactivity is more reliable than any other parameter.

This insight into fetal (patho-) physiology was recognized by Vintzileos and co-workers[24] in 1983.

Fetal movements and tone: the last to disappear

In 1983, Vintzileos and colleagues[24] published a paper – The fetal biophysical profile and its predictive value. In this study, fetal biophysical variables were assessed in order to determine the relationship between single and combined variables and the outcome of pregnancy. They added 'placental grading' to the 'list' of variables described previously by Manning and co-workers[23] in 1980.

In this study, the presence of normal biophysical activity indicated that the portion of the central nervous system responsible for controlling this activity was both intact and functioning. However, the absence of a given activity was much more difficult to interpret as a reflection of pathology or normal periodicity. The periodicity in biophysical activities, for example, could be of short-term circadian (diurnal) rhythms, as seen in extrauterine life. Respiratory movements, for instance, as well as sleep–wake cycles, are excellent examples of such a periodicity.

It also appeared that there was a certain order of disappearance of biophysical activities in the asphyxiation process. Those activities that became active first in fetal development were the last to disappear. For example, the fetal tone center in the cortical–subcortical area, functioning at 7–9 weeks' gestation, is the last to disappear during asphyxia. Indeed, in this study, the presence of poor or absent fetal tone was associated with the highest perinatal death rate (42.8%). The fetal movement center starting at about 9 weeks of development is more sensitive to hypoxia than the fetal tone center. The fetal heart reactivity center in the posterior hypothalamus and medulla is functional by the end of the second trimester and is, therefore, the most sensitive to hypoxia.

The above concept of 'grading' and 'time sequences' of fetal biophysical variables is of significant value for the interpretation of the biophysical assessment of fetal health.

Fetal breathing rediscovered

In 1888, Friedrich Ahlfeld was the first to report on intrauterine fetal respiratory movements at the IVth Meeting of the German Gynecological Congress in Halle.

He encountered considerable resistance within the society. His colleagues argued that the 'excursions' seen on the kymograph represented everything but fetal respiratory movements. This triggered Ahlfeld to 'rearrange his instrumentation during the vacation period of 1904 and to start a whole series of experiments'.

Observations

25. Ahlfeld, F. (1905). Die intrauterine Tätigkeit der Thorax- und Zwerchfellmuskulatur Intrauterine Atmung. *Monatschrift für Geburtsh., u. Gynäk.*, 21,143

As described in 1905 by Ahlfeld[25] and as shown in the following figures, the recordings comprise two 'lines', the upper trace representing time in seconds, and the lower trace, movements of the maternal abdomen. Ahlfeld demonstrated that these abdominal movements occurred at a rate of between 38 and 76 per min (mean = 61). In addition, by recording maternal respiratory movements and the radial pulse of the mother separately, Ahlfeld demonstrated that the excursions were not due to maternal, but rather to fetal thoracic movements.

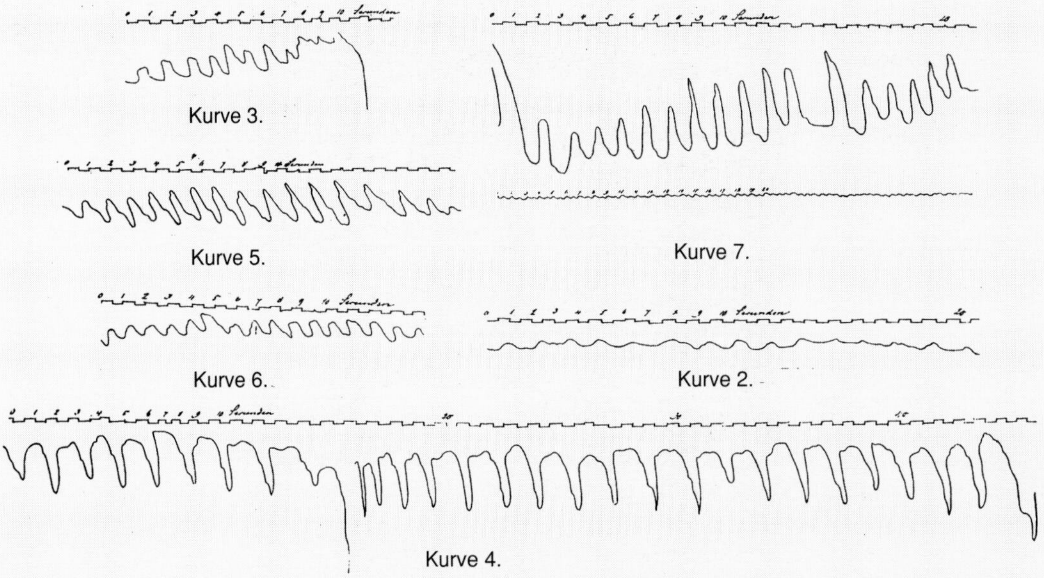

Kurve 3.

Kurve 5.

Kurve 7.

Kurve 6.

Kurve 2.

Kurve 4.

Kurve 2. Leichte wellige Erhebungen.
Kurve 3. Höhere Ausschläge bei intrauteriner Atmung.
Kurve 4. Sehr starke Erhebungen durch intrauterine Atmung.
Kurve 5. Intrauterine Atmung ohne mütterliche Atembewegungen.
Kurve 6. Fötale Atmung ohne mütterliche Atembewegungen.
Kurve 7. Intrauterine Atmung neben mütterlicher Pulskurve (Radialpuls).

Original observations made by Ahlfeld, the upper line in each 'kurve' representing time (seconds) and the lower trace, movements of the maternal abdomen.
Reproduced from Ahlfeld (1905)[25] with permission from Karger, Basel

Members of the 'Fetal Breathing Society', raised by Geoffrey Dawes in the 1970s, expected that further study of fetal breathing would yield results comparable to those on asphyxia in the neonate. However, this expectation was not fulfilled. Instead, insight was acquired as to the factors that could inhibit fetal breathing movements – quiet sleep, maternal hypoglycemia, smoking, narcotics and active labor, and also to the factors which could stimulate fetal breathing movements – rapid eye movement sleep and maternal hyperglycemia.

Apgar scores or blood gases?

As described in the summary of the paper – Do Apgar scores indicate asphyxia – published in *The Lancet* in 1982, Sykes and colleagues[26] studied the relationship between blood gas analyses performed on arterial and venous cord blood and the Apgar score. Their summary noted:

> In a prospective study of 1210 consecutive deliveries the relation between the Apgar scores and the acid-base status of the babies at birth was assessed. Only 21% of the babies with a 1 min Apgar score <7 and 19% of the babies with a 5 min Apgar score <7 had a severe acidosis (umbilical artery pH ≤7–10 and base deficit ≥13 mmol/l). 73% of the babies with a severe acidosis had an Apgar score ≥7 at 1 min, and 86% had an Apgar score ≥7 at 5 min. Because the Apgar score does not usually reflect the degree of acidosis at delivery, its value as an index for asphyxial assessment must be questioned.

A fall in pH can interfere with intracellular biochemical processes. It is remarkable that on observing pH values in umbilical cord arterial blood, even normal labor is accompanied by pH values of around 7.25 or even lower. These values can be lower still, depending on maternal–fetal risk factors during pregnancy and the mode of delivery[27].

Epilogue

The Apgar score is a rapid method of assessing the state of the newborn infant. Except for the monitoring of the heart rate, no instruments are needed. The score is also an excellent guide for the effectiveness of resuscitation. However, to equate a low Apgar score with asphyxia is a misuse of the score. For example, maternal sedation or analgesia may decrease tone and responsiveness. Indeed, neurological disease may decrease tone or interfere with respiration, and cardiorespiratory conditions may interfere with heart rate, respiration and tone. The 1-min Apgar score reflects immediate status rather than correlating with future outcome. A 5-min score is associated more with mortality or morbidity than the 1-min score but cannot be considered either as evidence for a consequence of asphyxia or hypoxia. Umbilical cord hypoxia or acidemia may provide much more evidence for asphyxia.

26. Sykes, G.S., Johnson, J., Ashworth, F., Molloy, P.M., Gu, W. and Stirrat, G.M. (1982). Do Apgar scores indicate asphyxia? *Lancet*, **1**, 494

27. Eskes, T.K.A.B., Jongsma, H.W. and Houx, P.C.W. (1983). Percentiles for gas values in human umbilical cord blood. *Eur. J. Obstet. Gynecol. Reprod. Biol.*, **14**, 341

Even a child with a low Apgar score has a 99% chance of not suffering from cerebral palsy at 7 years of age, and 75% of children with cerebral palsy have normal Apgar scores.

In order to resolve this 'dilemma', it is recommended that, in addition to the use of Apgar scores, cord blood gas values must be assessed, and also, that clinical procedures should be correctly documented.

It will also be clear, from the history of the Apgar score and the years thereafter, that studies using 'means' of scores of 'averages' should not be accepted in scientific reports because of the interdependency of the constituent variables. Only medians or grouping of scores and non-parametric testing are appropriate. Future research will undoubtedly concentrate on the development and function of the fetal brain, using methods such as magnetic resonance imaging and spectrometry, continuous measurements of vital signs, neurotransmission and oxygen free radicals in animals as well as in the human.

28. American College of Obstetricians and Gynecologists (1993). Fetal and neonatal neurologic injury. Technical Bulletin number 163, January 1992. *Int. J. Gynecol. Obstet.,* 41, 97

The concept that disturbances in the development and function of the embryonic and fetal brain can lead to asphyxia during labor, rather than the other way around[28], forces scientists to focus more acutely on cell biology, genetics and chemistry for fetal brain research.

Summary of references

1. Apgar, V. (1953). A proposal for a new method of evaluation of the newborn infant. *Curr. Res. Anesth. Analg.,* **32**, 260
2. Dawes, G.S. (1968). *Fetal and Neonatal Physiology*, p.149. (Chicago: Year Book Medical Publishers.)
3. Windle W. F. and Becker, R. F. (1943). Asphyxia neonatorum. An experimental study in the guinea pig. Am. J. Obstet. Gynecol., **45**, 183
4. Myers, R. E. (1972). Two patterns of perinatal brain damage and their conditions of occurrence. *Am. J. Obstet. Gynecol.,* **112**, 246
5. Niswander, K., Gordon, M. and Berendes, H. (1972). The Women *and Their Pregnancies*. (Philadelphia: W.B. Saunders Company)
6. Drage J.S., Kennedy, C. and Schwartz, B.K. (1965). The Apgar score as an index for neonatal mortality. *Obstet. Gynecol.,* **24**, 222
7. Drage, J.S., Kennedy, C. and Schwartz, B.K. (1966). The Apgar score as an index for neonatal morbidity. *Dev. Med. Child. Neurol.,* **8**, 141
8. Drage, J.S. and Berendes, H. (1969). Low Apgar scores and outcome of the newborn. *Pediatr. Clin. N. Am.,* **13**, 635
9. Little, W.J. (1862). On the influence of abnormal parturition, difficult labours, premature birth, and asphyxia neonatorum, on the mental and physical condition of the child, especially in relation to deformities. *Trans. Obstet. Soc. London,* **3**, 293

10. Nelson, K.B. and Ellenberg, J.H. (1986). Antecedents of cerebral palsy – multivariate analysis of risk. *N. Engl. J. Med.,* **315**, 81

11. Nelson, K.B. and Ellenberg, J.H. (1988). Antecedents of cerebral palsy: multivariate analysis of risk. In Kubli, F., Patel, N., Schmidt, W. and Linderkamp, O. (eds.) *Perinatal Events and Brain Damage in Surviving Children.* (Berlin, Heidelberg, New York, London, Paris, Tokyo: Springer Verlag)

12. Hagberg, B. and Hagberg, G. (1989). The changing panorama of infantile hydrocephalus and cerebral palsy over forty years. A Swedish survey. *Brain Dev.,* **11**, 368

13. Rosen, M.G. and Dickinson, J.C. (1992). The incidence of cerebral palsy. *Am. J. Obstet. Gynecol.,* **167**, 417

14. Illingworth, R.S. (1979). Why blame the obstetrician? A review. *Br. Med. J.,* **1**, 797

15. Hagberg, G., Hagberg, B. and Olow, I. (1976). The changing panorama of cerebral palsy in Sweden 1954–1970. *Acta Paediatr. Scand.,* **65**, 403

16. Penrose, L.S. (1949). Birth injury as a cause of mental defect: the statistical problem. *J. Ment. Sci.,* **95**, 373

17. Towbin, A. (1969). Cerebral hypoxic damage in fetus and newborn. Basic patterns and their clinical significance. *Arch. Neurol.,* **20**, 35

18. Nijhuis, J. G. Kruijt, N. and Van Wijck, J.A.M. (1988). Fetal brain death. Two case reports. *Br. J. Obstet. Gynaecol.,* **95**, 197

19. Prechtl, H.F.R. and Beintema, D. (1964). *The Neurological Examination of the Full-term Newborn Infant,* 1st edn. (London: W. Heinemann)

20. Prechtl, H.F.R. (1977). *The Neurological Examination of the Full-term Newborn Infant,* 2nd edn. (London: W. Heinemann)

21. Prechtl, H.F.R. (1967). Neurological sequelae of prenatal and perinatal complications. *Br. Med. J.,* **4**, 763

22. Brazelton, T.B. (1973). *Neonatal Behavioral Assessment Scale.* (Philadelphia: J.B. Lippincott)

23. Manning, F.A., Platt, L.D. and Sipos, L. (1980). Antepartum fetal evaluation: development of a fetal biophysical profile. *Am. J. Obstet. Gynecol.,* **136**, 787

24. Vintzileos, A.M., Campbell, W.A., Ingardia, C. J. and Nochimson, D. J. (1983). The fetal biophysical profile and its predictive value. *Obstet. Gynecol.,* **62**, 271

25. Ahlfeld, F. (1905). Die intrauterine Tätigkeit der Thorax- und Zwerchfellmuskulatur Intrauterine Atmung. *Monatschrift für Geburtsh. u. Gynäk.,* **21**, 143

26. Sykes, G.S., Johnson, J., Ashworth, F., Molloy, P.M., Gu, W. and Stirrat, G.M. (1982). Do Apgar scores indicate asphyxia? *Lancet,* **1**, 494

27. Eskes, T.K.A.B., Jongsma, H.W. and Houx, P.C.W. (1983). Percentiles for gas values in human umbilical cord blood. *Eur. J. Obstet. Gynecol. Reprod. Biol.,* **14**, 341

28. American College of Obstetricians and Gynecologists (1993). Fetal and neonatal neurologic injury. Technical Bulletin number 163, January 1992. *Int. J. Gynecol. Obstet.,* **41**, 97

FETAL HEART RATE

Classic
Paper
No.2

The development of vascular reflexes

SIR JOSEPH BARCROFT

Fellow of King's College, Cambridge; and Director of the Unit of Animal Physiology, Agricultural Research Council

1. Barcroft, J. (1946). *Researches on Pre-natal Life*, Chapter XII. (Oxford: Blackwell Scientific Publications)

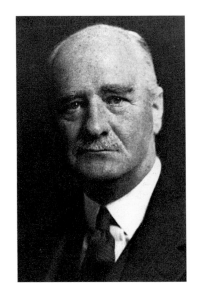

This chapter on fetal heart rate begins with the paper by Sir Joseph Barcroft which first described the development of vascular reflexes in the fetus. This study can be regarded as one of the classics in the field of fetal (patho-) physiology since it introduced the concept of fetal bradycardia and led to the description of early, variable and late decelerations in human fetal heart rate. The development of electronic fetal monitoring confirmed Sir Joseph's observations and brought with it the hope that, by monitoring fetal heart rate, mortality and morbidity of the fetus could be prevented. Unfortunately, this hope was not fully realized and randomized controlled trials failed to demonstrate a clear benefit associated with electronic fetal monitoring. Nevertheless, because of electronic fetal monitoring, much insight now exists into fetal regulatory mechanisms and the diagnosis of fetal stress and distress.

CHAPTER XII

The Development of Vascular Reflexes

AMONG the problems offered by foetal and neonatal physiology, perhaps none illustrates the danger of arguing from a single species better than the development of vascular reflexes. Whichever species had been first studied, had the picture so obtained been accepted as applying to the foetus generally, corrections would soon have become necessary.

Historically, the earliest work was that of G. A. Clark (1932), of Sheffield. on the embryo of the cat. Clark took a number of very beautiful tracings of arterial pressure. His principal conclusions were:

'1. Simultaneous records of maternal and foetal blood-pressure have been made in cats anaesthetized with chloralose.

2. Each uterine contraction causes changes in maternal and foetal blood-pressure:

(*a*) In the mother the pressure rises to reach a maximum at the height of contraction; this change occurs in the cat whether the vagi are cut or not.

(*b*) In the foetus a transient rise is followed by a well-defined fall, which lasts throughout the contraction; these changes are also seen whether the foetal vagi are cut or not and also after putting possible carotid sinus reflexes out of action. During the fall in pressure the foetal heart is slowed.

3. It is suggested that the fall in foetal blood pressure described is due, in the first place, to a reduced venous return to the heart and is in part maintained by cardiac slowing resulting from partial asphyxia.

4. The response of the foetal vaso-motor centre to asphyxia increases towards the end of pregnancy.'

Conclusions 3 and 4 above bring us to the question of vascular reflexes.

Next in chronological order came the goat. Here again the study centred round tracings of arterial pressure: such tracings showed that shortly after the ligature of the umbilical cord, at or near term, the foetal heart slows. This, of course, is a commonplace in obstetric practice, but the cause of the slowing still seemed to demand some investigation—this investigation was initiated in rather a curious way. At a meeting of the Physiological Society I chanced to give a demonstration of the recording of the effect on arterial pressure of temporary occlusion of the umbilical cord, and pointed out the bradycardia which took place after the occlusion and was abolished by the ensuing breath. On being asked what the mechanism of this slowing might be, I expressed ignorance (though I had given the matter some thought), at which a member of the Society said: 'Oh, of course, it's just asphyxial heart-block, there is no more in it than that'. Truth to tell I was just a little nettled by this remark, probably because having given this matter a good deal of thought, I had no reason to suppose that the speaker had given it any, or perhaps because I did not think it good for the Physiological Society that a great man should rap out so ill-considered a statement. However, as the demonstration was at an end, I wheeled the goat and the apparatus straight out of the room, cut the vagi, and repeated the experiment. Here is a graphic record of the two tracings (Figure 46). It is obvious, at least, that the two curves are not the same; in the first the fall is much more rapid than in the second, and that in itself gives some reason for exploring the possibility of a vagus bradycardia in addition to the slowing which must inevitably follow asphyxia as a step on the road to death.

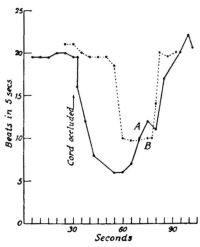

FIG. 46. Analysis of the effect of asphyxia on pulse rate. Goat foetus, 123 days. Thick line, vagi intact; A = first gasp. Broken line, vagi cut; B = first gasp. (Bauer.)

THE RABBIT

I therefore asked Bauer whether the phenomenon interested him; if so, whether he would take it up. I little realized the wealth of information which his beautiful research would produce. The principal points made by Bauer (1937) working on the sheep were, that the vagus will not produce cardiac slowing on occlusion of the cord before the 88th day, but it will by the 119th day. This slowing down commences, as in the above record, very soon after the occlusion—but if the vagi are cut a much longer interval elapses between the occlusion of the umbilical cord and the onset of the bradycardia. To record the heart beats Bauer used a string galvanometer, a very difficult thing to do considering that in the nature of the case the foetus made sundry movements on its own account, to say nothing of the disturbing effect of the maternal pulse. The method of recording was not the usual photographic one, but an adaptation of one devised by Winton by which the record was made on a smoked drum. There is a certain amount of distortion, but this method, which does not involve photographic records, can be used economically and simply for long experiments, and suffices to show that the asphyxial bradycardia was not due to heart-block but to a generally depressing action of the asphyxia upon the pacemakers. By the 140th day the slowing of the heart, consequent on asphyxia, comes on more rapidly than on the 119th, and Bauer showed that there was no sympathetic element involved. The position,

so far as the sheep and goat are concerned, may be stated quite simply. There
is a primary and secondary slowing, the former is immediate and sudden, it

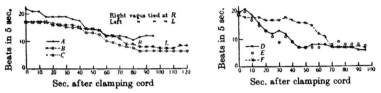

FIGS. 47 *a* and *b*.   Effect of occlusion of umbilical cord on pulse rate, sheep.
a = 88 days, *b* = 119 days. (Bauer.)
A = Vagi not ligatured.   B = Vagi ligatured.   C = Vagi released.
D and E = Successive clampings of cord with vagi intact.   F = Vagi cut.

depends upon the responsiveness of the central vagus mechanism and its
absence would argue impairment of the nervous system. The secondary
slowing is deferred and gradual (Figure 47). It is the effect of asphyxia on the
cardiac muscle and is not a heart-block.

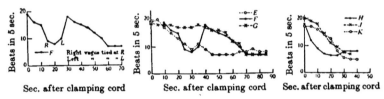

FIGS. 48 *a–c*.   Effect of occlusion of cord on pulse rate, sheep.
E = 119-day foetus, umbilical cord clamped at zero, vagi intact.   F = 119-day foetus,
umbilical cord clamped at zero, vagi ligatured at R and L respectively.   G = Repeat F,
both vagi cut from commencement.   H = 140 day foetus, umbilical cord ligatured at
zero time, vagi intact.   J = Repeat H, vagi cut.   K = Repeat J, but with stellat ganglia
removed on both sides.

Having given a general account of the relation of the cardiac slowing, which
takes place at birth by Caesarean section, to the central and peripheral elements involved, Bauer (1938, 1939) turned his attention from the sheep to
make a much more detailed analysis in the rabbit.

Electrocardiograms from the foetal rabbit showed a slowing of the heart
on occlusion of the cord, which commences a few seconds—perhaps ten—and
which takes about half a minute for its full development. This phenomenon
may be repeated without substantial alteration if the foetus be decapitated
and evidently involves no vagal factor, it is purely asphyxial: the vagus has
not yet got to work. In this respect, then, the rabbit resembles the cat and
differs from the sheep or goat at term. The rabbit, however, resembles the
88-day sheep foetus. Like the cat, of course, birth takes place at a very immature state. Any further study of the effect of asphyxia on the development
of vascular reflexes in the rabbit must clearly be carried out on the neonatal
creatures, and here it must be pointed out that the bradycardia incident on

occlusion of the trachea in the newly-born rabbit does not come on so rapidly as in the foetus of the same age. The reason seems simple, namely that the

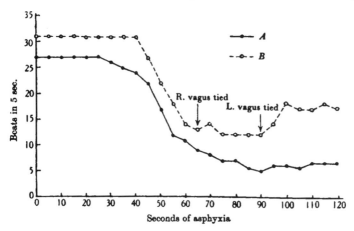

newly-born animal possesses stores of oxygen not at the disposal of the foetus: its lungs contain a certain quantity of the gas and its blood is more highly saturated, so that perhaps 30 to 40 seconds may elapse in case of the rabbit, once it has been well and truly born, from the ligature of the trachea to the on-

FIG. 49. Effect of asphyxia on pulse rate, rabbit, 4 days after birth. A = normal; B = vagi tied during asphyxia. (Bauer.)

set of the bradycardia, whereas in the same animal a few minutes earlier when it was a foetus, the slowing of the heart would have shown itself a few seconds after the occlusion of the umbilical cord.

The first signs of vagal slowing appear after the rabbit is four days old. The effect which the vagus produces at this time is not to usher in the bradycardia sooner but to deepen it somewhat when it does take place. This is shown in Figure 49.

By the 11th day, however (Figure 50), a great change takes place, an almost immediate slowing occurs on occlusion of the trachea as is shown by the fact that if the vagi are cut and the experiment repeated the curve reverts to the one-day type. It may be observed here that stimulation of the vagus with a faradic current does not produce its full inhibitory effect till the rabbit is eleven days old. Hitherto the curves have been very simple in character, after the onset of asphyxia, sooner or later the heart slows, and once having slowed it makes no attempt to revert to its original rate. But commencing on the 12th day (Figure 51) and reaching its full development by about the 20th day a new feature in the form of a

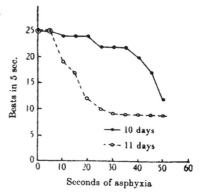

FIG. 50. Effect of asphyxia on pulse rate, rabbit, 10 and 11 days after birth respectively. (Bauer.)

spike appears on the curve. The curve starts, as have done the previous ones, with a rapid fall setting in about 10 seconds from the occlusion of the trachea, but in the second half-minute the heart quickens again and the curve attains a crest about a minute from the start; after this the pulse rate drops off again—this crest is not an escape from the vagus. If, after the first decline, that is when the vagi are inducing bradycardia, these nerves are cut the acceleration becomes even more marked than with the vagi intact: in fact the pulse rate may rise to beyond its orig-

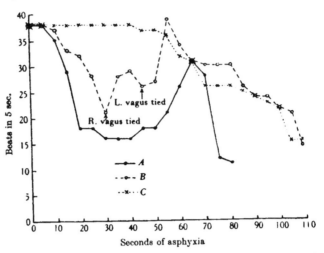

FIG. 51. Effect of asphyxia on pulse rate, rabbit, 20 days after birth. A = normal; B = vagi tied during asphyxia; C = vagi tied previous to asphyxia. (Bauer.)

inal value. The fact that the spike is abolished by ergotoxine seems to indicate that the acceleration of which it is the index is sympathetic in origin. The sequence, then, is as follows: the first effect of asphyxia at 20 days is to slow the heart due to a stimulation, which if it does not take place before the sympathetic is stimulated at least shows itself first. Later the sympathetic gets the upper hand and finally the effect of asphyxia on the node itself produces a permanent slowing of the pulse.

Though we have seen the advent of both the vagus and the sympathetic the story is by no means finished. From now onwards the vagus asserts itself more and more completely; the vagus

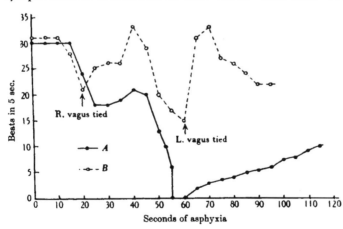

FIG. 52. Effect of asphyxia on pulse rate, rabbit, 32 days after birth. A = normal; B = vagi tied during asphyxia.

not only causes the initial depression in the curve, but as soon as the sympathetic spike appears the vagus influence increases and overrides the spike

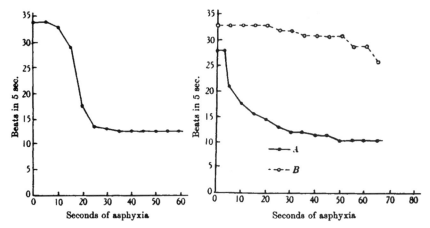

FIG. 53.   Effect of asphyxia on pulse rate, rabbit, 42 days after birth. (Bauer.)

FIG. 54.   Effect of asphyxia on pulse rate, adult rabbit. A = normal; B = after cutting vagi.

with such force that the heart may stop entirely for a moment. The reader can convince himself of the fact that this late slowing is a vagus effect by inspection of Figure 52, in which the curve is compared with one in which the vagi are cut at the appropriate moments. At the risk of anticipating what I shall discuss in detail later let me say that, in Bauer's view, the initial early vagus slowing is due to stimulation of the vagus centre, whilst the late effect, that of knocking down the sympathetic rise, is a manifestation of the depressor reflex which now appears for the first time, and is fully developed by the 36th day. The last phase, that of the increasing influence of the vagus, produces a type of curve (Figure 53) scarcely distinguishable from that which was obtained on the 11th day: the curve falls suddenly from the 10th second onwards and having once fallen never rises. The sympathetic spike is now entirely overwhelmed, any effort on its part to assert itself is overcome at the start. This final stage, according to Bauer, involves not only the depressor reflex but also the carotid sinus which latter appears before the 60th day, by which time the complete mechanism is at work (Figure 54).

Let us now turn to consider the reasons for supposing that the three possible ways in which the vagus may slow the heart—(1) to asphyxial action in the medullary vagus centre, (2) by evoking the depressor reflex, and (3) by calling into play the carotid sinus reflex—are all factors in the response of the heart to asphyxia and appear in the 1st, the 5th, and the 7th weeks respectively.

As regards the effect of asphyxia in the centre the following experiment may be performed: the depressors may be dissected out and loose ligatures put round them after a record has been made showing the effect of asphyxia on the pulse rate, the asphyxia having been produced by clamping of the

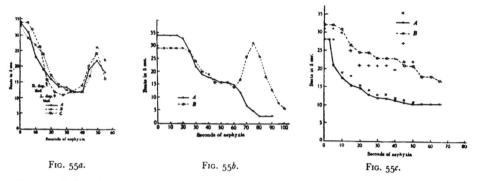

FIG. 55*a*. FIG. 55*b*. FIG. 55*c*.

FIG. 55*a*. Asphyxial curve, rabbit, 21 days after birth. A = normal; B = depressors tied during asphyxia. C = depressors tied previous to asphyxia. (Bauer.)

FIG. 55*b*. Asphyxial curves, rabbit, 34 days after birth. A = normal; B = depressors tied. (Bauer.)

FIG. 55*c*. Asphyxial curve, rabbit, adult. A = normal; B = depressors tied. (Bauer.)

trachea, the trachea is released, the ligatures are tied, conduction along the depressors is abolished and a second asphyxial record is taken. The second is not significantly different from the first: the depressors therefore have no action. This is true whether the curve was the simple fall in pressure typical of the 11th day, or whether it were the more complicated curve with the sympathetic spike which attains its full development by the 20th day (Figure 55*a*), but when the rabbit is about 32 days old the experiment has a different result. Up to about the 60th second the fall is the same whether the depressors are tied or not, but by the 60th second the effect of the depressor appears, if the depressors are intact the sympathetic spike does not take place, if, on the other hand, the depressors are cut the sympathetic spike in the asphyxial curve develops. Thus the influence which smothers the sympathetic spike at 34 days is a depressor one. As the days go on the depressor reflex comes in at an earlier stage, so that if the depressors be tied the pulse rate will rise at say 40 seconds, not at 60 as at 34 days (Figure 55*c*), and this is so whether or not the carotid sinus is in the circulation. Here, then, we revert to the carotid sinus; the easiest way of preventing these having influence, if, indeed, they can exert this, is to clamp the carotids just below the sinus. When the arteries are so clamped the sinus of the foetus appears to be sufficiently shielded from the possibility of a blood pressure to cut out its effect. By the 43rd day the clamping of the carotids produces a very marked difference on the curve, as may be seen from the subjoined Figure 56*b*.

Interesting as are the above facts, both in themselves and as evidence of the experimental skill and close reasoning by which they were elicited, there are some features about the development of the depressor and carotid sinus reflexes which seem to me even more interesting as evidence of the way in

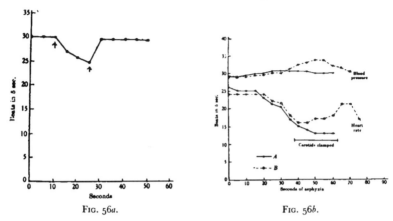

FIG. 56a.   FIG. 56b.

FIG. 56a. Stimulation of right carotid sinus at 14 days, effect upon heart rate. (Bauer.)
FIG. 56b. Asphyxial curve at 43 days, rabbit. (Ordinate, heart rate and blood pressure in arbitrary units.)   A = normal; B = carotid arteries tied during asphyxia. (Bauer.)

which development is organized in the body. The fact, I was going to say the astounding fact, is that the actual reflex machinery is developed at a considerably earlier stage than might be supposed from the experiments which I have described. It might be supposed that the 32nd day for the depressor reflex and the 60th day for the carotid sinus reflex were the days on which the machinery finally reached that stage of development and assembly before which it could not be used. The facts are far otherwise, the development and assembly took place at a much earlier stage in both cases and the reflex machinery has been waiting there ready for the day to come when the body should make use of it. Electrical stimulation of the central end of the depressor will produce a slowing of the heart as early as the 11th and of the carotid sinus as early as the 14th day (see Figure 56a).

What is the explanation of this mystery? What determines the date at which the machine, already there, shall be used for the first time? The answer, though experimentally not easy to come by, is actually very simple. The stimulus which invokes the reflex, both in the case of the depressor and of the carotid sinus, is the arterial blood pressure. The reflex is in a sense like a safety valve fitted to a boiler and set to blow off at a certain critical pressure. Bauer has determined that the critical pressure for the depressor reflex at this age is 65 mm. and for the carotid sinus 80 mm. Hg.; not until the arterial pressure reaches these thresholds do the respective reflexes operate. Now, the rabbit is born with a much lower blood pressure—about 30 mm. As the days pass the arterial pressure rises and it is not till it has risen to the values of 65 and 80 mm. respectively that the reflexes appear. Though this general statement covers the facts it does not complete the story. At birth asphyxia does not produce any rise in the arterial pressure, but as the sympathetic reflexes develop asphyxia tends more and more to raise the arterial pressure. There are therefore two factors involved in the appearance of the depressor and coronary sinus reflexes with age: firstly, the rise in the general level of arterial pressure from day to day: and secondly, superimposed on that, the rise due to asphyxia. The depressor reflex, when it first appears, is invoked at a rather late stage in the asphyxia, that is to say, when the general degree of sympathetic stimulation has reached a stage which shows itself on the pulse curve by the sympathetic spike. As the days pass and the general level of the arterial pressure rises the depressor reflex appears at an even earlier stage on the asphyxia pulse curve, because the blood pressure attains 65 mm. sooner after the asphyxia is imposed upon the rabbit.

The recording of arterial pressure in these young rabbits is not at all an easy affair. Bauer accomplished it by the introduction into the carotid of a cannula made from a hypodermic needle: it was necessary to hepatinase the rabbit and the actual record was made with a capsule which was calibrated against a mercurial manometer.

The thresholds for the reflex systems were determined in three ways, all of which give the same result:

1. If the depressor reflex is operating, ligature of the depressors will quicken the heart.
2. Asphyxia raises the arterial pressure. The point at which this rise induces slowing of the heart (65 mm.) is the threshold of the depressor, if the depressors be tied the pressure continues to rise and the slowing does not take place till a higher level is reached (80 mm.), which is the carotid sinus threshold.
3. As the age increases the normal pressure rises, but at first the pulse rate does not slow; however, when the rabbit becomes old enough for the pressure to reach 65 mm. the heart slows.

THE SHEEP

Experience of the rabbit has shown the necessity of distinguishing between the date at which the machinery of vascular reflexes is set up and that at which it is used. Moreover, in the case of any particular reflex, there is the interesting question of whether the machinery is all set up at the same time, or whether some parts appear before others. We are very far from being able to give a complete account of the dates at which the various items in the principal vasomotor reflexes come into being, are assembled into a complete arc and are first actually used, but neither are we without some body of information in the subject. Let us review what is known about dates of construction and later consider the dates of utilization.

THE CARDIO-INHIBITORY REFLEX

Stimulation of the Peripheral End of the vagus

By the term the 'peripheral end of the vagus' I mean the whole mechanism peripheral to a section in the neck of the vago-sympathetic trunk. So far as the true vagal components of this trunk are concerned the path stimulated involves the part of the pre-ganglionic mechanism peripheral to the cut, together with the post-ganglionic neurone and the actual nerve ending in the muscle.

The earliest date at which Bauer obtained slowing of the heart by peripheral vagus stimulation, was the 88th day, the following is his statement. 'Vagal stimulations were performed on all the foetuses, both nerves were able to slow the heart except in the case of the 88th day foetus, where the left vagus had no effect and the right vagus only a slight one.'

In the laboratory records of experiments on sheep, I have found a note in Barron's handwriting, that he had obtained slowing of the heart by stimulation of the peripheral end of the vagus on the 77th day.

More recently I myself (Barcroft and Barron, 1945) have obtained slowing as the result of stimulation of the peripheral end of the right vagus on the 77th day.

SHEEP 591, 77 DAYS. BEATS IN $\frac{1}{4}$ MINUTE STIMULATION

1. No stimulation	38
2. Peripheral end of right vagus	26
3. „ „ „	24
4. No stimulation	41

Whether the left vagus would have slowed the heart on the 77th day or not I do not know; it had been cut low down in the neck for another purpose but on the 81st day I obtained a suggestion of slowing, but a suggestion so slight as to be scarcely significant.

SHEEP 577, 81 DAYS.   BEATS IN $\frac{1}{2}$ MINUTE STIMULATION

1. No stimulation	84	6. Stimulation of peripheral end of right vagus	46
2. Stimulation of peripheral end left vagus	79	7. No stimulation	84
3. Stimulation of peripheral end left vagus	77	8. Stimulation of peripheral end of right vagus	50
4. No stimulation	83	9. Ditto	68
5. No stimulation	83	10. No stimulation	83

In essence, then, the implication in Bauer's statement is correct, namely, that cardiac inhibition along the right vagus is well established before it is along the left.

The corollary to the above experiment is, that in order to study the date at which the central machinery is elaborated, the correct procedure is the stimulation of the central end of the left vagus, the right vagus being intact.

So far as I have gone, this procedure has shown a central slowing as early as a peripheral one.

Stimulation of the Central End of the divided vagus

Pursuing the sequence indicated at the end of the last paragraph an answer may be sought to the question: What is the earliest date at which cardiac slowing, due to central vagal stimulation, can be obtained? This question is a little different from another which might be asked, namely: what is the earliest date at which the central mechanism is elaborated? Both questions are probably capable of an answer. The difference lies in the fact that in the first question actual slowing of the heart is taken as the index; therefore stimulation of the afferent end of the vagus, even were the central machinery elaborated earlier, could not slow the heart before the peripheral mechanism in the heart itself has developed. The answer to the second question might conceivably be obtained by using the nerve currents in the right vagus as a signal when the peripheral end of the left vagus is stimulated.

To clear the way to the answering of our first question we may ask a third, namely: can cardiac slowing as the result of peripheral vagus stimulation be obtained at an earlier date than that obtained by central stimulation? Or, tersely, can we obtain a bradycardia from excitation of the central end of the vagus on the 77th day? The following experiment gives the answer.

SHEEP 591.   77 DAYS

Stimulation of vagus		First quarter minute	Second quarter minute	Total half minute
1. None		39	39	78
2. Central end of left vagus.	Coil 60	34	30	64
3. Central end of left vagus.	Coil stronger	30	29	59
4. None—the half minute after (3)		36	28	64
5. None		45	—	—
6. Central end of left vagus		32	28	60
7. None		38	—	—
8. Distal end of right vagus		26	—	—
9. Distal end of right vagus		24	—	—
10. No stimulus		41	—	—

It is possible to obtain an appreciable slowing by stimulation of the central end of the vagus, of the heart at 77 days, which is as early as the direct effect has been obtained from the peripheral end of the right vagus and earlier than has been obtained from the peripheral end of the left vagus.

I need only add that the effect at 80 days seems to be greater, namely, the reduction of a pulse rate per half minute of 76 to one of 56 beats.

THE PULSE

Observations made at the London County Council Hospital, Hammersmith, by Dr. James Young and his staff, directed our attention to a much more complete study of the pulse of the foetus *in utero* than had previously taken place. I will not go too deeply into the errors from which he saved us. They are interesting enough as a practical warning of what may take place in research, but they would form a tortuous avenue to the established facts and these, after all, are the matters of importance.

Let me say at once that after the 93rd day in the sheep—and possibly before it—four levels of pulse rate may be recognized in the sheep.

(I)   The pulse *in utero*.
(II) The pulse on delivery.
(III) The pulse with both vagi severed.
(IV) The pulse driven as fast as adrenaline will drive it.

(1) *The pulse 'in utero'*

It is less easy to hear the foetal pulse through the uterine wall in the sheep than in man; towards the very end of gestation the foetal pulse may be counted in this way by the stethoscope, but earlier it is necessary to employ other methods. The two we have used involve an incision in the abdominal wall of the mother and either (*a*) listening to the pulse through the wall of the uterus or (*b*) passing the hand into the abdomen and feeling the pulse through the uterine wall. The obvious precaution must be taken of ensuring that it is the foetal and not the maternal pulse which is being counted, but a less obvious source of error is that of mistaking the respiration of the mother for the pulse of the foetus. The maternal respiration is often very rapid in the sheep and may press the foetus rhythmically up against the finger of the observer; we have discarded observations in which the apparent foetal pulse was within a few beats of the maternal respiration rate counted just previously or just subsequently.

The operation is as follows: the sheep, under spinal anaesthesia, is placed in the bath on its left side; the right leg is drawn out of the way and the right femoral artery of the mother is exposed sufficiently to render the counting of the maternal pulse easy. A longitudinal skin incision is made between the umbilicus and the mammary gland from the ends of which transverse incisions are made almost to the head of the femur and the crest of the ileum respectively—the flap of skin so formed is turned back. The body wall is then opened by two incisions along the insertions respectively of the superior and inferior oblique muscles. Working outwards from these the uterus is exposed and through its wall the foetal heart may easily be counted with the aid of the

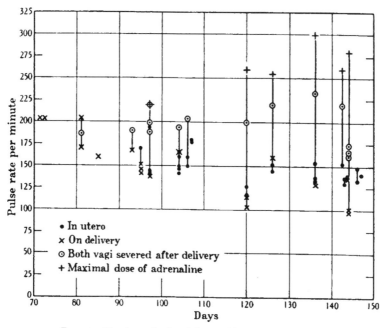

FIG. 57. Vagal tone in sheep's foetus. (Barcroft and Barron.)

stethoscope. This plan has been found successful about the 100th day, but later the foetus is too high up in the abdomen; it is then best, with the same incision, to pass the hand upwards and palpate.

As in the case of human adult pulses there seem to be individual differences, nevertheless certain points stand out in the sheep (see Figure 57).

1. There is a slight variation from minute to minute.
2. Apart from such slight variations the general trend, after the 93rd day, is for the pulse to become progressively slower as pregnancy proceeds (see Figure 57). Before 70 days the pulse quickens as gestation proceeds, as does the pulse of the chick embryo (Cohen and Wile, 1925; Bogue, 1933). In the 49 day sheep embryo it is 130.

(II) *The pulse on delivery*

The maximal normal rate *in utero* is therefore in the region of the 90th day and is about 180–200 beats per minute.

If the foetus is delivered through the uterine wall into the saline bath in which the mother is lying, if the delivery is rapid and easy, if there is no tension on the uterine wall, and once the immediate upset of delivery has passed off (say after three or four minutes)—the frequency of the heart is not very different from what it was in the uterus. As the foetus lies exposed in the bath, however great the precautions to preserve the tone of the umbilical vessels, the pulse tends to quicken as time goes on till it reaches or approximates to the heart rate with the vagi severed.

TABLE LXIX

RECOGNIZABLE LEVELS OF FOETAL PULSE IN SHEEP

Serial Number	Foetal age (days)	Mean pulse rate per minute			
		A in utero	B just after delivery	C immediately after observations in Column B Vagi cut	D maximal rate maintained for 15 seconds adrenaline heavy dose
590	90	170	—	—	—
604	97	143	138	200	220
593	104	152	166	—	194
589	106	154	—	208	—
584	108	155[1] 134[2]	138	227	248
599	120	129	104	200	260
592	126	155	162	220	256
598	136	—	112	—	—
610	143	134	130	—	—
605	144	107	102	165	280
611	146	141[1] 134[2]	118	—	—

[1] Before putting mother in bath.   [2] With mother in bath.

(III) *The pulse with both vagi severed*

The figures in Table LXIX show clearly that at any time after the 97th day, and perhaps before that date, the heart of the intra-uterine foetus is under vagal control. This period embraces the last third of the gestation period in the sheep.

A feature presented by the data is the comparative uniformity of the degree of control as represented by the intra-uterine rate considered as a percentage of the rate with the vagi severed. Individual animals may have more or less rapid pulses, but expressed as a percentage of the rate when freed from vagal control they become more uniform, though the tendency is for the vagal control to increase, which would suggest:

1. A relatively uniform degree of vagal control at any specific age, but one with a tendency to increase as gestation proceeds.
2. That the control is seen against some background, such as idiosyncrasy of the individual heart, or hormonal control, which affects the pulse rate proportionately in the same degree whether or no the vagi be cut.

TABLE LXX

Sheep	Foetal age (days)	A Intra-uterine pulses	B Pulse with vagi cut	$\frac{A}{B} \times 100$
604	97	143	200	71
589	106	154	208	73
599	120	129	200	65
592	126	155	230	70
584	137	154	234	66
605	143	107	165	65

(IV) *The pulse driven as fast as adrenaline will drive it*

After section of both vagi, it is still possible to increase the pulse rate by the injection of large doses of adrenaline (see Figure 57).

Let me emphasize again, that if the phenomena which have just been described are to be observed they must be observed at once on the delivery of the foetus—a delivery which must be carried through with no strain on the uterine and umbilical vessels and no exposure of the cord or foetus. It is the absence of these precautions which has hitherto obscured the facts. The natural tendency to economy prompts the operator, when using valuable material, to observe one or two other things before he cuts the vagus irrevocably. It is a false economy, the only right policy in work on foetal physiology is for the operator to make up his mind on the precise point on which he seeks to be informed and to sacrifice everything to it. It may seem wasteful to do an experiment on a sheep which only takes ten minutes and produces but a single lesion, but it is less wasteful than for him to misinform himself on three or four matters.

Mere exposure of the foetus produces in time sufficient deterioration, presumably of the medulla, to free the heart from vagus control. Thus in foetus 598 (136 days) the pulse on delivery was 112, the foetus was prepared for a record of the blood pressure, involving some degree of manipulation and a lapse of time of perhaps 15 minutes. At the commencement of the tracing the pulse rate was 192 and was not further quickened by section of the vagi.

The foetus, however, becomes 'tougher' as term approaches. Vagal tone therefore will survive a degree of manipulation in older foetuses that would abolish it in younger ones   For instance, foetus 610 (143 days):

TABLE LXXI

Time Hour Min.		Condition (Half Min.)	Pulse	Remarks
11	17	in utero	67	
11	20	—	—	Foetus delivered
11	21	in saline bath	65	
11	32	,, ,,	65	
11	45	,, ,,	79	
11	52	,, ,,	80	
11	53	,, ,,	77	
12	13	,, ,,		Kymograph tracing commenced
12	14	,, ,,	89	
12	16	,, ,,	101	Both vagi cut

In the above experiment full vagal control was maintained for at least 12 minutes and it was not entirely abolished at the end of nearly an hour.

This is where Dr. Young saved me; a year ago I would have said, and indeed in a draft of this chapter written then I did say, that vagal control did not appear till about the 120th to 130th day, up to which time the normal pulse gradually rose to about 200 per minute and was unaffected by section of the vagi, and that then it fell rather suddenly till at term it was in the region of 100–120 rising to the neighbourhood of 200 on section of the vagi. This picture was based on blood pressure records taken with the mercurial manometer. The data in question are shown in Figure 58. When Dr. Young

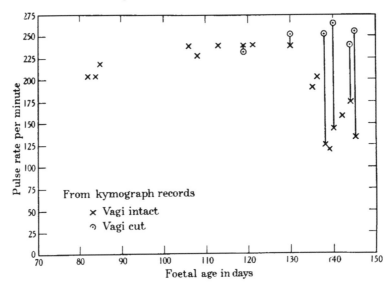

FIG. 58. Vagal slowing of the foetal pulse as shown by manometer tracings.

saw this figure he said to me, 'That corresponds to nothing that I can hear with the stethoscope in the wards'. So it became clear that before making any statement I had to devise some method of studying the pulse rate *in utero*, and that event showed that in foetuses younger than about 120 days the degree of manipulation involved in the insertion of the cannula and the other preliminaries contingent in the taking of the tracing had involved a (medullary?) deterioration sufficient to free the heart from vagal tone.

Let me go further: in a book, *The Brain and its Environment*, I made a statement on the basis of a couple of experiments under full urethane anaesthesia and on the basis of a kymograph record of blood pressure that the foetal heart was not under vagal control at 123 days. Well, in the animals in question it was not, but I have learned a good deal in the school of adversity since those days.

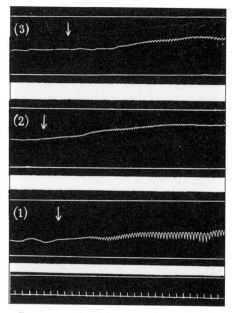

FIG. 59. 1–3. Arterial pressure, sheep 143. Effect of intravenous injection of 1 c.c. 1/50,000 adrenaline. (1) Vagi not blocked; (2) vagi blocked by ice-cooled plates; (3) vagi not blocked. Lower horizontal time 50 mm., upper time 100 mm. (Barcroft and Barron.)

BLOOD PRESSURE

In this period of toughness which occurs during the last ten days of pregnancy a number of the standard vasomotor reflexes have been demonstrated. Presumably they could be demonstrated at an earlier foetal age by more delicate methods, but we do not know what the earliest age may be.

1. That adrenaline will raise the blood pressure in the foetus is already known. Clark (1932), Schlossmann (1932). The records so far published show no clear indication of the effects on the heart.

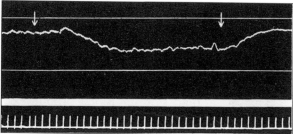

FIG. 60. Arterial blood pressure. Sheep 606. Arrows denote commencement and end of stimulation of central end of left vagus, with left vagus cut. (Barcroft and Barron.)

Figure 59 shows three tracings. The arrow marks the point of injection of 1 c.c. 1-50,000 adrenaline which was injected intravenously in each case. In No. 1, after a slight rise of blood pressure,

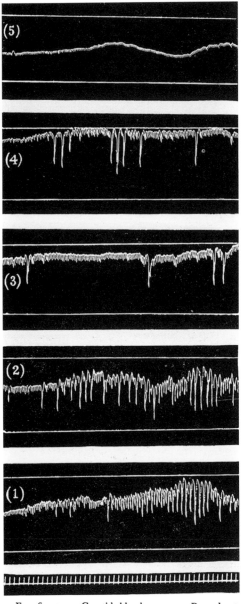

FIG. 61. 1–5. Carotid blood pressure. Records at intervals of about 3 mins. The lower horizontal time in end tracing corresponds to 50 mm., the upper time to 90 mm. Between 4 and 5 both vagi cut. Seconds. (Barcroft and Barron).

the heart commences to slow, the bradycardia becoming more pronounced as the pressure rises. In No. 2 the dose is repeated but the vagi are blocked with a strip of copper the end of which is plunged in a freezing mixture. If there is any slowing it is almost inappreciable. In No. 3 the original procedure is repeated, the bradycardia reappears but the effect is less marked than in tracing 1 presumably because the medulla of the foetus is by that time in less good condition.

2. Figure 60 is the classical fall of blood pressure caused by stimulation of the central end of one vagus (in this case the left) with the other cut, showing the existence of sympathetic tone. (This tracing also shows signs of respiratory movement, though, being under saline, no air went into or out of the chest.)

3. Figure 61 shows the gradual rise in blood pressure which occurs for some time after the delivery of the foetus. At first the rise is associated, as in Figure 59, with a bradycardia, by the time the end of the fourth tracing is reached (about 12 minutes) the pressure has risen from about 70 to just under 90 mm., as described earlier in this chapter and the cardiac slowing is less pronounced, either because the preparation has become less sensitive or because the threshold has risen. Even so a good deal of vagal tone

remains as shown by the comparison between tracings 4 and 5; in the latter the vagi are cut.

The following may now be said with considerable confidence about the sheep.

1. Rid of vagus control the pulse tends to quicken throughout pregnancy.
2. Actually, *in utero*, during the last third of pregnancy the tendency is for the pulse gradually to become slower.
3. The discrepancy between the actual slowing (§2) and the potential quickening (§1) is due to vagus control.
4. That up to the 120th day, or later, the central nervous system is so delicate that exposure of the foetus, even under carefully guarded experimental conditions, may easily abolish vagal tone.
5. That at about the 120th to 130th day the foetus 'toughens' to a degree which enables it better to withstand exposure.

MAN

Man at birth is intermediate in development between the sheep on the one hand and the rabbit on the other. It is therefore impossible to prophesy, with any degree of confidence, whether the cardio-inhibitory reflex will exist at birth or not. If it does exist, however, it will probably be less developed than in the sheep.

It is possible to approach the subject in this way. If the vagus reflex is not developed the pulse rate may be expected to rise to the end of the gestation, if towards the end of gestation the pulse rate remains level or commences to fall it is probably on the analogy with the sheep that the cardio-inhibitory reflex has commenced to operate. Figure 62 shows the results of a number of cases observed by Professor Young (1945) and his staff which he has kindly allowed me to quote. Irrespective of the inferences drawn from them the results are of great interest.

In the new-born babe the pulse is consistently faster when awake than when asleep, and faster when crying than in a placid wakeful condition. This fact alone shows that by birth the nervous mechanism for the adjustment of the heart to the activity of the organism is already developed. This is an important contribution.

The outlying questions, then, are:

1. At what stage in foetal life were these mechanisms developed? and
2. Granting that they were developed during foetal life were they operating at that time?

About these matters it is difficult to say a great deal because of lack of uniformity of the individual tracings; two are relatively smooth, Palmer and Gregg; four, Rook, Exton, James, and Praess, tend to get less smooth towards the end of pregnancy. Mitchell and Dowett show considerable variations

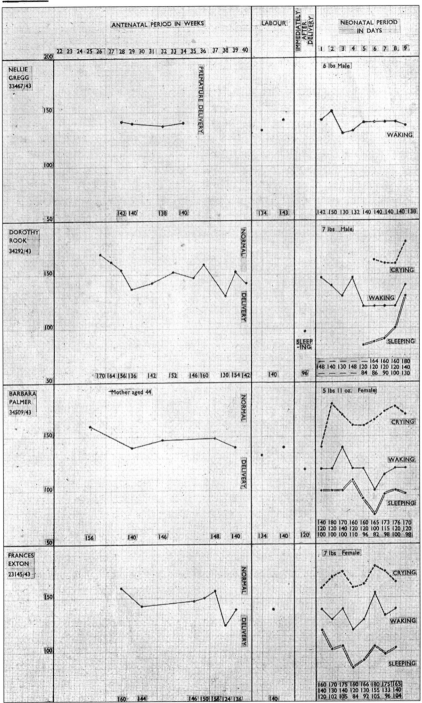

FIG. 62. Foetal pulse rate during pregnancy and after birth, human. (Young and Kenny.)

142

'T' CASES

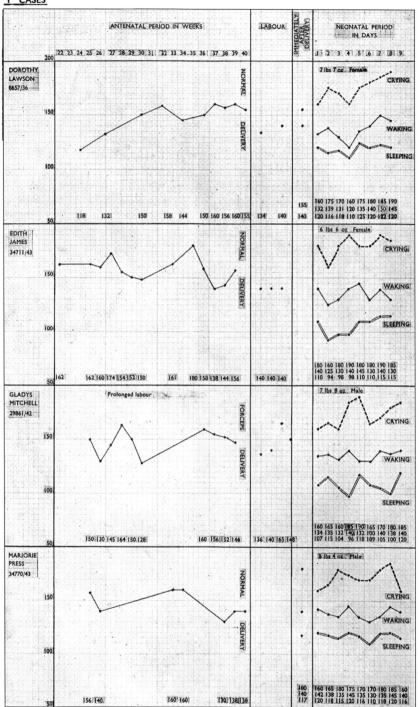

	ANTENATAL PERIOD IN WEEKS	LABOUR	IMMEDIATELY AFTER DELIVERY	NEONATAL PERIOD IN DAYS

DOROTHY LAWSON 8657/36 — NORMAL DELIVERY

7 lbs 7 oz Female — CRYING, WAKING, SLEEPING

118	132	150	158 144	150 160 156 160 155	134	140	140	155

160 175 170 160 175 180 185 190
132 139 131 120 135 140 150 145
120 116 118 110 125 120 122 120

EDITH JAMES 34711/43 — NORMAL DELIVERY

6 lbs 6 oz Female — CRYING, WAKING, SLEEPING

162	162 160 174 154 152 150	161	180 158 138 144 156	140 140 140

180 160 180 190 180 180 190 185
140 125 130 140 145 130 140 130
110 94 98 98 110 110 115 115

GLADYS MITCHELL 29861/42 — FORCEPS DELIVERY

Prolonged labour

7 lbs 8 oz Male — CRYING, WAKING, SLEEPING

150 130 145 164 150 128	160 156 152 144	136 140 165 148

160 165 160 185 190 165 170 180 185
134 135 132 140 132 190 140 138 140
107 115 104 96 118 109 105 100 120

MARJORIE PRESS 34770/43 — NORMAL DELIVERY

3 lbs 4 oz Male — CRYING, WAKING, SLEEPING

156 140	160 160	130 138 138	180 140 117

160 165 180 175 170 170 180 185 160
142 138 135 135 130 135 135 145 140
120 118 115 120 116 110 118 120 116

143

throughout, whilst Lawson is quite anomalous. Taking the general run of the curve and neglecting, in so far as we can neglect, the local fluctuations, there seems to be a suggestion that (apart from Gregg which proved to be prematurely born) the normal pulse rate at 25 weeks is 150–170 beats to the minute and at term in most cases under 150, that is, the general tendency is for the pulse to fall. If there were no vagus control it would tend to rise. All we can say at present is that the betting on there being some vagus control before birth is rather more than 'fifty-fifty on'. If, however, half a dozen smooth cases like that of Palmer were forthcoming in which there was a gradual fall of pulse rate with age, and no smooth cases in which there was a rise, the chances in favour of vagus control would look much better.

It would seem likely, that local undulations are due to evanescent causes, associated with movement of the foetus. The study of the movements of the foetus whilst still in the uterus is a very fascinating one, but it must wait for the second volume of this book.

REFERENCES

BARCROFT, J., and BARRON, D. H. (1945). *J. exp. Biol.* 22, 63.
BAUER, D. J. (1937). *J. Physiol.* 90, 25P.
BAUER, D. J. (1937). *J. Physiol.* 90, 27P.
BAUER, D. J. (1938). *J. Physiol.* 93, 90.
BAUER, D. J. (1939). *J. Physiol.* 95, 187.
BOGUE, I. Y. (1933). *J. exp. Biol.* 9, 351.
CLARK, G. A. (1932). *J. Physiol.* 74, 391.
COHN, A. E. (1925). *J. exp. Med.* 42, 291.
SCHLOSSMANN, H. (1932). *Arch. exp. Path. Pharmak.* 166, 74.
YOUNG, J., and KENNY, M. (1945). Personal communication.

*This paper has been reproduced by kind permission of
Blackwell Scientific Publications Ltd., Oxford.*

Commentary on Classic Paper No. 2

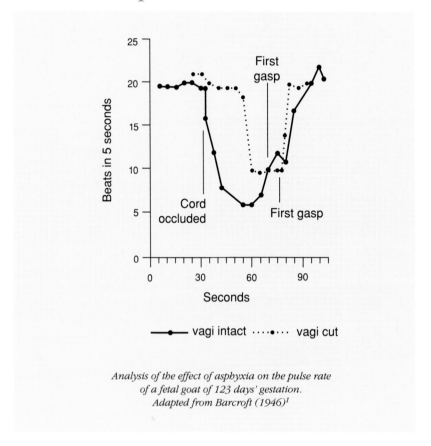

Analysis of the effect of asphyxia on the pulse rate of a fetal goat of 123 days' gestation. Adapted from Barcroft (1946)[1]

In *Researches on Pre-natal Life*[1], Sir Joseph Barcroft used the illustration above (taken from the work of Bauer) to describe an experiment in the fetal goat, in which the effect of umbilical cord compression on the pulse rate of a goat fetus was analyzed.

The authors of this commentary had the privilege of sitting next to Sir Joseph's amanuensis during dinner at the Sir Joseph Barcroft Centenary Symposium in Cambridge in 1972. He told us how these studies were performed – counting heart beats by hand, calculating beats per minute with chronometers, making graphs by hand and wrestling with smoked drums – the atmosphere of a typical physiological laboratory in those days.

Sir Joseph even had to convince his colleagues of the Physiological Society that the delayed bradycardia following vagotomy was not merely due to a heart block. Nevertheless, the concept of fetal bradycardia being due to reflectory vagal activity as well as hypoxic myocardial depression was born. (Later they would be classified as 'early' and 'late' decelerations.)

1. Barcroft, J. (1946). *Researches on Pre-natal Life*, Chapter XII. (Oxford: Blackwell Scientific Publications)

Mount Everest *in utero*

2. Eastman, N.J. (1954).
Mount Everest *in utero*.
Am. J. Obstet. Gynecol.,
67, 701

The unique environment in which the fetus lives was brought to the attention of clinicians by the Presidential Address of Nicholson J. Eastman[2] from Johns Hopkins in Baltimore (Maryland, USA). In this Address to the American Association of Obstetricians, Gynecologists and Abdominal Surgeons, the fetus was compared to a mountain climber ascending to high altitudes; emphasis was placed on hypoxia as a possible cause for perinatal mortality and morbidity, particularly cerebral palsy.

Fetal physiology

Low oxygen in the fetus

3. Huggett, A.St.G. (1927).
Foetal bloodgas tensions
and gas transfusion
through the placenta of the
goat.
J. Physiol. London, **62**, 373

In 1927, Huggett[3] had found that fetal goat blood had a low partial pressure of oxygen (po_2: 20–30 Torr). This was also observed in cord blood of the human neonate by Eastman[4] in 1930.

A different oxygen dissociation curve for fetal blood

4. Eastman, N.J. (1930).
Foetal blood studies. *Bull.
Johns Hopkins Hospital,*
47, 221

5. Roos, J. and Romijn, C.
(1938). Some conditions of
foetal respiration in the
cow. *J. Physiol.,* **92**, 249

A great deal of time and effort was devoted to elucidating how the fetus could survive at these low oxygen pressures and much attention was given to the finding that fetal blood *in vitro* has a greater oxygen-binding capacity at a given pressure than adult blood – the so-called 'oxygen-dissociation curve' (see figure below).

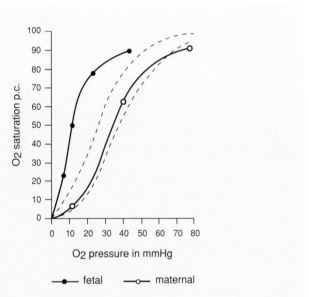

Dissociation curves of a pregnant cow (about 8 months' gestation) and the fetus. CO_2 pressure, 43–45 mmHg; temperature, 38.50. Adapted from Roos and Romijn[5] with permission

Fetal oxygenation is guaranteed

It is now recognized that, despite the oxygen tension in fetal blood being only 25% that of the adult, a combination of factors guarantees that a more than adequate oxygen supply to the fetus is maintained. These factors are:

a) A relatively high hemoglobin concentration, and thus oxygen capacity. Therefore, despite the lowered oxygen tension, the oxygen content equals that of adult blood.

b) The relatively high oxygen affinity of fetal blood.

c) The hemoglobin–circulatory flow (probably the most important factor of all) in placenta and fetal organs including fetal economy, such as cessation of movements, preferential circulation and anerobic metabolism when necessary.

The historical development of ideas concerning the po_2 difference between mother and fetus and other aspects of fetal oxygenation were reviewed by Hellegers (1970)[6] and Longo (1987)[7].

Unique fetal bloodstreams

In 1939, Barclay and colleagues[8] published the results of a radiographic demonstration of the fetal circulation in sheep 100–145 days in age delivered by Cesarean section. The intrauterine conditions were preserved by leaving the umbilical cord attached to the placenta and covering the snout of the fetus with a rubber bag containing amniotic fluid to prevent respiration.

The elegant studies from the Nuffield Institute for Medical Research at Oxford, the Physiological Laboratory and the School of Anatomy at Cambridge – a very early form of interdisciplinary research – clearly demonstrated the 'parallel' bloodstreams from the superior caval blood into the right ventricle, through the pulmonary valve into the pulmonary arteries or via the ductus arteriosus into the aorta, and from the inferior caval vein through the foramen ovale, left auricle and ventricle into the aorta.

The authors concluded: 'Hence, the heart and brain are given preferential treatment with respect to the supply of oxygenated blood coming from the placenta.' These organ-flow preferences were later confirmed by Rudolph and Heymann[9] in a series of studies using radio-labelled microspheres.

The anatomical features of the foramen ovale and the ductus arteriosus had been described in the second century AD by Galen. In 1628, Harvey[10] first described the circulation of the blood and also hypothesized about the course of the circulation in the fetus.

6. Hellegers, A.E. (1970). Some developments in opinions about the placenta as a barrier to oxygen. *Yale J. Biol. Med.*, **42**, 180

7. Longo. L. D. (1987). Respiratory gas exchange in the placenta. In Fishman, A.P., Farhi, L.E. and Tenney, S.M. (eds.) *Handbook of Physiology*, *Section 3: The Respiratory System*, Vol. IV, *Gas Exchanges*, p. 351. (Washington, DC: Am. Physiol. Society)

8. Barclay, A.E., Barcroft, J., Barron, D.H. and Franklin, K.J. (1939). A radiographic demonstration of the circulation through the heart in the adult and in the foetus and the identification of the ductus arteriosus. *Br. J. Radiol.*, **12**, 505

9. Rudolph, A.M. and Heymann, M.A. (1967). The circulation of the fetus in utero. Methods for studying distribution of blood flow, cardiac output, and organ blood flow. *Circ. Res.*, **21**, 163

10. Harvey, W. (1628). *Exercitatio Anatomica de Motu Cordis et Sanguinis in Animalibus*. (Frankfurt: Sumptibus Gulielmi Fitzeri)

11. Born, G.V.R., Dawes, G.S., Mott, J.C. and Widdicombe, J.G. (1954). Changes in the heart and lungs at birth. Cold Spring Harbor Symposium. *Quant. Biol.*, **19**, 102

12. Ramsey, E.M., Corner, G.W. and Donner, M.W. (1963). Serial and cineangiographic visualization of maternal circulation in the primate (hemochorial) placenta. *Am. J. Obstet. Gynecol.*, **86**, 213

13. Ramsey, E.M. and Donner, M.W. (1980). *Placental Vasculature and Circulation.* (Stuttgart: Thieme Verlag)

14. Moll, W., Künzel, W., Stolte, L.A.M., Kleinhout, J., Jong, de P.A. and Veth, A.F.L. (1974). The blood pressure in the decidual part of the uteroplacental arteries (spiral arteries) of the rhesus monkey. *Pflügers Archiv.*, **346**, 291

15. Longo, L.D., Power, G.G. and Forster II, R.E. (1967). Respiratory function of the placenta as determined with carbon monoxide in sheep and dogs. *J. Clin. Invest.*, **46**, 812

16. Longo, L.D., Hill, E.P. and Power, G.G. (1972). Theoretical analysis of factors affecting placental O_2 transfer. *Am. J. Physiol.*, **222**, 730

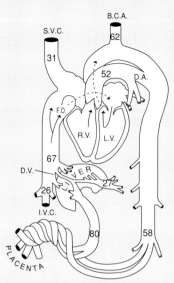

The fetal circulation in the lamb. I.V.C., inferior vena cava; S.V.C., superior vena cava; R.V., right ventricle; L.V., left ventricle; D.V., ductus venosus; F.O., foramen ovale; D.A., ductus arteriosus; B.C.A., brachiocephalic artery. The numbers indicate the mean percentage oxygen saturation of blood withdrawn simultaneously and averaged from estimations on six lambs. Adapted from Born et al. (1954)[11] with permission

Subsequently, a picture of the fetal circulation could be drawn including measurements of oxygen saturations at various points (see above figure).

The placental circulation

In a series of studies in the primate with Samuel Reynolds, Elisabeth Ramsey[12,13] described the circulation of maternal and fetal blood in the placenta (see figure over) based on anatomical and radio-angiographic techniques.

The radio-angiographic pictures gave the impression of 'jet' streams emerging from the spiral arteries into the intervillous space. However, as shown by Moll and colleagues[14] in 1974, accurate measurement using glass capillaries in monkeys demonstrated a pressure head of only 20mmHg. This favors the concept of the maternal placental circulation being more 'marsh-like'.

The placental barrier

The hemochorial placental membrane in the human has a thickness of 2–3 μm and a total surface area of $10m^2$.

Longo and colleagues[15,16] demonstrated that in the epitheliochorial placenta of the sheep, a relatively small oxygen pressure difference of 8–12 Torr is necessary for the normal role of oxygen transfer (8ml min^{-1} kg^{-1}) to supply fetal requirements. Thus for the respiratory gasses the placenta does not constitute a significant barrier to diffusion.

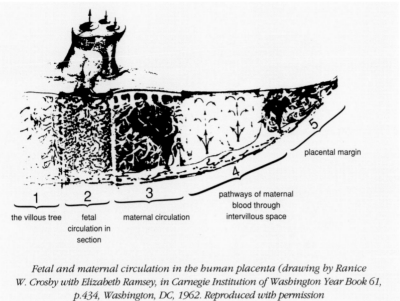

1 the villous tree 2 fetal circulation in section 3 maternal circulation 4 pathways of maternal blood through intervillous space 5 placental margin

Fetal and maternal circulation in the human placenta (drawing by Ranice W. Crosby with Elizabeth Ramsey, in Carnegie Institution of Washington Year Book 61, p.434, Washington, DC, 1962. Reproduced with permission

Indwelling catheters

It is interesting to note that since the 1930s, when the animal fetus was studied in experiments under anesthesia with manual compression of the umbilical cord, and recordings were made on smoked drums, so much more insight now exists on the regulation of fetal circulation, oxygenation, growth and metabolism.

To a great extent this scientific gain has been due to a number of factors, including the development of techniques for the study of the fetus under conditions free from anesthetic and surgical stress by using indwelling fetal catheters permitting long-term studies, as described by Meschia and colleagues[17].

Human studies

Intrauterine pressure

The development of techniques during and after the Second World War for detecting and processing biophysical signals led to the possibility of conducting studies in the human fetus.

In 1950, Alvarez and Caldeyro[18], working in Montevideo, Uruguay recorded intrauterine pressure by indwelling fluid-filled catheters. In addition, they described the patterns of the fetal heart rate, recorded by direct scalp electrodes, classifying type I and type II dips.

17. Meschia, G., Cotter, J.R., Breathnach, C.S. and Barron, D.H. (1965). The hemoglobin, oxygen, carbon oxide and hydrogen ion concentration in the umbilical bloods of sheep and goats as sampled via indwelling catheters. *Q. J. Exp. Physiol.*, **50**, 185

18. Alvarez, H. and Caldeyro, R. (1950). Contractility of the human uterus recorded by new methods. *Surg. Gynecol. Obstet.*, **91**, 1

19. Hon, E.H. (1968). *An Atlas of Fetal Heart Rate Patterns.* (New Haven, Connecticut: Harty Press Inc.)

20. Hammacher, K. (1962). Neue Methoden zur selektiven Registrierung der fetalen Herzschlagfrequenz. *Geburtsh. Frauenheilk.,* **22**, 1542

21. Haan, J. de, Bemmel, J.H. van, Versteeg, B., Veth, A.F.L., Stolte, L.A.M., Janssens, J., and Eskes, T.K.A.B. (1971). Quantitative evaluation of fetal heart rate patterns. I. Processing methods. *Eur. J. Obstet. Gynecol. Reprod. Biol.,* **3**, 95

22. Haan, J. de, Bemmel, J.H. van, Stolte, L.A.M., Janssens, J., Eskes, T.K.A.B., Versteeg, B., Veth, A.F.L. and Braaksma, J.T. (1971). Quantitative evaluation of fetal heart rate patterns. II. The significance of the fixed heart rate during pregnancy and labor. *Eur. J. Obstet. Gynecol. Reprod. Biol.,* **3**, 103.

23. Wulf, K.H. (1985). The history of fetal heart rate monitoring. In Künzel, W. (ed.) *Fetal Heart Rate Monitoring.* (Berlin, Heidelberg: Springer-Verlag)

24. Timor-Tritsch, I.E., Dierker, L.J., Hertz, R.H., Deagan, N.C. and Rosen, M.G. (1978). Studies of antepartum behavioral state in the human fetus at term. *Am. J. Obstet. Gynecol.,* **132**, 524

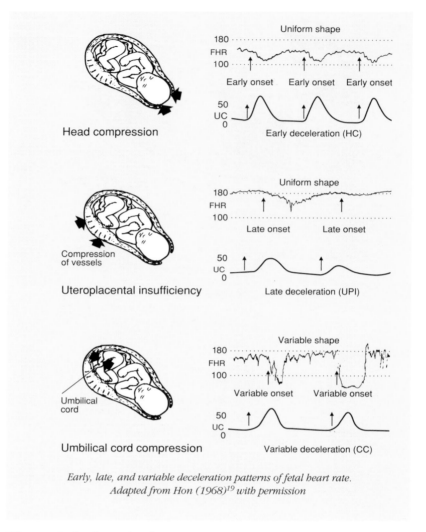

Early, late, and variable deceleration patterns of fetal heart rate.
Adapted from Hon (1968)[19] with permission

Electronic fetal monitoring

Almost simultaneously, Edward Hon[18] and colleagues in New Haven, Connecticut published their interpretation of the various fetal heart rate patterns that could be observed, such as early, variable and late decelerations, as illustrated (see figure above). Hon and his colleagues did much to popularize electronic heart rate monitoring.

The importance of the beat-to-beat variation of fetal heart rate tracings was first recognized by Hammacher[20] in 1962, and the influence of sedatives and analgesics recognized by de Haan and colleagues[21,22], in 1971.

The history of electronic fetal monitoring was described by Wulf[23] in 1985.

Fetal behavior

Timor-Tritsch and colleagues[24] in 1978 and Nijhuis and co-workers[25] in 1982 reported that the interpretation of the fetal heart rate tracings could

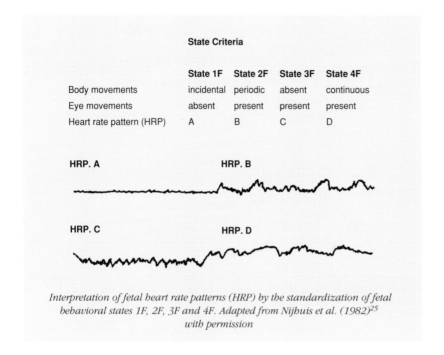

State Criteria

	State 1F	State 2F	State 3F	State 4F
Body movements	incidental	periodic	absent	continuous
Eye movements	absent	present	present	present
Heart rate pattern (HRP)	A	B	C	D

HRP. A   HRP. B

HRP. C   HRP. D

Interpretation of fetal heart rate patterns (HRP) by the standardization of fetal behavioral states 1F, 2F, 3F and 4F. Adapted from Nijhuis et al. (1982)[25] with permission

further be improved, particularly during late pregnancy, by the insight and standardization of fetal behavioral states (see figure above). The finding of Bots and colleagues[26] in 1981 that eye movements of the fetus could be recorded by ultrasonography enabled rapid eye movement (REM) sleep to be distinguished from non-REM sleep.

The finding that deep sleep is accompanied by a 'flat' tracing (up to 45 min at term), changing into REM sleep with sporadic accelerations or transitions to other states is now clinically recognized as belonging to a 'happy' fetus.

Microblood investigation of the human fetus

It was Erich Saling[27] from Berlin who recognized that heart rate tracings would never be able to cover the whole area of 'fetal condition'. He first described fetal sampling by using vaginal specula; the fetus could be reached during labor when the cervix was dilated. A small quantity of capillary blood from the presenting part of the fetus permitted the analysis of fetal blood gases (pH, po_2, pco_2, base deficit). Early detection and prevention of fetal acidosis were now possible[28].

Sensitivity and specificity

Obstetricians were not the first to embrace 'two-by-two' tables and statistics. Indeed, for a long time they relied only on case histories and experience, but gradually they came to use these techniques. Indeed, use of the tables enabled 'true false-positives' and 'false true-negatives' to be inter-

25. Nijhuis, J.G., Prechtl, H.F.R., Martin, C.B. Jr. and Bots, R.S.G.M. (1982). Are there behavioural states in the human fetus? *Early Hum. Dev.*, **6**, 177

26. Bots, R.S.G.M., Nijhuis, J.G., Martin, C.B. Jr. and Prechtl, H.F.R. (1981). Human fetal eye movements: detection *in utero* by ultrasonography. *Early Hum. Dev.*, **5**, 87

27. Saling, E. (1962). Erstmalige Blutgasanalysen und pH – messungen an Feten unter der Geburt und die Klinische Bedeutung dieses neuer Verfahrens. *Arch. f. Gynäkologie*, **198**, 82

28. Rooth, G. (1964). Early detection and prevention of foetal acidosis. *Lancet*, **1**, 290

29. Enkin, M. and
Chalmers, I. (1982).
*Effectiveness and
Satisfaction in Antenatal
Care. Clinics in
Developmental Medicine
No. 81/82.* (London:
MacKeith Press)

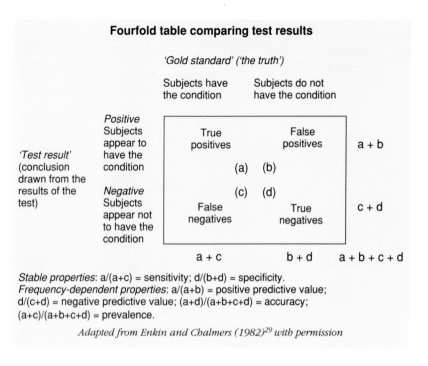

Fourfold table comparing test results

'Gold standard' ('the truth')

		Subjects have the condition	Subjects do not have the condition	
'Test result' (conclusion drawn from the results of the test)	*Positive* Subjects appear to have the condition	True positives (a)	False positives (b)	a + b
	Negative Subjects appear not to have the condition	(c) False negatives	(d) True negatives	c + d
		a + c	b + d	a + b + c + d

Stable properties: a/(a+c) = sensitivity; d/(b+d) = specificity.
Frequency-dependent properties: a/(a+b) = positive predictive value;
d/(c+d) = negative predictive value; (a+d)/(a+b+c+d) = accuracy;
(a+c)/(a+b+c+d) = prevalence.

Adapted from Enkin and Chalmers (1982)[29] with permission

30. Chalmers, I., Enkin,
M.W. and Keirse, M.J.N.C.
(1989). *Effective Care in
Pregnancy and Childbirth.*
(Oxford, New York,
Toronto: Oxford University
Press)

preted in terms of percentages of sensitivity and specificity (stable propeties) and predictive values, accuracy and prevalence (frequency-dependent properties)[30]. This 'decision-matrix' is now widely used for technological assessment.

In 1979 Banta and Thacker[31] first assessed the costs and benefits of electronic fetal monitoring. They searched the literature, subsequently categorizing the diagnostic precision of fetal heart rate monitoring using the Apgar score or acidosis as the measure of outcome.

31. Banta, H.D. and
Thacker, S.B. (1979).
Assessing the costs and
benefits of electronic fetal
monitoring.
Obstet. Gynecol. Surv.,
34, 627

They calculated a specificity (true-negative ratio), being the extent to which 'normals' were correctly classified. Sensitivity (true-positive ratio) was defined as the extent to which 'abnormals' were correctly classified. Next to this correct classification, false-positives and false-negatives were calculated in terms of percentages. Also, the predictive value of electronic fetal monitoring was calculated, which related sensitivity and specificity to the occurrence of the disease in the population studied. The predictive value of a positive test is the percentage of time that a positive test denotes a true abnormality – positive predictive value. Similarly, the predictive value of a negative test is the percentage of time that a negative test will detect a person who is actually unaffected by the disease or condition.

Using the Apgar score as the measure of outcome, they calculated that the sensitivity ranged from 32.4 to 84.2%, the specificity from 43.7 to 93.2%, the false-positives from 18.5 to 79.6% and the false-negatives from 0.7–19.9%. These percentages for specificity (84.1–92.4%) were better when using fetal scalp blood sampling.

Randomized controlled trials

The introduction of concepts such as 'gold standard' sensitivity, specificity, predictive values, odd ratios and cost–benefit analysis prompted randomized controlled trials, the largest ever performed being the Dublin trial conducted by MacDonald and colleagues[32] in 1985.

In this trial, 12 964 women were randomized to continuous electronic intrapartum fetal monitoring or intermittent auscultation, fetal blood scalp pH being available in both groups.

The trial size was calculated prior to the study. The anticipated trial size of 10 000 women had an 80% chance (power beta) of observation of a statistically significant difference at the 5% level (alpha) if adverse outcomes were actually reduced by 50%.

Cases of neonatal seizures were twice as frequent in the intermittent auscultation group, and the occurrence of forceps delivery was higher in the electronic fetal heart monitoring group.

Epilogue

An overview of some aspects of fetal respiratory and cardiovascular physiology in animals and the human reveals great interest in perinatal mortality and morbidity, particularly of the central nervous system of the fetus/neonate.

The fetus grows and develops in an adequate oxygen environment despite its low arterial oxygen tension. In particular, electronic fetal monitoring and microblood investigations of the human fetus have given more insight into fetal reactions to stress and the ability of the fetus to adapt, particularly during labor.

Nevertheless, consumer associations and increased litigation seem to be in conflict with the rather technical approach of the obstetrician 'performing unnecessary interventions cool heartedly[33]. Randomized controlled trials demonstrated that, although not everything could be predicted, unnecessary interventions could be recognized.

It follows that human touch, research intelligence and empathy have to go hand-in-hand in order to guide the fascinating process of investigating the growth and development of the intrauterine existence of the human embryo and fetus.

32. MacDonald, D., Grant, A., Sheridan-Pereira, M., Boylan, P. and Chalmers, I. (1985). The Dublin randomized controlled trial of intrapartum fetal heart rate monitoring. *Am. J. Obstet. Gynecol.*, 152, 524

33. World Health Organization (1980). Having a Baby in Europe. *Report on a Study Public Health in Europe* 26. (Copenhagen: World Health Organization)

Summary of references

1. Barcroft, J. (1946). *Researches on Pre-natal Life*, Chapter XII. (Oxford: Blackwell Scientific Publications)

2. Eastman, N.J. (1954). 'Mount Everest *in utero*'. *Am. J. Obstet. Gynecol.*, **67**, 701

3. Huggett, A.St.G. (1927). Foetal bloodgas tensions and gas transfusion through the placenta of the goat. *J. Physiol. (London)*, **62**, 373

4. Eastman, N.J. (1930). Foetal blood studies. *Bull. Johns Hopkins Hospital*, **47**, 221

5. Roos, J. and Romijn, C. (1938). Some conditions of foetal respiration in the cow. *J. Physiol.*, **92**, 249

6. Hellegers, A.E. (1970). Some developments in opinions about the placenta as a barrier to oxygen. *Yale J. Biol. Med.*, **42**, 180

7. Longo, L. D. (1987) Respiratory gas exchange in the placenta. In Fishman, A.P., Farhi, L.E. and Tenney, S.M. (eds.) *Handbook of Physiology*, Section 3: *The Respiratory System, Vol. IV, Gas Exchanges*, p.351. (Washington, DC: Am. Physiol. Society)

8. Barclay, A.E., Barcroft, J., Barron, D.H. and Franklin, K.J. (1939). A radiographic demonstration of the circulation through the heart in the adult and in the foetus and the identification of the ductus arteriosus. *Br. J. Radiol.*, **12**, 505

9. Rudolph, A.M. and Heymann, M.A. (1967). The circulation of the fetus in utero. Methods for studying distribution of blood flow, cardiac output, and organ blood flow. *Circ. Res.*, **21**, 163

10. Harvey, W. (1628). *Exercitatio Anatomica de Motu Cordis et Sanguinis in Animalibus.* (Frankfurt: Sumptibus Gulielmi Fitzeri)

11. Born, G.V.R., Dawes, G.S., Mott, J.C. and Widdicombe, J.G. (1954). Changes in the heart and lungs at birth. Cold Spring Harbor Symposium. *Quant. Biol.*, **19**, 102

12. Ramsey, E.M., Corner, G.W. and Donner, M.W. (1963). Serial and cineangiographic visualization of maternal circulation in the primate (hemochorial) placenta. *Am. J. Obstet. Gynecol.*, **86**, 213

13. Ramsey, E.M. and Donner, M.W. (1980). *Placental Vasculature and Circulation.* (Stuttgart: Thieme Verlag)

14. Moll, W., Künzel, W., Stolte, L.A.M., Kleinhout, J., Jong, de P.A. and Veth, A.F.L. (1974). The blood pressure in the decidual part of the uteroplacental arteries (spiral arteries) of the rhesus monkey. *Pflügers Archiv.*, **346**, 291

15. Longo, L.D., Power, G.G. and Forster II, R.E. (1967). Respiratory function of the placenta as determined with carbon monoxide in sheep and dogs. *J. Clin. Invest.*, **46**, 812

16. Longo, L.D., Hill, E.P. and Power, G.G. (1972). Theoretical analysis of factors affecting placental O_2 transfer. *Am. J. Physiol.*, **222**, 730

17. Meschia, G., Cotter, J.R., Breathnach, C.S. and Barron, D.H. (1965). The hemoglobin, oxygen, carbon oxide and hydrogen ion concentration in the umbilical bloods of sheep and goats as sampled via indwelling catheters. *Q. J. Exp. Physiol.*, **50**, 185

18. Alvarez, H. and Caldeyro, R. (1950). Contractility of the human uterus recorded by new methods. *Surg. Gynecol. Obstet.*, **91**, 1

19. Hon, E.H. (1968). *An Atlas of Fetal Heart Rate Patterns*. (New Haven, Connecticut: Harty Press Inc.)

20. Hammacher, K. (1962). Neue Methoden zur selektiven Registrierung der fetalen Herzschlagfrequenz. *Geburtsh. Frauenheilk,* **22**, 1542

21. Haan, J. de, Bemmel, J.H. van, Versteeg, B., Veth, A.F.L., Stolte, L.A.M., Janssens, J. and Eskes, T.K.A.B. (1971). Quantitative evaluation of fetal heart rate patterns. I. Processing methods. *Eur. J. Obstet. Gynecol. Reprod. Biol.*, **3**, 95

22. Haan, J. de, Bemmel, J.H. van, Stolte, L.A.M., Janssens, J., Eskes, T.K.A.B., Versteeg, B., Veth, A.F.L. and Braaksma, J.T. (1971). Quantitative evaluation of fetal heart rate patterns. II. The significance of the fixed heart rate during pregnancy and labor. *Eur. J. Obstet. Gynecol. Reprod. Biol.*, **3**, 103

23. Wulf, K.H. (1985). The history of fetal heart rate monitoring. In Künzel, W. (ed.) *Fetal Heart Rate Monitoring*. (Berlin, Heidelberg: Springer-Verlag)

24. Timor-Tritsch, I.E., Dierker, L.J., Hertz, R.H., Deagan, N.C. and Rosen, M.G. (1978). Studies of antepartum behavioral state in the human fetus at term. *Am. J. Obstet. Gynecol.*, **132**, 524

25. Nijhuis, J.G., Prechtl, H.F.R., Martin, C.B. Jr. and Bots, R.S.G.M. (1982). Are there behavioural states in the human fetus? *Early Hum. Dev.*, **6**, 177

26. Bots, R.S.G.M., Nijhuis, J.G., Martin, C.B. Jr. and Prechtl, H.F.R. (1981). Human fetal eye movements: detection *in utero* by ultrasonography. *Early Hum. Dev.*, **5**, 87

27. Saling, E. (1962). Erstmalige Blutgasanalysen und pH – messungen an Feten unter der Geburt und die Klinische Bedeutung dieses neuer Verfahrens. *Arch. f. Gynäkologie,* **198**, 82

28. Rooth, G. (1964). Early detection and prevention of foetal acidosis. *Lancet,* **1**, 290

29. Enkin, M. and Chalmers, I. (1982). *Effectiveness and Satisfaction in Antenatal Care. Clinics in Developmental Medicine No. 81/82.* (London: MacKeith Press)

30. Chalmers, I., Enkin, M.W. and Keirse, M.J.N.C. (1989). *Effective Care in Pregnancy and Childbirth.* (Oxford, New York, Toronto: Oxford University Press)

31. Banta, H.D. and Thacker, S.B. (1979). Assessing the costs and benefits of electronic fetal monitoring. *Obstet. Gynecol. Surv.,* **34**, 627

32. MacDonald, D., Grant, A., Sheridan-Pereira, M., Boylan, P. and Chalmers, I. (1985). The Dublin randomized controlled trial of intrapartum fetal heart rate monitoring. *Am. J. Obstet. Gynecol.,* **152**, 524

33. World Health Organization (1985). Having a Baby in Europe. *Report on a Study Public Health in Europe* 26. (Copenhagen: World Health Organization)

BRAXTON HICKS CONTRACTIONS

Classic
Paper
No.3

On the contractions of the uterus throughout pregnancy

JOHN BRAXTON HICKS

Lecturer on Midwifery and Diseases of Women, and Physician Accoucheur to Guy's Hospital; Physician to the Royal Maternity Charity; Examiner in Midwifery at the Royal College of Physicians, London

1. Braxton Hicks, J.
(1872). On the
contractions of the uterus
throughout pregnancy:
their physiological effects
and their value in the
diagnosis of pregnancy.
*Trans. Obstet. Soc.
London,* **13**, 216

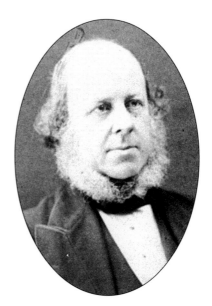

John Braxton Hicks' paper is a fine example of careful observations of the pregnant human uterus. There are not many clinicians who would take the time to sit with a pregnant woman, holding their hands on the uterus for more than 20–30 minutes. These original observations of uterine contractions, meticulously recorded by John Braxton Hicks, were later confirmed by intrauterine pressure recordings. As to their purpose, with great insight, Braxton Hicks suggested a number of physiological effects of the contractions that could help trigger the fetus to prepare for extrauterine survival and labor. Because the factors that precipitate labor in the human are virtually unknown, it remains unclear when prelabor contractions do lead to delivery, and this gap in our knowledge has led to considerable overtreatment with utero-inhibitory drugs in cases of threatening premature labor.

ON THE CONTRACTIONS OF THE UTERUS THROUGHOUT PREGNANCY: THEIR PHYSIOLOGICAL EFFECTS AND THEIR VALUE IN THE DIAGNOSIS OF PREGNANCY.

By J. Braxton Hicks, M.D. Lond., F.R.S.

LECTURER ON MIDWIFERY AND DISEASES OF WOMEN, AND PHYSICIAN
ACCOUCHEUR TO GUY'S HOSPITAL ; PHYSICIAN TO THE ROYAL
MATERNITY CHARITY ; EXAMINER IN MIDWIFERY AT
THE ROYAL COLLEGE OF PHYSICIANS, LONDON,
PRESIDENT OF THE SOCIETY, ETC. ETC.

I AM anxious to direct the attention of the profession to a point connected with the pregnant uterus, which has been almost entirely and surprisingly overlooked, as far as my researches into authors lead me to believe. Perhaps the following quotation from Dr. Tanner's work 'On the Signs and Diseases of Pregnancy,' p. 118, 1860, will best show the state of our knowledge and the authors who have alluded to the subject:

" More than twenty years since Mr. Ingleby observed that 'in advanced pregnancy the uterus, when moderately grasped and rubbed, slightly hardens and almost instantly regains its yielding condition.' Dr. Oldham has since pointed out that this power of contraction possessed by the uterus may be taken as a trustworthy characteristic of pregnancy; for he states that the large gravid uterus alters in a marked manner, under the influence of pressure, from a state of flaccidity to one of tension. Thus, if we expose a pregnant woman, the outline of the tumour is seen to be less defined before manual examination than it becomes afterwards ; for on applying the hand, the tumour which at first is felt soft and ill-circumscribed, rapidly assumes a tense rounded form, becoming firm and resisting. According to Dr. Oldham no other tumour but the pregnant uterus possesses the power of altering its form when irritated by palpation; but I must here beg to differ in opinion from this gentleman. Only a short time since I was examining the abdomen of a poor woman suffering from an attack of flooding, caused by the presence of a very large polypus in the uterus. The loss of blood had been very great, so that all the tissues were relaxed and flabby; and on placing my hands—which were very cold—over the tumour, I distinctly felt an increased rigidity of the walls of the uterus. The truth, indeed, appears to me to be this— that the uterus, in common with other hollow viscera, has, when enlarged through the presence of any substance in its cavity, a regular peristaltic movement consisting in slight contractions and dilatations. Under the influence of the former the outline of the organ can be easily appreciated, other conditions being favorable, and these contractions are undoubtedly the more evident the greater the size of the womb, and the more it is irritated by external manipulation. But as it seems that the peristaltic motions occur whenever the uterine cavity becomes enlarged from any cause, it necessarily appears objectionable to instance such movements as a trustworthy sign of pregnancy."

To these remarks of Dr. Tanner's I may add a remark of Dr. Montgomery's in his work ' On the Signs of Pregnancy,' p. 100. He says :—" The uterus within the first four months has a feel of a soft, though pretty firm, fleshy tumour, not sensitive when pressed, of a uniform smooth surface, and of such a size as would be without difficulty grasped in the hollow of the hand. After this period, that is, from the fifth month, it loses somewhat of its firmness and distinct feel, owing to the greater expansion and consequent lengthening out of its fibres, which continuing to increase as pregnancy advances towards its termination, the circumscribed organ becomes less and less distinguishable; though generally to be detected by making pressure with one hand while we examine with the other, in doing which we also ascertain some degree of obscure fluctuation, but in the same proportion as the parietes of the organ become indistinct, its solid contents are more easily felt, and even separate limbs may be recognised and traced; the firmness of the tumour as well as the degree of fluctuation which it affords will very much depend on the size it has acquired or the natural firmness or suppleness of its structure, and on the quantity of liquor amnii. Owing to the variation in these causes a corresponding degree of difference will be recognised in its consistence in different instances, so that, while in some persons it is so soft and yielding as hardly to be felt, in others it presents a degree of solidity amounting to absolute hardness, though still healthy, and retaining its round or oval form and its uniform smooth surface."

Dr. Priestley* remarks only thus far, p. 83 :—"There can be no doubt, I believe, that it possesses contractile properties (before impregnation), as it expels blood-clots, dysmenorrhœal membranes, and intra-uterine polypi.   During the extrusion of these we may sometimes distinctly recognise the alternate hardening and relaxation of the organ by placing the hand over the hypogastric region.   Its muscularity at the full term of pregnancy scarcely admits of room for controversy."   He then instances the pressure felt on your hand during a pain, &c.   He thus passes over the contractility during pregnancy.

It is evident that Dr. Montgomery did not recognise inter-mittent contractile power in the uterus, but thought the difference he had noticed was owing to an inherent difference in the tonicity of the tissues in different persons.   It does not appear how far Dr. Tanner's opinion as to the peristaltic movements was based on facts observed by himself in the different stages of pregnancy, because he gives no further information on this point, or whether his opinion was formed by a consideration of the analogy which the uterus distended bears to other hollow contractile organs.

Dr. Tyler Smith is much more clear regarding the con-tractions of the uterus, and foreshadowed in a measure the substance of this paper ; but the contractions he instances are those which are caused by excitation, as the context shows. In discussing the position of the fœtus in utero he considers that the peristaltic action of the uterus has as much influence as the movements of the fœtus itself on its position.   These movements he attributes to reflex irritation, derived from various causes of excitation.   He believes very strongly in

* 'Lectures on the Development of Gravid Uterus,' 1860.

these movements as being of even greater frequency than the movements of the fœtus within it. Thus: "I have no doubt of the frequent movements of the fœtus in utero, but wish to insist upon the equal or even still greater frequency of the movements of the uterus itself."

Again: "With this change of shape the uterus acquires more power of muscular contraction, and becomes the subject of reflex and peristaltic movements."*

These passages from Dr. Tyler Smith's thoughtful work on 'Midwifery' show that he had a very clear perception of the movements of the uterus, but I gather from them that he looked upon them as being excited by various accidental causes of a reflex kind, which he enumerates at p. 197. It may be that the frequent and almost regular movements I shall describe are really due to reflex action, but they are best observed in complete passiveness of the woman. It may be that the semi-stagnant state of the blood in the uterine sinuses, &c., may provoke contraction, but certainly there is some other excitor than either the fœtal movements or the irritation of the various nerves in sympathetic communication with the uterus. These remarks of Dr. Tyler Smith were made two years before the appearance of Dr. Tanner's, but probably they had not arrested his attention. In any case subsequent authors are silent on the subject so far as I can find, both at home and abroad.

It was a source of difficulty to the older obstetricians to explain how that, at a certain time, namely, at the full period of pregnancy, the uterus, passive up till then, began all at once to acquire a new power, that of contracting; forgetful that, long before the full period had arrived, the uterus has the power to expel the fœtus, and under mental excitement or local stimulation, attempted to do so frequently.

But after many years' constant observation, I have ascertained it to be a fact that the uterus possesses the power and habit of spontaneously contracting and relaxing from a very early period of pregnancy, as early, indeed, as it is possible

* 'Manual of Midwifery,' p. 217, 1858.

to recognise the difference of consistence—that is, from about the third month.

When the uterus is normally placed it is, of course, difficult to make it out till a little after that time, but in the case of retroversion accompanying pregnancy, then the fundus being readily felt per vaginam, the contractions can without any difficulty be perceived.

Up to the end of the second month the walls are still dense, but after this time the fundus, as can be noticed if the uterus be retroverted, will begin to be elastic, and variation in its consistence is recognisable as the end of the third month is approached.

If, then, the uterus be examined without friction or any pressure beyond that necessary for full contact of the hand continuously over a period of from five to twenty minutes, it will be noticed to become firm if relaxed at first, and more or less flaccid if it be firm at first. It is seldom that so long an interval occurs as that of twenty minutes; most frequently it occurs every five or ten minutes, sometimes even twice in five minutes. However, in some cases I have found only one contraction in thirty minutes. The duration of each contraction is generally not long, ordinarily it lasts from two to five minutes. When the uterus is irritable or has been irritated it lasts longer than this; under particular circumstances, to be alluded to again, it may assume an almost continuous action analogous to that which is noticed after long obstructed labour.

Supposing, then, we commence our examination when the uterus is contracted, we find the organ firm and solid, somewhat like the uterus affected by a fibrous tumour. Gradually this state alters, the walls becoming softer and ultimately so flaccid that their outline can be hardly made out, unless the other hand be placed on the os uteri per vaginam, and even then sometimes with difficulty. So also, if we commence our examination when the uterus is in its flaccid state, it will at first be very ill-defined, so that, if we are careless or too rapid, we might readily say that there was no pregnancy; but shortly the shape of the organ gradually becomes more and more distinct, till we have no doubt but that we have an enlargement of the uterus to deal with; after a time the firmness abates, and gradually the original condition of relaxation is complete.

If we more carefully investigate the uterus after the fourth month of pregnancy we shall further notice the phenomenon, which has been well described by authors, that during the period of relaxation the fœtus (if one be there) is generally to be detected by external palpation or by external ballotment. By internal ballotment also, in consequence of the increased impressibility of the uterine wall, we can make out the fœtal presence, its contour, often its movements, and its capability of being moved. But it is interesting also to notice, during the gradual increase of solidity, how the presence of the fœtus, quite distinct before, slowly becomes more indistinct, whilst the outline of the uterus becomes more clearly marked, till instead of the fœtus we find a hard globular swelling, which we could at the time we recognised the fœtus, scarcely, if at all, feel. That this phenomenon extends from the early period I have already mentioned, to the time of labour, is a fact to which I have never seen but one exception during a course of observations extending over about eight years; and this apparent single exception might have been none at all had a more prolonged examination been carried out at a time. It occurred in a case of paraplegia. Although she was under my care some time, and was subjected to frequent examination, yet the uterus was never found to contract. She went out of the hospital before labour arrived, but the labour was natural.

The constancy with which these contractions of the uterus have always occurred to me leaves no doubt on my mind but that it is a natural condition of pregnancy irrespective of external irritation.

In a general way the pregnant woman is not conscious of these contractions of the uterus, but sometimes she will remark that she has a tumour in her lower abdomen, thinking it a constant thing; but another will observe that she has a swelling sometimes, but which vanishes at other times. But occasionally it happens that the uterus is more than usually sensitive, and that the contractions are accompanied by pain; and then on examination it is found that each pain she complains of is coincident with a contraction.

Again, when the uterus has been excited by any cause, and these contractions are more than usually powerful, the woman is conscious of their presence, and by watching these we shall convince ourselves that the contractions, which were before unnoticed by her, are really the same as the so-called "pains" of premature expulsion of the fœtus and also of true labour.

Sometimes I have found the contractions last a considerable time, longer often than the intervals; and this is more frequently the case if the uterus contain a diseased ovum, and particularly a solid or carneous mole; but in general the contraction from its commencement to final recession lasts about five minutes. The duration both of contraction and interval varies very considerably.

But it is not only in healthy pregnancy that this phenomenon exists; it is well marked, as just mentioned, where the fœtus is dead; it is also to be found where the fœtus is absent, as in the case of hydatiniform degeneration of the chorion (vesicular mole).

How far this action is the same as the peristaltic or vermicular movement observed in the lower animals one can hardly say, but one can hardly doubt a close analogy to it if not identity with it. But when excited into a more vigorous state there can be no doubt but they are of the same character and identical with "labour pains." And this serves to explain how it is that at a short notice we can bring on labour, and how it is that the uterus shall respond in a few hours (I have seen labour artificially induced accomplished without any traction in two hours) so as to expel the fœtus at the sixth month as well as it does at the ninth month.

By our manipulation we simply exaggerate the action already going on to such an extent that the natural process exhibited by the uterus at labour at full term continues till the fœtus is expelled. In other words, we supply that stimulus which nature herself supplies at the beginning of labour at full term. The rest of the process is precisely similar. We need not, with the cognizance of this intermittent action, any longer wonder how it is that suddenly a new function is given to the uterus at the end of the ninth month; it is already in active exercise, not perceptible to the pregnant woman, though it is to the examining hand. We also find in this frequent contraction an explanation of the change of note in the uterine souffle. Every one conversant with the sounds of pregnancy has noticed how that while listening to the sounds formerly called *placental,* but now acknowledged to be uterine, the loud sonorous sound has become gradually higher till it is almost a shrill piping musical one. It has puzzled many authors to explain this, but one sees no difficulty in it; the diameters of the uterine sinuses are slowly reduced by the contraction of the walls, the rapidity of the rush of the blood increased, and the pitch of the sound consequently heightened. It also explains the phenomenon of "after pains," in which we see a continuation of the same intermittent movements after the removal of the exciting cause. It is probable that the enlarged state of the cavity after labour allows the exhibition of the action, and the uterus being more sensitive than before labour sets in, the contractions are more productive of pain than during pregnancy. As the cavity becomes smaller, and the walls relatively thicker, and as the uterus resumes its natural state of insensitiveness, the contractions are not any longer recognised unless exaggerated during suckling.

It is not impossible that a something akin to this is going on in the unimpregnated uterus; at least, we find not unfrequently that mental emotions and other exciting causes do bring on a forcing sensation in the empty womb.

In the case mentioned by Dr. Tanner already described, and in cases where I have removed intra-uterine polypi, there is clear evidence of the contractility of the uterus in the intermittent manner, but these cases occurred upon handling and irritating the organ. That of pregnancy is spontaneous.

The only other conditions at all resembling pregnancy are those which occur from retention of the menses in utero, collections of pus, or of serum.   I am sorry I have not been able to observe whether in these states the uterus spontaneously or upon irritation has the power of contracting.   It would be highly desirable to obtain information upon this point.   To these we shall again allude.

Let me next consider the effects or uses of these contractions.   It is possible that there are others, but two appear to be tolerably clear.

In the *first* place, *it will provide for the frequent movement of the blood in the uterine sinus and decidual processes,* for as the sinuses of the uterus are so much larger than the supplying arteries, the current is more slow in them than in the ordinary systemic veins.   The contraction of the walls through which the sinuses meander tends to send the current onward, and to act somewhat as a supplementary heart.

Besides this, *it facilitates the movement of the fluid in the intervillal space* of the placenta, or in that which is called the placental sinuses.   Whatever view we may hold of the structure of the placenta, whether, on the one hand, there be blood amongst the villi in maternal sinuses, or, on the other, merely a serous fluid, in any case it is through one or the other medium the villi absorb the material for the aëration, &c., of the fœtal blood; and there can be no doubt that from its position it must be more or less in a stagnant state, for even if it be blood, this entering in by small openings into a much larger area, and making its exit also by small openings, must necessarily proceed at a very much slower rate, as has been pointed out by Dr. A. Fare, article Uterus, 'Cyclopædia of Anatomy and Physiology.'   It is not difficult, therefore, to recognise the effect which the change in the solidity and shape must produce on the fluids in the placenta as well as on that of the uterine walls; in other words, the contractions act as a kind of supplementary heart to the fluids in the uterine walls and the placenta.

In the *second* place, the uterine action *adapts the position of the fœtus to the form of the uterus.*   There has been, as is well known, much dispute as to the cause of the head presenting so frequently in labour as it does.   There can be little doubt but the more recent opinion is the correct one, namely, that the motions of the fœtus combined with the preparatory pains of labour to secure the head to present. For it has been also well shown that the head of the fœtus when folded up in utero is not really the larger end, but that the body with the limbs forms the greater portion; and as the uterus is larger at its fundal end than below, the fœtus folded up corresponds to the shape of the uterus only when the head presents at the os.

But this explanation has been weak in one point, namely, that the head presents in all the later months of pregnancy (although not quite so regularly) long before the pains of labour have set in.

The feebleness of the explanation seems to be corrected in part, if not altogether, by the recognition of these contractions to which I am endeavouring to draw attention. During the whole of pregnancy this silent power is being exerted, so that, be there little or much liquor amnii, in other words, be the child freely floating or closely pressed by the uterus on the approach of full term labour, yet there is a time, even so early as the fifth or sixth month, when the uterine contractions must act on the fœtus in a manner similar to that in which it is supposed to act on it during the last stage of pregnancy. The remarks and quotation above given show how clearly Dr. Tyler Smith had pointed out this effect of the uterine contractions.

Let us now discuss of what value in the diagnosis of pregnancy is the intermittent action of the uterus.

In the before quoted passage Dr. Tanner says, " But it seems that as the peristaltic motions occur whenever the uterine cavity becomes enlarged from any cause, it necessarily appears objectionable to instance such movements as a trustworthy sign of pregnancy."

To these remarks I would make this rejoinder. For the last six years and upwards I have made use of the intermittent action of the uterus as the principal symptom upon which I have depended in the diagnosis of pregnancy. I

am not aware that I have been less successful than others
in determining the existence of pregnancy ; on the contrary,
I have felt myself at an advantage in the possession of an
additional sign to make up the deficiency or temporary inapplicability of the others ; as, for instance, when external
noise prevents the heart sounds from being heard.

But leaving egotistical expressions, let us consider what
are the other causes of enlargement of the uterine cavity, in
order that we may see how far they are practically liable to
impede our diagnosis.

They are five in number : 1, retained menses ; 2, hydrometra ; 3, collections of pus ; 4, polypus ; 5, large fibroids,
nearly polypoid.

We will dispose of these *seriatim*, and first, *retained
menses*.

In the first place it would be very rare to find a case of
retained menses, without severe periodical monthly pains.
If such a case presents itself we always examine per vaginam,
and then the obstruction is detected.   But it is possible that
a case may present itself to us—indeed, I have met with one
such—where an obstruction exists in the vagina almost in-
superable to the escape of the menses from the very small
opening, and yet a pregnancy ensues. Now, in this case,
of course much obstacle to diagnosis must arise, because of
the difficulty of exploring the lower portion of the uterus.
In such an event we should, independently of the stethoscope,
be enabled in almost every case to make out the presence of
the fœtus within the tumour, which we should recognise as
being the uterus by its power of contractility. The fœtal
presence, detected by the hand and stethoscope, would
point out the true state of the case. But also in almost
every case of occlusion occurring in those who have already
borne children, there is a history of severe labour, or some
sign which would lead us at once to institute a vaginal ex-
ploration.

But supposing that a girl fell pregnant before the appearance of menstruation, of which I have known one case, then

under these circumstances we should, of course, always institute an internal examination, because in any case it is necessary to make out the actual condition.

Almost always retention of menses in early life results from *vaginal* obstruction, and the majority of those after also; in these cases the uterus itself does not become distended by the secretion till the vagina above the obstruction is dilated to the utmost, and then gradually the uterus enlarges. But this distension is not gradual as in pregnancy, but at each monthly " period " it becomes rapidly larger, subsiding to a certain degree after the " period " has subsided. The decrease in all cases is very well marked. Thus we can feel through the parietes two swellings, the upper one the smaller; and as this is so unlike the pregnant uterus, we can scarcely, with any ordinary amount of attention, mistake one for the other; even supposing, which has not yet been proved, that the uterus distended by menses contracts intermittently, as does the pregnant uterus.

2nd, *hydrometra*, and 3rd, *retention of pus* in the uterus.— Both of these conditions are very rare; both require an occlusion of the os or cervix uteri. The causes of this occlusion would be sufficiently well marked to place the probability of pregnancy aside; but if any doubt existed, vaginal examination would show occlusion, or the state of a developed uterus as in pregnancy. And supposing that vaginal examination were unattainable, then the absence of any solid within (assuming that the uterus in these diseases presented the same phenomena as in pregnancy, which, as I said before, is still unproved), would be sufficient to distinguish these conditions. When hydrometra attains a great size, it possibly might be confused with hydrops amnii; but collections of pus in the cavity of the uterus, seldom, if ever, become larger than the uterus in the fourth month of pregnancy.

Practically their infrequency during the menstrual epoch might permit us to ignore them as a source of difficulty in the diagnosis of pregnancy.

The *fourth* cause of uterine distension is polypus. In the first place, it is very rare to find a polypus in utero so large as to be confounded with pregnancy, without metrorrhagia. This latter was a very prominent symptom in Dr. Tanner's case above quoted. It would not interfere therefore with the diagnosis of normal, but of abnormal pregnancy; and principally with that form where carneous mole was present,

For if there were a pregnancy coupled for some time with hæmorrhages, if the ovum were not converted into a solid form, the fœtus would be felt during the interval of relaxation; and it is in these cases where very frequently, the fœtus being already dead, we are deprived of the employment of the stethoscope, that the advantage of the alternate relaxation and contraction in diagnosis is well shown. Because not only does it show that the tumour is wholly uterine, but by the flaccidity we can tell that the contents are not of a solid nature, for although when the organ is fully contracted over an ordinary ovum the density is as great as if there were a fibroid or polypus within it, yet when it relaxes it is seldom that the laxity is not sufficiently complete but that we can at once satisfy ourselves that a solid of the size of the uterus is not contained within.

Again, it would be a very rare case of polypus where the uterus had by its distension grown as rapidly as it would have done in pregnancy; certainly a polypus so large as to be like a seven months' pregnancy must have taken a long time to grow, and it would be very rare that it should have been unnoticed till within that period.

In the case of a carneous mole, however, there may be some difficulty in distinguishing it from a polypus, especially in a patient seen only lately; because by physical signs they are scarcely distinguishable. By the history, however, we may generally glean information that the menses had absented themselves for a greater or less time. However, the difficulty always has been great, but it is not increased by the knowledge of the intermittent contractility of the uterus.

Taking, however, only the tactile symptom in distinguishing

polypus from pregnancy, we may say that the uterus in pregnancy, when relaxed, becomes quite flaccid, and that a moveable solid is felt floating readily about in it, whereas with polypus, although possibly we may feel the difference between the contracted and relaxed conditions, yet it is so very slight that there is no likelihood of their being confused.

But of course we do not always tie ourselves to only one symptom; and the other symptoms of pregnancy, amenorrhœa, the size of uterus compared with the date of the absence of menses, the state of os uteri, &c., will assist us in our diagnosis, even if the auscultatory signs be absent.

The above remarks apply to the *fifth* cause of distension of the uterine cavity, namely, to fibroid tumours of the uterus, when these project polypus-like into the cavity, except that it is highly improbable that we should find any sensible amount of contraction. In any way it would only be in the case of carneous mole that any difficulty could possibly arise; from this the long standing hæmorrhages, frequently the want of symmetry and persistent solidity, with absence of changes about the os uteri, would enable us to distinguish the fibroid tumour.

Thus it appears to me that the difficulties which would seem at first sight to be caused by the assumption that the uterus distended by diseases contracts intermittently as when distended by pregnancy, readily vanish on closer acquaintance, so far as is required in practice. The knowledge of the fact does not add to our difficulty, whilst it gives us another sign which adds materially to our ease in the diagnosis of pregnancy.

But not only are we assisted in our diagnosis of pregnancy from other uterine tumours, but still further are we helped to distinguish uterine from non-uterine enlargements.

Because if we find a tumour varying in consistence at

intervals, it is quite clear that it must be the uterus, as far as our present information guides us.

There is only one doubt on my mind, derived from the absence of information as to whether the bladder in retention of urine possesses a perceptible intermittent action. That it contracts periodically under accumulation of urine there can be no doubt, but how far this is palpable remains yet open to observation. Of course there is no difficulty in clearing up the question between bladder and uterus, either by vaginal examination or passing the catheter; still, the absence of any solid within will clearly distinguish the vesical from the uterine tumour.

There is one form of abnormal pregnancy which, possessing a consistence between carneous mole and ordinary pregnancy, and being without the presence of the fœtus, may be liable to give rise to difficulty—I mean the vesicular mole or hydatiniform degeneration of the chorion. In this form I have distinctly found the intermittent contractions of the uterus, yet in the state of relaxation no fœtus can be found. Of course, if we examine per vaginam we shall find a more or less patulous os uteri, history of rapid growth, with, most probably, some short suspension of the menses, succeeded by sero-sanguineous discharges. The absence of all fœtal signs, the want of complete fluidity, coupled with the intermittent contraction, will point out that a pregnancy without a fœtus exists, and will, sufficiently with the other signs, show the absence of other diseases distending the uterus.

There is also great advantage to be found in the facility with which in many cases we can obtain an approximative diagnosis. Whilst engaging the patient in conversation the abdominal examination can be carried on without arresting attention such as auscultation would do. If we found a swelling which relaxed at one time and became firm at another, this would be quite sufficient to guide us as to the advisability of insisting on a more complete examination. And then, supposing also there was amenorrhœa, the patient having been " regular " before, the general health being at the same time good, with or without sickness, we may be quite assured that we may extend the examination to a more complete degree without committing ourselves unnecessarily.

In conclusion I may add that, whilst endeavouring to point out the proper position, as a diagnostic sign, of this intermittent action of the uterus, I do not wish to underrate the value of the auscultatory signs of the fœtal presence, but rather when these, from circumstances, are unattainable or impeded, then this sign proves itself of much more value than authors have, as yet, attributed to it.

I have not added any cases to illustrate the above remarks, because, as the phenomenon is so constant and so easily recognised, and its applicability to diagnosis self-apparent, it would be unnecessarily occupying the attention of the Society to relate instances.

Dr. BARNES called attention to the work of Dr. Tyler Smith, in which the peristaltic movements of the pregnant uterus were well described, not only as forming the basis of the expelling force during labour, but also as characteristic of pregnancy.

The PRESIDENT, in answer to Dr. Barnes, replied that the extract he quoted from Dr. Tyler Smith had escaped his notice. He should be pleased to add it to his paper.* But Dr. Tyler Smith had referred to the peristaltic movements, the result of external excitation, while that which had been just described occurred spontaneously. It was not necessary to use cold hand or friction, and it could be obtained before the uterus could be recognised through the abdominal parietes. Both the text-books and other works at home and abroad were silent on the subject of the paper except so far as the quotations showed.

* N.B.—This has consequently been done in the body of the paper.—ED.

This paper has been reproduced by kind permission of the Royal Society of Medicine, London.

Commentary on
Classic Paper No. 3

In the days prior to sophisticated biological and chemical pregnancy tests, the early diagnosis of pregnancy presented difficulties. The 'Braxton Hicks' sign[1], of intermittent, painless uterine contractions palpable by manual examination from the third month on, published in 1872, proved a useful indicator of pregnancy in these early days. Hicks wrote, 'After many years' constant observation, I have ascertained it to be fact that the uterus possesses the power and habit of spontaneously contracting and relaxing from a very early period of pregnancy, as early, indeed, as it is possible to recognise the difference of consistence - that is, from about the third month.' He continued, 'The constancy with which these contractions of the uterus have always occurred leaves no doubt in my mind but that it is a natural condition of pregnancy, irrespective of external irritation.' With great insight, Hicks considered the physiological effects of these contractions, concluding that 'In the first place, it will provide for the frequent movement of the blood in the uterine sinus and decidual processes, for as the sinuses of the uterus are so much larger than the supplying arteries, the current is more slow in them than in the ordinary systemic veins. The contractions of the walls through which the sinuses meander tends to send the current onward, and to act somewhat as a supplementary heart. Besides this, it facilitates the movement of the fluid in the intervillal space of the placenta, or in that which is called the placental sinuses... In the second place, the uterine action adapts the position of the fetus to the form of the uterus...' Finally, he testified to the value of these contractions in the diagnosis of pregnancy. 'For the last six years and upwards I have made use of the intermittent action of the uterus as the principal symptom upon which I have depended in the diagnosis of pregnancy. I am not aware that I have been less successful than others in determining the existence of pregnancy; on the contrary, I have felt myself at an advantage in the possession of an additional sign to make up the deficiency or temporary inapplicability of the others; as, for instance, when external noise prevents the heart sounds from being heard.'

1. Braxton Hicks. J. (1872). On the contractions of the uterus throughout pregnancy: their physiological effects and their value in the diagnosis of pregnancy. *Trans. Obstet. Soc. London*, **13**, 216

The concept of 'uterine contractions'

It is remarkable to read that Braxton Hicks observed these contractions simply by 'full contact of the hand continuously over a period of from five to twenty minutes' . . . 'observations extending over about eight years'. He was probably unaware of the fact that, at the same time, German colleagues had developed techniques for recording uterine activity by internal or external methods (tocodynamometers).

Methods to record uterine contractions

2. Schatz, F. (1872).
Beitrage zur physiologis-
chen Geburtskunde.
Arch. Gynäk., **5**, 58

In 1872, Schatz[2] used an internally placed fluid-filled bag (kolpeurynter) connected through fluid-filled tubes with a mercury manometer and a smoked drum (see figure below).

An internally placed fluid-filled bag connected through fluid-filled tubes with a mercury manometer and a smoked drum, as used by Schatz for recording uterine contractions. Adapted from Schatz, F. (1872)[2]

3. Alvarez, H. and
Caldeyro, R. (1948).
Estudios sobre la fisiología
de la actividad contractil
del útero humano. Primera
communicacion: nueva
técnica para registrar la
actividad contractil del
útero humano gravido.
*Arch. Ginecol. Obstet.
Urug.*, **7**, 7

A turning point in the approach to the study of uterine physiology occurred in Montevideo (Uruguay) in June 1947 when Alvarez and Caldeyro Barcia[3] introduced the transabdominal intrauterine needle fluid-filled catheter and modern, electrically heated pen recorders. Their first publications were in Uruguayan journals, but soon the work was published in the Anglo-American literature[4].

4. Alvarez, H. and
Caldeyro, R. (1950).
Contractility of the human
uterus recorded by new
methods.
Surg. Gynecol. Obstet.,
91, 1

From prelabor to labor

5. Hendricks, C.H., Eskes,
T.K.A.B. and Saameli, K.
(1962). Uterine
contractility at delivery and
in the puerperium.
Am. J. Obstet. Gynecol.,
83, 890

In 1962, Hendricks and colleagues[5], using the technique of Alvarez and Caldeyro, described the intrauterine pressure curves during prelabor (and 2–4 h postpartum) in the human as 'incoordinate contractility patterns' (see figure below).

It is remarkable to note that Braxton Hicks contractions can actually be recorded shortly after implantation[6] (see figure over).

6. Eskes, T.K.A.B. (1993). Uterine contractions and their possible influence on fetal oxygenation. *Gynäkologe*, **26**, 39

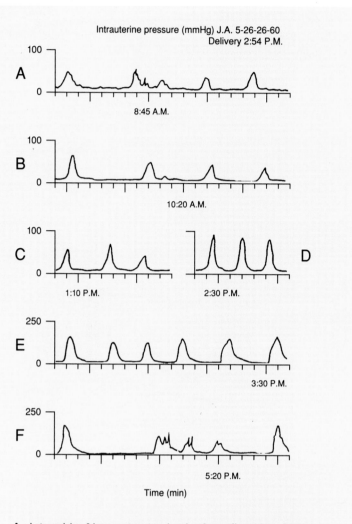

A – Late prelabor 6 hours antepartum (cervix x 2 cm, effaced 50%, Station –2)
B – Early labor 5 hours antepartum
C – Active labor 2 hours antepartum (cervix x 3 cm, effaced 70%, Station 0)
D – Late labor, predelivery (cervix x 9 cm, Station 0+)
E – Spontaneous activity ½ hour postpartum
F – Spontaneous activity 2½ hours postpartum

Segments of intrauterine pressure curves during prelabor, labor and 2–4 h postpartum in a laboring woman. Adapted from Hendricks et al. (1962)[5] with permission

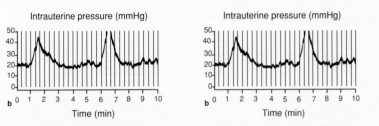

(a) Intrauterine pressure measured with open-tip sponge catheter 2 days before conception. Note high frequency (± 4 contractions/min) and low amplitude (5–30 mm Hg) of uterine contractions. (b) Arterial pulsations are still observed despite high basal pressure (above 30 Torr). Intrauterine pressure measured with open-tip sponge catheter on 11th day after conception in the same woman. Note 'Braxton Hicks' contractions and arterial pulsations even in pressure ranges of 20–55 Torr. Adapted from Eskes (1993)[6] with permission

Possible impact of Braxton Hicks contractions

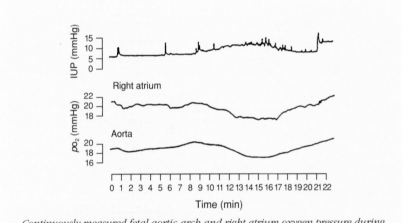

Continuously measured fetal aortic arch and right atrium oxygen pressure during a spontaneously occurring prelabor uterine contraction in a sheep. IUP, intrauterine pressure. Adapted from Jansen et al. (1979)[7] with permission

7. Jansen, C.A.M., Krane, E.J., Thomas, A.L., Beck, N.F.G., Lowe, K.C., Joyce, P., Parr, M. and Nathanielsz, P.W. (1979). Continuous variability of fetal po, in the chronically catheterized fetal sheep. *Am. J. Obstet. Gynecol.*, **134**, 776

8. Smits, T.M., Aarnoudse, J.G., De Wolf, B.T.H.M., Posma, A.L. and Zijlstra, W.G. (1986). pH and blood gas variations in the chronically catheterized fetal lamb : effect of uterine contractions. *Eur. J. Obstet. Gynecol. Reprod. Biol.*, **22**, 263

Braxton Hicks speculated on the possible impact of prelabor contractions, stating 'it facilitates the movement of the fluid in the intervillous space of the placenta' and 'the uterine action adapts the position of the fetus to the form of the uterus'.

These suggestions are substantiated in the chronically catheterized fetal sheep (see figure above), which demonstrates a temporary fall in fetal po_2 during a uterine contraction.

Also fetal pH can fall during contractions in sheep while pco_2 is increasing[8].

Cabalum and Nathanielsz[9] showed that approximately 70% of prelabor contractions were associated with decreases in uterine blood flow of at least 10%, and in 1980, Nathanielsz and colleagues[10] demonstrated a change from rapid eye movement (REM) sleep to quiet sleep. Rapid irregular breathing changed to absent or sporadic breathing, and prelabor contractions changed to contractions associated with full labor. One study in the human has shown that Braxton Hicks contractions coincide with a specific clustering of fetal body movements and cause an increase in fetal heart rate variability[11]. It seems that the resistance to the uteroplacental blood flow has little effect on fetal hemodynamics, as demonstrated in the internal carotid and umbilical artery when blood flow is measured with Doppler velocimetry in the near-term fetus[12].

Uterine contractility

The basic mechanism of uterine contractions involves the following processes:

a) Depolarization and repolarization of the uterine cell provide the action potential, the excitability of the cell being dependent on the membrane potential, which in turn is dependent on ion fluxes across the membrane (especially sodium, potassium, calcium and chloride);

b) In the contraction process, cyclic adenosine monophosphate (cAMP), intracellular calcium, phosphorylation of myocin and the interaction of actin and myosin are involved;

c) Braxton Hicks contractions may be due to coincidental contractions of a large group of cells.

Work by Garfield and colleagues suggests that Braxton Hicks contractions may represent coincidental contractions of a large number of cells[13].

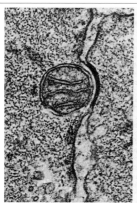 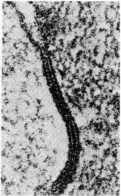

(a) Electron micrograph of gap junction between two smooth muscle cells of the longitudinal muscle layer of rat myometrium fixed by intra-arterial perfusion during parturition (scale bar, 0.1 μm). (b) Gap junction between muscle cells from tissue similar to that in (a), as shown at higher magnification (scale bar, 0.1 μm). Reproduced from Garfield et al. (1977[13] with permission. Copyright (1977) by the AAAS

9. Cabalum, T. and Nathanielsz, P.W. (1981). The effect of episodes of tonic myometrial activity on common uterine artery blood flow in the pregnant sheep at 100 to 135 days gestation. *J. Physiol.*, **320**, 104P

10. Nathanielsz, W.P., Bailey, A., Poort, E.R., Thorburn, G.D. and Harding, R. (1980). The relationship between myometrial activity and sleep state and breathing in fetal sheep throughout the last third of gestation. *Am. J. Obstet. Gynecol.*, **138**, 653

11. Mulder, E.J.H. and Visser, G.H.A. (1987). Braxton Hicks' contractions and motor behavior in the near-term human fetus. *Am. J. Obstet. Gynecol.*, **156**, 543

12. Oosterhof, H., Dijkstra, K. and Aarnoudse, J.G. (1992). Fetal Doppler velocimetry in the internal carotid and umbilical artery during Braxton Hicks' contractions. *Early Hum. Dev.*, **30**, 33

13. Garfield, R.E., Sims, S. and Daniel, E.E. (1977). Gap junctions: their presence and necessity in myometrium during parturition. *Science*, **198**, 958

Cervical dilatation

14. Friedman, E.A. (1954). The graphic analysis of labor. *Am. J. Obstet. Gynecol.*, **68**, 1568

15. Hendricks, C.H., Brenner, W.E. and Kraus, J. (1970). Normal cervical dilatation pattern in late pregnancy and labor. *Am. J. Obstet. Gynecol.*, **106**, 1065

16. Philpott, R.H., Sapire, K.E. and Axton, J.H.M. (1977). *Obstetrics, Family Planning and Paediatrics. A Manual of Practical Management for Doctors and Nurses.* (Pietermaritzburg: University of Natal Press)

The first stage of labor, being the interval between the onset of labor and full cervical dilatation, has been described by Friedman[14]. Plotting cervical dilatation against time, he described a latent phase, an acceleration phase and a deceleration phase, leading to a S-shaped curve. However, taking into account the many interventions which can occur during labor, such as analgesia, there is some doubt about the S-curve representing normal labor. It seems more likely that uterine work and cervical dilatation both increase in an exponential fashion, as documented by Hendricks and colleagues[15] in 1970. In 1977, Philpott and colleagues recognized this dilation curve when they published their study on 'alert' and 'action' lines[16].

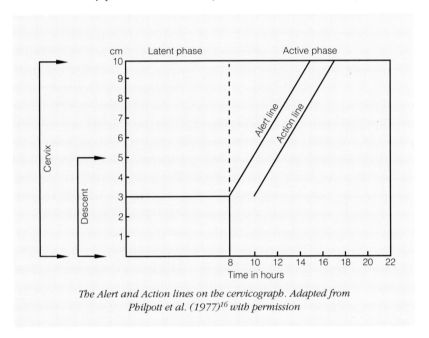

The Alert and Action lines on the cervicograph. Adapted from Philpott et al. (1977)[16] with permission

Braxton Hicks: prelabor or premature delivery?

In distinguishing between Braxton Hicks contractions and (pre-)labor contractions, electrohysterography can show characteristic differences (see figure below).

17. Wolfs, G.M.J.A. and Van Leeuwen, M. (1979). Electromyographic observations on the human uterus during labour. *Acta. Obstet. Gynecol. Scand.*, Suppl. 90.

Wolfs and Van Leeuwen[17], working with an intrauterine pressure catheter and bipolar electrodes, found that in spontaneous as well as in mechanically or chemically induced labor, uterine activity progressed with gradual synchronization. This is reflected in the pressure curves by an increasing regularity of the pressure waveform, an increasing slope of the curve and increasing amplitude. The corresponding electromyogram was at first of low voltage and irregular, without any time relationship with the pressure waveform, but gradually the electrical activity became grouped into bursts almost preceding the uterine pressure wave curve.

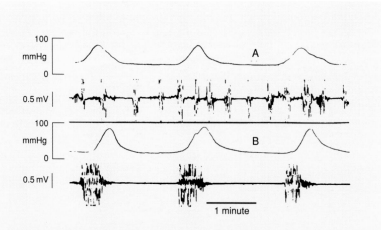

Secundipara, 32 years of age. Mechanical induction. Mechanical and electrical activity during the first phase of labor. A) Early stage of the dilatation period. B) The end of the dilatation period. Upper tracings: intrauterine pressure via open-end catheter. Lower tracings: electrical activity via intrauterine, extra-ovular, bipolar electrodes. Reproduced from Wolfs and Van Leeuwen (1979)[17] with permission

In 1978, Zahn[18], with the aid of tocodynamometry, investigated uterine contractions in ambulatory subjects and found that above 2–6 contractions per hour, and increasing with advanced gestation, there was a higher risk of premature delivery (see figure below). A circadian rhythm was also found, with marked peaking of the frequency of uterine contractions between 8.30 p.m. and 2.00 a.m.[19].

Uterine activity monitoring at home

In recent years, considerable attention has been given to uterine activity monitoring at home. This technique has the potential to reduce preterm birth in high-risk populations, but prospective randomized blind clinical trials remain necessary to confirm such a benefit[20].

18. Zahn, V. (1978). Physiologie der Uterus Kontraktionen. *Z. Geburtsh. u. Perinat.*, **182**, 263

19. Zahn, V. and Hattensperger, W. (1993). Circadiane Rhythmik von Schwangerschafts-kontraktionen. *Z. Geburtsh. u. Perinat.*, **197**, 1

20. American College of Obstetricians and Gynecologists (1993). Committee opinion. Home uterine activity monitoring. *Int. J. Gynecol. Obstet.*, **41**, 203 .

What number of uterine contractions per hour can be tolerated during pregnancy?

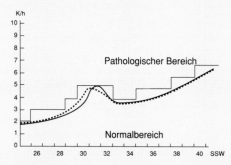

External tocodynamometric observations in women during pregnancy. The normal frequency of uterine contractions was found to be 2–6 per hour, increasing with advanced gestation. Adapted from Zahn (1978)[18] with permission

Tocolysis

21. Ahlquist, R.P. (1948). Study of adrenotropic receptors. *Am. J. Physiol.*, **153**, 586

22. Hendricks, C.H., Cibils, L.A., Pose, S.V. and Eskes, T.K.A.B. (1961). The pharmacologic control of excessive uterine activity with isoxsuprine. *Am. J. Obstet. Gynecol.*, **82**, 1064

When the stage of fetal immaturity is reached or passed at around 24–26 weeks, and when uterine contractions are present, the obstetrician has in his or her armamentarium a range of beta-adrenergic drugs that can inhibit uterine contractions. For many years it has been known that catecholamines are able to stimulate (noradrenaline) or inhibit (adrenaline) uterine contractions. In 1948, Ahlquist[21] clearly distinguished the effects of catecholamines and their derivatives, and introduced the concept of alpha (stimulating) and beta (relaxing) receptors. One of the first derivatives to be tested and shown to be an inhibitor of uterine contractions was isoxsuprine[22] (see figure below)

The effect of isoxsuprine infusion on spontaneous uterine activity and intra-arterial femoral blood pressure. Note the inhibition of uterine contractions. Reproduced from Hendricks et al. (1961) [22] with permission

23. Ariëns, E.J., Simonis, A.M. and Van Rossum, J.M. (1964). In Ariëns, E.J. (ed.) *Molecular Pharmacology*, p.224. (New York: Academic Press)

24. King, J.F., Keirse, M.J.N.C., Grant, A. and Chalmers, I. (1985) Tocolysis – the case for and against. In Beard, R. W. and Sharp, F. (eds.) *Proceedings of the 13th Study Group of the Royal College of Obstetricians and Gynaecologists.* (London: RCOG)

25. The Canadian Preterm Labor Investigators Group (1992). Treatment of preterm labor with the beta-adrenergic agonist ritodrine. *N. Engl. J. Med.*, **327**, 308

Ariëns[23] carried out *in vitro* studies using the tracheal muscles of the calf, which only contain beta-receptors. He studied the percentage relaxation of the calf muscle after adding dichloroarterenol (DCA) and found that it led to a parallel shift in the curves (see figure opposite). The concept of competitive antagonism was born and this led to the development of more specific beta-agonists, among them Ritodrine. Randomized controlled trials were performed and these demonstrated that beta-adrenergics are capable of postponing delivery for 24–48 hours[24].

Despite this, a recent report on beta-adrenergic agonists in the treatment of preterm labor (The Canadian Preterm Labor Investigators Group 1992)[25] found no significant beneficial effect on perinatal mortality, the frequency of prolongation of pregnancy to term, or birth weight.

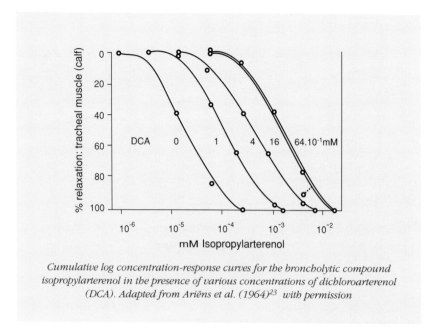

Cumulative log concentration-response curves for the broncholytic compound isopropylarterenol in the presence of various concentrations of dichloroarterenol (DCA). Adapted from Ariëns et al. (1964)[23] with permission

In the approach to the problem of preterm labor, one is still hampered by the fact that the multiple factors that cause the initiation of labor in the individual patient remain not precisely known. In the meantime, we must wait for further studies into fetal and maternal factors such as corticoreleasing factor (CRF) and fibronectine, and the use of other drugs for inhibition of unwanted uterine activity like prostaglandin-synthase inhibitors, calcium antagonists and oxytocin analogues.

Epilogue

Careful observations revealed the existence of uterine contractions during pregnancy.

Prelabor contractions appear to 'trigger' the fetus for extrauterine survival. From studies in pregnant sheep conducted by Parer and colleagues[26], one might conclude that these contractions can be associated with small reductions in uterine blood flow, decreases in fetal oxygen content and transient fetal arousal. It is still not easy to distinguish clinically between prelabor and real labor contractions, an important factor in the timely diagnosis of threatening premature labor.

Prelabor contractions are also efficient in terms of preparatory activity for labor. These mild contractions develop into slow, painful contractions leading to cervical dilatation and delivery. Nature seems to choose an exponential rather than a linear process in this regard. This knowledge is of use to obstetricians, as it helps them to distinguish between normal and abnormal labor.

26. Parer, J.T., Court D.J., Block, B.S.B. and Llanos, A. (1981).Variability of basal oxygenation of the fetus – causes and associations. *Eur. J. Obstet. Gynecol. Reprod. Biol.*, **18**, 1

Summary of references

1. Braxton Hicks, J. (1872). On the contractions of the uterus through-out pregnancy: their physiological effects and their value in the diagnosis of pregnancy. *Trans. Obstet. Soc. London,* **13**, 216

2. Schatz, F. (1872). Beitrage zur physiologischen Geburtskunde. *Arch.Gynäk.,* **5**, 58

3. Alvarez, H. and Caldeyro, R. (1948). Estudios sobre la fisiología de la actividad contractil del útero humano. Primera communicacíon: nueva técnica para registrar la actividad contractil del útero humano gravido. *Arch. Ginecol. Obstet. Urug.,* **7**, 7

4. Alvarez, H. and Caldeyro, R. (1950). Contractility of the human uterus recorded by new methods. *Surg. Gynecol. Obstet.,* **91**, 1

5. Hendricks, C.H., Eskes, T.K.A.B. and Saameli, K. (1962). Uterine contractility at delivery and in the puerperium. *Am. J. Obstet. Gynecol.,* **83**, 890

6. Eskes, T.K.A.B. (1993). Uterine contractions and their possible influence on fetal oxygenation. *Gynäkologe,* **26**, 39

7. Jansen, C.A.M., Krane, E.J., Thomas, A.L., Beck, N.F.G., Lowe, K.C., Joyce, P., Parr, M. and Nathanielsz, P.W. (1979). Continuous variability of fetal po_2 in the chronically catheterized fetal sheep. *Am. J. Obstet. Gynecol.,* **134**, 776

8. Smits, T.M., Aarnoudse, J.G., De Wolf, B.T.H.M., Posma, A.L. and Zijlstra, W.G. (1986). pH and blood gas variations in the chronically catheterized fetal lamb : effect of uterine contractions. *Eur. J. Obstet. Gynecol. Reprod. Biol.,* **22**, 263

9. Cabalum, T. and Nathanielsz, P.W. (1981). The effect of episodes of tonic myometrial activity on common uterine artery blood flow in the pregnant sheep at 100 to 135 days gestation. *J. Physiol.,* **320**, 104P

10. Nathanielsz, W.P., Bailey, A., Poort, E.R., Thorburn, G.D. and Harding, R. (1980). The relationship between myometrial activity and sleep state and breathing in fetal sheep throughout the last third of gestation. *Am. J. Obstet. Gynecol.,* **138**, 653

11. Mulder, E.J.H. and Visser, G.H.A. (1987). Braxton Hicks' contractions and motor behavior in the near-term human fetus. *Am. J. Obstet. Gynecol.,* **156**, 543

12. Oosterhof, H., Dijkstra, K. and Aarnoudse, J.G. (1992). Fetal Doppler velocimetry in the internal carotid and umbilical artery during Braxton Hicks' contractions. *Early Hum. Dev.,* **30**, 33

13. Garfield, R.E., Sims, S. and Daniel, E.E. (1977). Gap junctions: their presence and necessity in myometrium during parturition. *Science,* **198**, 958

14. Friedman, E.A. (1954). The graphic analysis of labor. *Am. J. Obstet. Gynecol.,* **68**, 1568

15. Hendricks, C.H., Brenner, W.E. and Kraus, J. (1970). Normal cervical dilatation pattern in late pregnancy and labor. *Am. J. Obstet. Gynecol.,* **106**, 1065

16. Philpott, R.H., Sapire, K.E. and Axton, J.H.M. (1977). *Obstetrics, Family Planning and Paediatrics. A Manual of Practical Management for Doctors and Nurses.* (Pietermaritzburg: University of Natal Press)

17. Wolfs, G.M.J.A. and Van Leeuwen, M. (1979). Electromyographic observations on the human uterus during labour. *Acta Obstet. Gynecol. Scand.*, Suppl. 90

18. Zahn, V. (1978). Physiologie der Uterus Kontraktionen. *Z. Geburtsh. u. Perinat.*, **182**, 263

19. Zahn, V. and Hattensperger, W. (1993). Circadiane Rhythmik von Schwangerschaftskontraktionen. *Z. Geburtsh. u. Perinat.*, **197**, 1

20. American College of Obstetricians and Gynecologists (1993). Committee opinion. Home uterine activity monitoring. *Int. J. Gynecol. Obstet.*, **41**, 203

21. Ahlquist, R.P. (1948). Study of adrenotropic receptors. *Am. J. Physiol.*, **153**, 586

22. Hendricks, C.H., Cibils, L.A., Pose, S.V. and Eskes, T.K.A.B. (1961). The pharmacologic control of excessive uterine activity with isoxsuprine. *Am. J. Obstet. Gynecol.*, **82**, 1064

23. Ariëns, E.J., Simonis, A.M. and Van Rossum, J.M. (1964) In Ariëns, E.J. (ed.). *Molecular Pharmacology.* p.224. (New York: Academic Press)

24. King, J.F., Keirse, M.J.N.C., Grant, A. and Chalmers, I. (1985). Tocolysis – the case for and against. In Beard, R. W. and Sharp, F. (eds.) *Proceedings of the 13th Study Group of the Royal College of Obstetricians and Gynaecologists.* (London: RCOG)

25. The Canadian Preterm Labor Investigators Group (1992). Treatment of preterm labor with the beta-adrenergic agonist ritodrine. *N. Engl. J. Med.*, **327**, 308

26. Parer, J.T., Court D.J., Block, B.S.B. and Llanos, A. (1981). Variability of basal oxygenation of the fetus – causes and associations. *Eur. J. Obstet. Gynecol. Reprod. Biol.*, **18, 1**

OXYTOCIN

The action of extracts of the pituitary body

SIR HENRY DALE

Wellcome Physiological Research Laboratories, Herne Hill, London

1. Dale, H.H. (1909). The action of extracts of the pituitary body.
Biochem. J., **4**, 427

Sir Henry Dale's discovery, that extracts of the posterior lobe of the pituitary gland stimulate uterine contraction, represented the starting point for research that led to an understanding of the role of oxytocin, its purification, and its widespread use for the induction of labor. Once it was appreciated that pituitary extract contained both vasopressin and oxytocin, it was possible for the latter to be sequenced as a nonapeptide (or octapeptide taking cystine as one) and for the industrial preparation of synthetic oxytocin to begin. It took years, however, to recognize that a dose of 2 International Units (IU) of oxytocin intramuscularly was far too high and for the intravenous drip- or pump-infusion of milli-Units/min to be accepted. The aim of current research remains to achieve fast delivery, with the fetus and mother working in concert to initiate labor, and many lessons can still be learnt from the history of oxytocin.

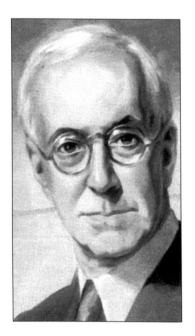

THE ACTION OF EXTRACTS OF THE PITUITARY BODY

By H. H. DALE, M.A., M.D.

*From the Wellcome Physiological Research Laboratories,
Herne Hill, London, S.E.*

(*Received October 1st, 1909*)

I. INTRODUCTORY

Though the activity of pituitary extracts was discovered by Oliver
and Schäfer (1) almost simultaneously with that of suprarenal extracts,
the conceptions of the nature of the action of the former are as yet far less
precise. A comparison of the two was inevitable, and it has more than once
been suggested that their action, at least as regards vaso-constriction, is
of the same kind and produced by stimulation of the same structures.
Herring (2) advanced this view as regards the arteries: a more recent
observation by Cramer (3), of the action of pituitary extract on the pupil
of the frog's eye (enucleated), lends support to the same idea: still more
recently an account given by Bell and Hick (4) of the action on the uterus
emphasised the similarity between the action of extracts from the two
organs. I thought it worth while, therefore, to bring together a number
of observations, made at different times and in different connexions,
which appear to me to indicate that such correspondence as exists is wholly
superficial and illusory. In the first place it must be admitted that the
actions of pituitary and suprarenal extracts have superficially several
points of suggestive similarity. Both raise the blood-pressure, peripheral
vaso-constriction being a principal factor in the effect (Oliver and Schäfer):
in both cases the active principle is limited to a small, morphologically
independent portion of the gland, developmentally related to the central
nervous system in the one case, as to the sympathetic system in the other.
Attention is drawn to these points of similarity by Schäfer and
Herring (5), who state that 'here the parallelism ends': but the
divergence of which they make specific mention is that the pituitary
extract has an additional effect on the kidney. Since they attribute this
to a separate active principle, no true divergence is indicated between
the *pressor* principles of the two organs. It has been shown (Langley (6),
Brodie and Dixon (7), Elliott (8)) that the action of adrenaline reproduces
with striking accuracy the effects of stimulating nerves of the true

sympathetic or thoracico-lumbar division of the autonomic system. An examination of the action of pituitary extract on various organs and systems containing plain muscle and gland-cells will indicate whether its action has more than a superficial resemblance to that of adrenaline by showing whether its effects, or any group of them, can be similarly summarised by relating them to a particular element of the visceral nervous system. Incidentally evidence will be discussed which throws light on the contention of Schäfer and Herring that two active principles exist in the extract, one acting on the circulatory system, the other specifically on the kidney.

The extract used in my experiments, except where otherwise stated, was a 5 per cent. decoction of the fresh posterior lobes of ox pituitaries. The posterior lobes were dissected clean from the rest of the gland and from dura water, weighed in the moist condition, pounded with sand, and boiled with water faintly acidulated with acetic acid to produce coagulation. The extract, filtered from coagulum, is a clear colourless fluid giving a faint biuret reaction. For experiments on isolated organs the extract was prepared with Ringer's solution and carefully neutralised before use.

II. The Effect on the Circulatory System

It has been mentioned that pituitary extract causes a striking rise of blood-pressure, chiefly due to arterial constriction. If the action had any relation to innervation by the sympathetic system we should expect to find that the effect on the arteries was accompanied by an increased frequency and force of the heart-beat, corresponding to the effect of the cardio-accelerator nerves. It was pointed out by Schäfer and Oliver that this was not the case: the beat of the heart usually becomes slower, even after exclusion of vagus action, though it may be somewhat augmented. Reference will be made later to the action of the extract on the isolated heart, which enables the effect to be studied in its least complicated form.

We should further expect to find, if the action were like that produced by sympathetic nerve-impulses, that the action on the arteries showed irregularities of distribution corresponding to that of sympathetic nerves. It was of special interest, therefore, to examine the action on those arteries which have been shown to be exceptional in their innervation and in their reaction to adrenaline.

The pulmonary arteries. Brodie and Dixon showed that the peripheral branches of the pulmonary artery are exceptional in that their muscular coats are not under the control of sympathetic nerves, and made the interesting parallel observation that adrenaline, perfused through the pulmonary vessels, produces no vaso-constrictor but a small vaso-dilator effect. With segments of the main branches of the pulmonary artery, treated as isolated organs, others have obtained definite constrictor effects with adrenaline (Meyer (9), Langendorff (10)). It is clear that there is no real discrepancy between the two sets of observations: the only conclusion justified by the evidence is that the sympathetic nerves send motor fibres to the muscular walls of the pulmonary artery and its main branches, but that the innervation stops short of the peripheral arterioles, the calibre of which is alone concerned in determining the rate of perfusion under constant pressure, as measured by Brodie and Dixon.

In a few experiments with isolated rings of large branches of the pulmonary arteries of large dogs and goats, I observed contraction on adding small quantities of the pituitary extract to the Ringer's solution in which the rings were suspended. Since these experiments were made similar observations have been published by de Bonis and Susanna (11). Since, however, I obtained even more pronounced constriction of the strips of pulmonary artery on adding adrenaline, these results only add another to the cases already known in which adrenaline and pituitary extract both cause constriction of an artery, and are of no significance for our present enquiry. I owe to Professor Dixon the opportunity of making with him observations on the effect of pituitary extract on the peripheral pulmonary arterioles. The observations were made in connection with experiments concerning action on these arterioles of certain organic bases. The lungs were perfused with Ringer's solution, or defibrinated blood diluted therewith, according to the method described by Brodie and Dixon. After it had been shown that either adrenaline or p. hydroxyphenyl-ethylamine caused only a slight acceleration of the rate of perfusion, 1 c.c. of the pituitary extract was introduced into the circulating fluid. As soon as the extract reached the lungs there was a pronounced retardation of the outflow. The observation was repeated several times, in different experiments, with uniform result. Here, then, is a clear case of vaso-constriction produced by pituitary extract on a system in which no such constriction is produced by adrenaline or substances of similar action.

The coronary arteries. The innervation of the coronary arteries cannot be regarded yet as definitely settled, even the more recent observations being by no means concordant. Maas (12) found that the vagus supplies vaso-constrictor fibres to this system: Dogiel and

Archangelsky (13) found that vaso-constrictor fibres are contained in the accelerator nerves: on the other hand Schäfer (14) could not find any evidence for vaso-motor nerves to these arteries, and observed no constriction of them under the influence of adrenaline. The last observation was confirmed by Elliott (8), who found the outflow from a perfused segment of ventricle increased by adrenaline. Langendorff observed that adrenaline caused relaxation of an isolated ring of coronary artery, and this has been confirmed by de Bonis and Susanna. Still more recently Wiggers (15) has found evidence of vaso-constriction when adrenaline is added to a fluid perfusing the coronary arteries. From all this conflicting evidence emerge the facts that the coronary arteries are slightly, if at all, controlled by vaso-motor nerves, and that the constrictor effect of adrenaline on the peripheral branches, if it exist at all, is very weak compared with the effect of that principle on other arteries.

In this instance I made no experiments with isolated rings of artery, but such have recently been published by Pal (16) and by de Bonis and Susanna. These observers agree in finding that pituitary extract causes a marked constriction of a ring cut from a large coronary artery. De Bonis and Susanna also confirmed Langendorff's observation that adrenaline causes relaxation of such a ring, so that in this case the action of the two principles is again contrasted.

My own experiments were made with the isolated heart of the rabbit, perfused with oxygenated Locke-Ringer solution, by Langendorff's method as modified by Locke. There are several errors involved in the measurement of the coronary outflow from such a preparation. These have recently been discussed by Wiggers. The outflowing Ringer's fluid always accumulates to a certain extent in the right auricle and ventricle, and, as Schäfer pointed out, a certain amount may pass the semi-lunar valves and so reach the left ventricle. With small hearts I have not found that these defects seriously disturb the *average* rate of outflow: the principal drawback is that the dripping of the fluid from the heart is rendered irregular by the accumulation of fluid in the right side of the heart during diastole, and its ejection by the systole. With a small, rapidly-beating heart the quick and irregular succession of small drops which results can be averaged and converted into a regular series of large drops by a simple device. I used a large glass funnel, placed immediately beneath the recording lever. A skein of threads, hanging loosely from the heart and lever into the mouth of the funnel, ensured the delivery into it of all the fluid leaving the heart, without at all interfering with the record of the contractions. The funnel was fixed in an inclined position and over the lower opening of the stem was drawn a short length of rubber tubing, the diameter of which could be reduced by a clip. This device converts an irregular series of drips and splashes into a regular series of large drops, which fall at a constant rate so long as the average rate of the drippings from the heart remains constant. These large drops were recorded on the smoked drum by the ordinary arrangement of receiving and recording tambours. When the beat of the heart and the rate of the coronary outflow, as shown by the drop recorder, had become constant, a small quantity of the filtered and warmed pituitary extract was introduced into the bulb of the heart-cannula by means of a hypodermic syringe, the needle being thrust through the wall of the rubber tube leading to the cannula. Fig. 1 shows a typical effect. It will be seen that the outflow from the coronary sinus becomes very much slower as soon as the extract reaches the heart. The effect shown in the figure is quite typical, and I know of no other drug which, in doses not immediately fatal to the heart-muscle itself, will produce so pronounced a constriction of the coronary arteries. That the effect is genuinely due to constriction, and not to viscosity or mechanical accident, can easily be ascertained from the fact that a second dose, introduced when the effect of the first has subsided, produces a very small change in the rate of outflow. This is quite in accordance with the observation, first made by Howell (25), that a second dose of the extract, given intravenously when the effect of a first large dose has passed off, produces hardly any rise of arterial blood-pressure.[1]

One other point needs mention. It is clear from what has been said above that a weakening or stoppage of systole might lead to an apparent temporary retardation of the coronary outflow by allowing accumulation in the right side of the heart. The phenomenon illustrated is not of that kind. It is a prolonged effect, which persists to some degree for upwards of half an hour after the injection, and its maximum coincides with a phase of increased ventricular activity. There is no room for doubt, therefore, that the coronary arterioles afford another example of an arterial area slightly, if at all affected by adrenaline, stimulated to intense constriction by pituitary extract.

The effect on the ventricular beat of the isolated heart

---

1. It is of interest to note that Dr. W. H. Harvey, to whom I communicated my observation of the constricting effect of pituitary extract on the coronary arteries, has produced sclerotic changes in these arteries by repeated injections of the extract.

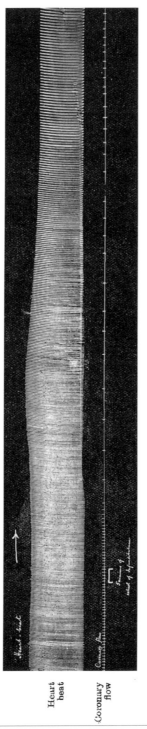

Heart beat

Coronary flow

5 minims of
extract of infundibulum

Figure 1.—Ventricular beat and flow through coronary vessels of the isolated heart of a rabbit. Effect of adding 5 minims of pituitary extract to the perfusing Locke-Ringer solution. Scale $\frac{1}{2}$ linear.

can also be studied in fig. 1. It will be seen that, immediately after the injection, it becomes slightly slower and considerably more vigorous: later, with persistent retardation, it becomes weaker than before the injection. Similar effects, in the same order, have been previously described by Hedbom (17) and by Cleghorn (18). It is difficult, however, to decide how far these changes in ventricular activity are due to primary action on the cardiac muscle, how far to reduction of the oxygen supply by coronary constriction. Neither effect is modified by previous atropinisation, so that there can be no question of the peripheral vagus-mechanism being concerned. There is further, in the case of the effect on the heart-beat, as in that of the coronary constriction, no resemblance whatever to the effect of accelerator nerves or of adrenaline. The safest conclusion is to regard the action on the coronary arteries as certainly a primary effect of the extract, that on the heart-beat as probably in part due to direct effect on the heart-muscle, and in part secondary to the altered rate of coronary perfusion. It should be noted, in this connection, that under conditions of natural circulation, in which the effect of coronary constriction would be antagonised by the great rise of systemic pressure, the secondary weakening of the beat is not usually observed.

The renal arteries. Schäfer with Magnus (19), and later with Herring (5), found that the kidney expanded when pituitary extract was injected intravenously. It was of interest, therefore, to examine the effect of pituitary extract on the rate of perfusion through the renal vessels. The perfusion was made with oxygenated Ringer's solution under constant pressure, as for the isolated heart, the outflow from the renal veins being measured by the drop-counter. The kidneys used were those of cats and dogs. Both kidneys of the cat were perfused, the cannulae being inserted into segments of aorta and vena cava. From the dog one kidney was used, with cannulae in the renal artery and vein. The pituitary extract was added by injection into the circulating Ringer's fluid. The following results were obtained:—

INJECTION OF PITUITARY EXTRACT			RATE OF OUTFLOW IN DROPS PER 20 SECONDS	
			Before injection	After injection
Experiment I.—Cat.		5 minims	34	20
Experiment II.—Cat.	1st.	5 minims	39	27
	2nd.	10 minims	29	31
Experiment III.—Dog.	1st.	5 minims	24	20
	2nd.	10 minims	20	22

It will be seen that the first injection causes in each case a decided though small constriction. The genuineness of the phenomenon is again shown by the failure of second injections, which even slightly reduce the resistance of the constricted arteries. Similar results were obtained by Houghton and Merrill (24), in the course of experiments made to determine whether the extract locally excites the renal epithelium to secretion. On the other hand Pal states that isolated rings of the proximal portion of the renal artery were constricted, while rings from more peripheral portions were relaxed by the extract. On the whole the evidence obtained with isolated organs suggests that the marked swelling of the kidney in its natural relations must be chiefly due to a relative insensitiveness of the renal arteries towards the vaso-constrictor effect of the extract. It might seem, at first sight, that even this implied, as Pal concludes, an action of the vaso-constrictor principle on some nervous structure, and not on the muscular coats of the arteries themselves. This, however, is by no means the only instance of an exceptional reaction of the renal arteries towards general stimulants of plain-muscle contraction. The various drugs of the digitalis series, for example, injected in small doses, cause expansion of the kidney and diuresis, especially in the rabbit; but the result of most experiments on the artificial perfusion of these drugs through the vessels of the excised kidney, especially of the dog and the cat, has been to demonstrate a marked constrictor action even on the vessels of that organ. There is no reason at all for supposing that these drugs act on nervous structures, and there is as little in the case of the pituitary extract. The anomalous reaction of the kidney vessels in their natural relations is clearly a similar phenomenon to their reaction to the digitalis series; but since the pituitary extract acts more powerfully on the arterioles and less on the heart than digitalis and its allies, the phenomenon is presented by the former in an exaggerated form.

The Spleen. The spleen may be regarded, in so far as its contractile activity is concerned, as belonging to the circulatory system. Schäfer and Magnus showed that pituitary extract caused contraction of the muscular capsule. I have repeated this observation with a like result. A plethyomographic record of the effect is shown in fig. 2.

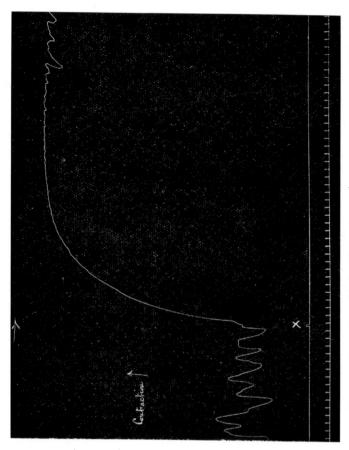

Figure 3.—Contractions of isolated horn of cat's uterus (not pregnant). At × 3 drops of pituitary, extract were added to the 200 c.c. of Ringer's solution in the bath. Time = 10 seconds. Scale, ⅓ linear.

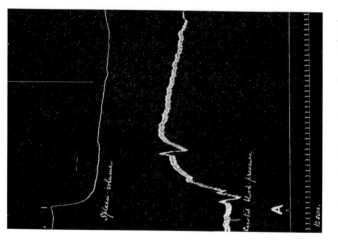

Figure 2.—Spleen volume and carotid blood-pressure of pithed cat. At A, 1 c.c. of pituitary extract injected intravenously. Signal line = zero of blood-pressure. Scale, ⅓ linear.

III. The Uterus

In a paper on another subject (22) I mentioned incidentally the powerful uterine contraction produced by pituitary extract. I have since extended the observation, finding, as expected, that the action, like that on the arteries, is possessed by extracts of the posterior lobe only.

Bell and Hick, working with the extract which I myself used, appear to have obtained a comparatively small effect on the rabbit's uterus in the resting (i.e., non-pregnant and non-oestrous) condition. This is quite contrary to my own experience. They worked exclusively with the rabbit. This animal is not really suitable, however, for our present enquiry, since its uterus responds, under all conditions, to the stimulus of sympathetic nerves or adrenaline, by contraction. In the cat, on the other hand, as was shown independently and almost simultaneously by Cushny (20), by Kehrer (21), and by myself (22), the uterine tone and contractions are inhibited in the non-pregnant, stimulated in the pregnant animal, by sympathetic nerves or supra-renal preparations. I regard it, then, as of great significance that in the uterus of the cat, as well as in that of the dog, the guinea-pig, the rat, and the rabbit, I have always observed, in all functional conditions, powerful tonic contraction as the effect of applying pituitary extract. The results were obtained by intravenous injection into the anaesthetised or brainless animal, and also by Kehrer's method of adding the extract to a bath of warm oxygenated Ringer's solution, in which the isolated horn of the uterus was so suspended as to pull on a recording lever. The effect, under these conditions of adding a few drops of pituitary extract to the 200 c.c. of Ringer's solution in the bath, is illustrated in figs. 3 and 4. So little, in my experience, is the effect dependent on the condition of the uterus as regards oestrum or pregnancy, that the uterus of a virgin, half-grown cat responded to the pituitary extract by as marked a tonic contraction as was given by any of the numerous pregnant or multiparous organs examined.

The effect of pituitary extract on the uterus, then, shows again the absence of parallelism to the effects of sympathetic nerves, the effect of the extract being always tonic contraction, even when stimulation of the hypogastric nerves produces pure inhibition of tone and rhythm.

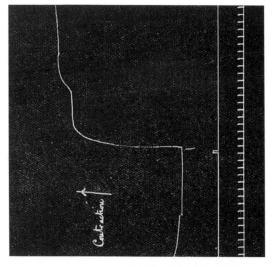

Figure 5.—Isolated retractor penis of the dog. Effect of adding 0·5 c.c. pituitary extract to the bath. Scale, ½ linear.

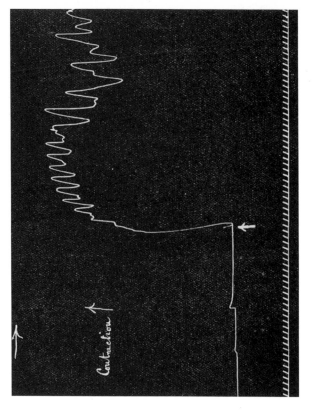

Figure 4.—A record, similar to that of Fig. 3, from the uterus of a pregnant guinea-pig. At ∧ 3 drops of pituitary extract were added to the bath. Scale, ½ linear.

IV. Other Organs Containing Plain Muscle

The intestines and the urinary bladder give no such marked response to the pituitary extract as the organs hitherto mentioned. In a dog anaesthetised with A.C.E. mixture I observed, indeed, a distinct inhibition of intestinal movements when the extract was given intravenously, even when the splanchnic nerves were cut. This might be regarded as indicating a similarity of action to sympathetic nerves. An isolated loop of intestine, however, the rhythm and tone of which are immediately inhibited by adrenaline, contracts, though but feebly, when pituitary extract is added to the bath. It is probable, therefore, that the inhibition, seen under normal conditions of circulation, is due to the intense anaemia which the vaso-constrictor action of the extract produces.

The bladder of the cat, when the extract is injected intravenously, usually exhibits a temporary weakening, followed by more prolonged increase of tone. Neither is of any great extent. A guinea-pig's bladder, suspended in the Ringer-bath, contracted feebly when pituitary extract was added.

The plain muscular coats of the intestines and the bladder contract, then, like other plain muscle, in response to pituitary extract, but their sensitiveness thereto is small in comparison to that of some organs. The retractor penis of the dog, a convenient sheet of plain muscle for examination in the Ringer bath, contracts, as might be expected, when the extract is added (fig. 5).

No effect could be detected on pilo-motor muscles or on the mammalian pupil.

V. Gland Cells

Schäfer and Herring found that the extract caused secretion neither of saliva nor pancreatic juice, which observations I have confirmed. In its failure to evoke salivary secretion the extract is again contrasted to adrenaline. The profuse flow of urine which the extract causes, as first shown by Schäfer, in conjunction with Magnus (13) and with Herring (3), can hardly be regarded as a true glandular secretion.

VI. The Action after Ergotoxine

I have shown (23) that the specific ergot alkaloid ergotoxine, when injected intravenously in certain doses, annuls all motor effects of sympathetic nerves and adrenaline, so that the latter produces, in the cat, a fall of blood-pressure and relaxation of the pregnant uterus in place of the customary rise and contraction. Ergotoxine may be given, however, in any quantity without affecting the contraction of arterial and uterine muscle produced by a subsequent injection of pituitary extract (fig. 6).

ACTION OF ENZYMES, ETC., ON THE EXTRACT

Schäfer and Herring (5) state that peptic digestion reduces the action of the extract on the blood-pressure without affecting the action on the kidney, but that neither action is affected by tryptic digestion. They also obtained results which they regarded as indicating that oxidation by H_2O_2 destroys the pressor action more quickly than the diuretic action. Certain obvious precautions seem to have been omitted: there is no indication that they controlled the activity of their enzymes or the response of their animal. A negative result should obviously not be accepted as indicating destruction of the agent unless a positive effect could subsequently be obtained with the untreated extract. Adopting these precautions I have failed to confirm them on all points. Digestion for twenty-four hours with a peptic extract of proved activity and 0·2 per cent. HCl failed to alter in any perceptible degree the pressor or diuretic action of my extract. I can only conclude that the peptic extract used by Schäfer and Herring contained some antagonistic depressor substance, or that their animal was for some reason unresponsive to the pressor effect. On the other hand every active preparation of trypsin which I have tried has reduced the action on the blood-pressure and on the urinary flow practically to *nil* after a few hours' digestion. Commercial trypsin, 'liquor pancreaticus,' pure pancreatic juice obtained by secretin and activated by enterokinase—all gave the same result. In all cases a subsequent injection of the original extract produced the usual rise of blood-pressure and acceleration of the flow of urine (figs. 7 and 8). It may be suggested, in the absence of evidence for control on that point, that Schäfer and Herring were using an inactive preparation of trypsin: at least it is clear that the tryptic preparations used by me contained something which was not present in theirs. In my experience oxidation with H_2O_2 failed likewise to discriminate between the pressor and diuretic activities. Both effects were smaller after oxidation than those produced by a subsequent injection of the original extract; but that either had suffered greater change than the other was not apparent.

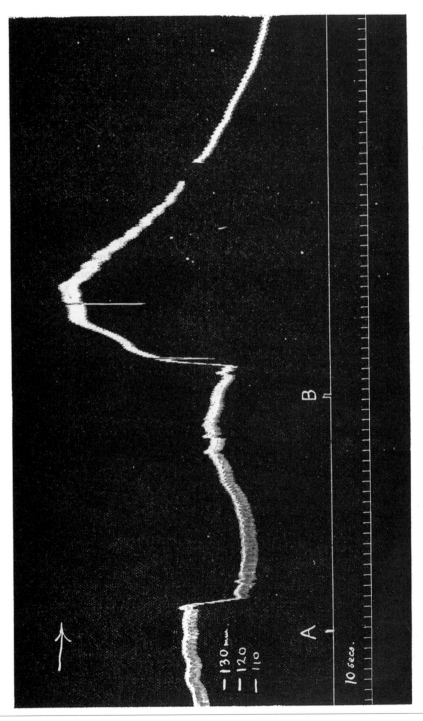

Figure 6.—Carotid blood-pressure of pithed cat. 5 mgms. ergotoxine phosphate injected previously.   Injections :
At A—0·1 mgm. adrenaline.
At B—2 c.c. pituitary extract.
Scale, ½ linear.

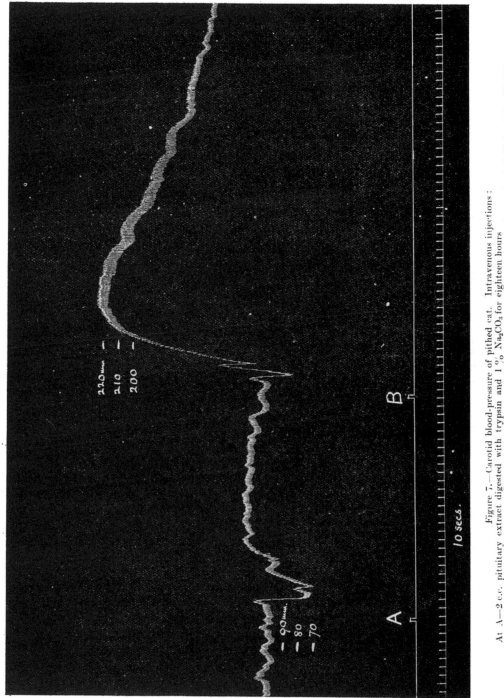

Figure 7.—Carotid blood-pressure of pithed cat. Intravenous injections :
At A—2 c.c. pituitary extract digested with trypsin and 1 % Na₂CO₃ for eighteen hours
At B—2 c.c. of the same extract digested for the same time with the same amount of trypsin *previously boiled* and 1 % Na₂CO₃.
Scale, ½ linear.

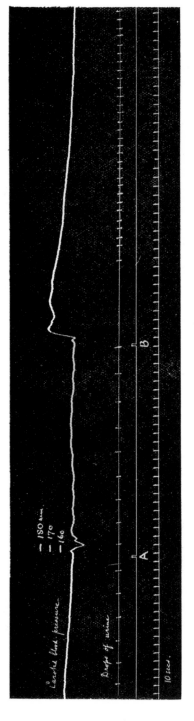

Figure 8.—Carotid blood-pressure and drop-record of urine (bladder cannula) of cat (ether). Injections as in Fig. 7 :

At A—1 c.c. extract digested with trypsin.

At B—1 c.c. extract incubated with boiled trypsin.

Scale, $\frac{1}{2}$ linear.

EXCRETION. ATTEMPT TO PRODUCE IMMUNITY

The fact, discovered by Howell, that second doses are relatively ineffective, suggests that the active principle is not readily destroyed or rendered inactive in the body   I found that the urine of a cat, excreted in response to an injection of the extract, had a pressor action, like a dilution of the extract, when tested on another cat (fig. 9). Probably the active principle, therefore, is at least to some extent excreted unchanged.

The refractory state to further injections has nothing to do with a true ' immune ' reaction. In the serum of a rabbit, treated for a month with increasing injections of the extract, I could distinguish no trace of a body neutralising the physiological activities of the extract.

DISCUSSION OF THE RESULTS

It is clear from the foregoing that the characteristic action of extracts of the posterior lobe of the pituitary body is stimulation of plain muscle fibres. Different organs containing plain muscle show a varying sensitiveness of response to the extract, the arteries, the uterus and the spleen being conspicuously affected. This unequal distribution of effect cannot, however, in any way be related to inequalities of innervation by nerves of the true sympathetic or of the autonomic system as a whole. Ergotoxine, which excludes motor effects of true sympathetic nerves, and of drugs acting through those nerves or like them, leaves the action of pituitary extract intact. Neither atropine nor curare affects its direct action in any degree. The muscle of the mammalian heart is possibly affected to some extent by the extract, apart from effects secondary to constriction of the coronary arterioles: Herring's observations on the frog's heart render this most probable. No effect could be detected on the response of voluntary muscles, either to direct or indirect stimulation. The active principle is then essentially a stimulant of involuntary, and especially of plain muscle.

The question of the diuretic effect needs some further discussion Houghton and Merrill (24) have recently taken the somewhat extreme view that this is entirely secondary to the rise of blood-pressure. They state that the rise of blood-pressure produced by adrenaline is accompanied by a similar diuresis. This latter observation is directly opposed to the experience of others, and I have never myself been able to confirm it. Further it was shown quite clearly by Schäfer and Herring that a second injection of pituitary extract may cause distinct

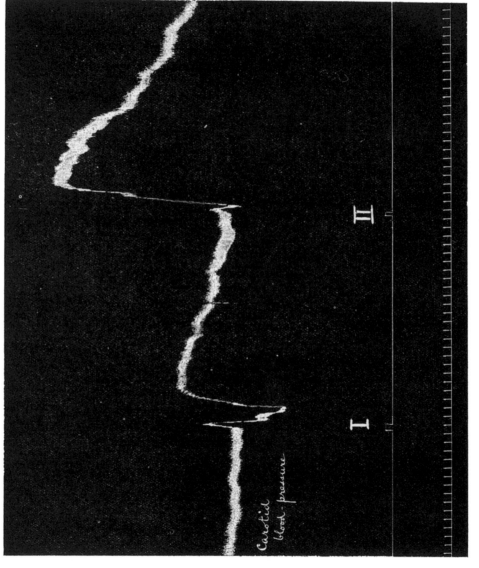

Figure 9.—Carotid blood-pressure of pithed cat. Intravenous injections :

At I.—8 c.c. of normal cat's urine.
At II.—8 c.c. of urine collected after injection of 4 c.c. pituitary extract. (50 c.c. in all collected during 2 hours).

diuresis without any perceptible rise of blood-pressure. While such an observation, which I have been able repeatedly to confirm, sufficiently disproves the statement that the diuresis is secondary to and runs parallel to the actual rise of systemic pressure, it does not remove the possibility of the dependence of the diuresis on vascular effects. A redistribution of the blood in the system, caused by the comparative irresponsiveness of the renal arterioles, is conceivable without actual rise of general systemic pressure, especially if the arterial constriction is accompanied by weakening of the heart's action, due to the depressor constituent which the extract always contains, the action of which, moreover, is much more evident in the case of a second injection.

The differential action of enzymes and oxidation on the supposed pressor and diuretic principles, alleged by Schäfer and Herring, has not been confirmed in my experiments. On the contrary I have found that whatever destroyed one action destroyed both. Their other evidence for the existence of two principles seems to me also inadequate. They lay stress on the difference in the time relations between the two effects and the relatively greater effect of second injections on diuresis. The difference in time-relations of a diuretic and pressor effect is, however, a familiar phenomenon in cases where there can be no question of the presence of more than one active principle. If strophanthin, for example, be injected intravenously into a dog or cat, the immediate effect on the diuresis is usually a distinct retardation: later, as the rise of arterial blood-pressure passes off, there is generally a secondary acceleration which often persists after the blood-pressure has regained its original level. A similar sequence of events was recently observed by P. P. Laidlaw and myself in experiments, in course of publication, on the action of a pure, crystalline active principle from Apocynum. Such a difference in time-relations cannot, therefore, be accepted as necessitating the presence of two principles. The relatively greater efficacy of a second injection in causing diuresis as compared with its pressor effect can also be interpreted in another way, as indicated above. The blood-pressure tracing is complicated by the presence of the heart-depressing principle: it is not a fair index of the degree of vaso-constriction in this instance. An apparently greater relative efficacy of second injections can also be observed in the case of the uterus, when the effect on that organ is compared with that on the arterial pressure. I have frequently seen, as the result of a second injection, marked contraction of the uterus accompanying a very slight or no rise of blood-pressure.

It does not seem justifiable, however, to draw from this observation the conclusion that the principle acting on the plain muscle of the uterus is different from that which acts on the plain muscle of the arteries. It is, of course, true that nothing short of the isolation of a single pure principle, producing both pressor and diuretic effects, would make the view that two principles exist untenable. While awaiting further evidence, however, the conception of both effects as due to one principle seems to me adequate and simpler.

Conclusions

1. The action of extracts of the posterior lobe of the pituitary body is a direct stimulation of involuntary muscle, without any relation to innervation. The action is most nearly allied to that of the digitalis series, but the effect on the heart is in this case slight, that on plain muscle intense.

2. The active principle is excreted in the urine.

3. No true immune reaction is produced by repeated injections of the extract.

4. The evidence advanced in proof of the existence of separate pressor and diuretic principles is inadequate.

REFERENCES

1. Oliver and Schäfer, *Journ. of Physiol.*, XVIII, p. 277, 1895.
2. Herring, *Journ. of Physiol.*, XXXI, p. 429, 1904.
3. Cramer, *Quart. Journ. of Exper. Physiol.*, I, p. 189, 1908.
4. Bell and Hiok, *B.M.J.*, 1909 (I), p. 777.
5. Schäfer and Herring, *Phil. Trans.*, 1906.
6. Langley, *Journal of Physiol.*, XXVII, p. 237, 1901.
7. Brodie and Dixon, *Ibid.*, XXX, p. 476, 1904.
8. Elliott, *Ibid.*, XXXII, p. 401, 1905.
9. Meyer, *Zeitschr. f. Biol.*, XLVIII, 1906.
10. Langendorff, *Zentralbl. f. Physiol.*, XXI, p. 551, 1907.
11. De Bonis and Susanna, *Zentralbl. f. Physiol.*, XXIII, p. 169, 1909.
12. Maas, *Pflüger's Arch.*, LXXIV, p. 281, 1899.
13. Dogiel and Archangelsky, *ibid.*, CXVI., p. 482, 1906.
14. Schäfer, *Arch. de Sci. biol. de St. Petersbourg (Pawlow Festschrift)*, p. 251, 1904.
15. Wiggers, *Amer. Journ. of Physiol.*, XXIV, p. 391, 1909.
16. Pal, *Wien med. Wochenschr.*, No. 3, 1909.
17. Hedborn, *Skand. Arch. f. Physiol.*, VIII., 1898.
18. Cleghorn, *Amer. Journ. of Physiol.*, II, p. 273, 1899.
19. Schäfer and Magnus, *Journ. of Physiol.*, XXVII, p. ix (*Proc. Phys. Soc.*).
20. Cushny, *Journ. of Physiol.*, XXXV, p. 1, 1906.
21. Kehrer, *Arch. f. Gynäkol.*, LXXXI, p. 160, 1906.
22. Dale, *Journ. of Physiol.*, XXXIV, p. 163, 1906.
23. Barger and Dale, *Bio-Chem. Journal*, II, p. 240, 1907.
24. Houghton and Merrill, *Journ. of the Amer. Med. Assoc.*, LI, p. 1849, 1908.
25. Howell, *Journ. of Exper. Med.*, III, p. 2, 1898.

Commentary on Classic Paper No.4

The discovery of oxytocin and its subsequent synthesis owe much to the original work of Sir Henry Dale[1], who demonstrated that crude extracts of the posterior lobe of the pituitary gland stimulated the uterus. Nearly 20 years later, Kamm and colleagues[2] succeeded in obtaining a posterior pituitary extract which existed mainly of oxytocin, i.e. largely free from vasopressin. This extract was called Pitocin. Finally, after more than 40 years of experimental work, Du Vigneaud's long interest in the chemistry of the neurohypophysial hormones culminated in the announcement of the structure of oxytocin[3].

1. Dale, H.H. (1909). The action of extracts of the pituitary body. *Biochem. J.*, **4**, 427

2. Kamm, O., Aldrich, T.B., Grote, I.W., Rowe, L.W. and Bugbee, E.P. (1928). The active principles of the posterior lobe of the pituitary gland. I. The demonstration of the presence of two active principles. II. The separation of the two principles and their concentration in the form of potent solid preparations. *J. Am. Chem. Soc.*, **50**, 573

3. Vigneaud, V. Du., Ressler, C., Swan, J.M., Roberts, C.W., Katsoyannis, P.G. and Gordon, S. (1954). The synthesis of an octapeptide amide with the hormonal activity of oxytocin. *J. Am. Chem. Soc.*, **75**, 4879

4. Berde, B. (1959). *Recent Progress in Oxytocin Research.* (Springfield, Illinois: Charles C. Thomas)

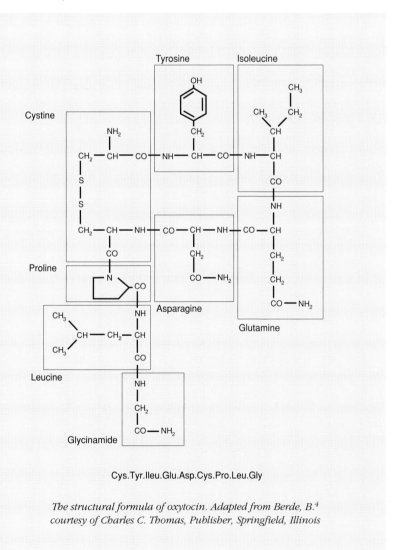

Cys.Tyr.Ileu.Glu.Asp.Cys.Pro.Leu.Gly

The structural formula of oxytocin. Adapted from Berde, B.[4] courtesy of Charles C. Thomas, Publisher, Springfield, Illinois

5. Stein, A. (1917). Geburtshilfliche Tagesfragen uber die Anwendung minimaler Dosen von Pituitrin zur Einleitung der Geburt am Ende der Schwangerschaft. *Zentralbl. Gynäkol.*, **41**, 1152

6. Theobald, G.W., Graham, A., Campbell, J., Gange, P.D. and Driscoll, W.J. (1948). The use of post-pituitary extract in physiological amounts in obstetrics. *Br. Med. J.*, **2**, 123

7. Theobald, G.W., Kelsey, H.A. and Muirhead, J.M.B. (1956). The pitocin drip. *J. Obstet. Gynaecol. Br. Emp.*, **63**, 641

8. Caldeyro-Barcia, R., Sica-Blanco, Y., Poseiro, J.J., Gonzalez-Panizza, V., Mendez-Bauer, C., Fielits, C., Alvarez, H., Pose, S.V. and Hendricks, C.H. (1957). A quantitative study of the action of synthetic oxytocin on the pregnant human uterus. *J. Pharmacol. Exp. Ther.*, **121**, 18

The activity of hormones was tested in a range of bio-assays: the rat uterus *in vitro*, blood pressure in the fowl, milk ejection in rabbits, blood pressure in the rat and diureses in the dog. Results from these tests demonstrated that the biological activities of oxytocin and vasopressin were markedly different, although the difference between the molecules was just two amino acids (isoleucine in the ring structure for phenylalanine and leucine in the side-chain for arginine).

Paralleling the work to identify, understand the physiological processes and synthesize the pituitary hormones was a separate but associated research line into clinical applications.

Clinical applications

In 1917, less than 10 years after Sir Henry Dale's original work, Stein[5] reported on the use of 'minimal' doses of pituitrin for the induction of labor. It took quite some time, however, for obstetricians to realize that 2 IU of oxytocin i.m. were not a minimal dose at all!

In 1948, Theobald and colleagues[6] described the use of oxytocin, administered by intravenous drip, for the induction of labor and went on to introduce the concept of physiological amounts of oxytocin[6,7]. The intravenous administration of diluted Pitocin by drip infusion was heavily promoted, but it took years to convince obstetricians to avoid the intramuscular administration of the huge doses originally advocated by Stein.

The pioneering studies of Alvarez and Caldeyro-Barcia in Montevideo (Uruguay) launched the possibility of the quantification of uterine activity by invasive fluid filled catheters in contact with the amniotic fluid (see figure below). Uterine activity was quantified as the product of the intensity of intrauterine pressure (minus tone) in mmHg and the frequency of the uterine contractions per 10 min. This product became known as the Montevideo unit[8].

The induction of labor by intravenous administration of oxytocin has now become a widely applied methodology in obstetric practice. Nevertheless, the obstetrician always has to ask: 'Is it really necessary to intervene and if so what is the safest method for mother and baby?' Some help in answering these questions has been gained by studying nature, namely the factors that initiate labor and the circadian rhythms of mother and fetus.

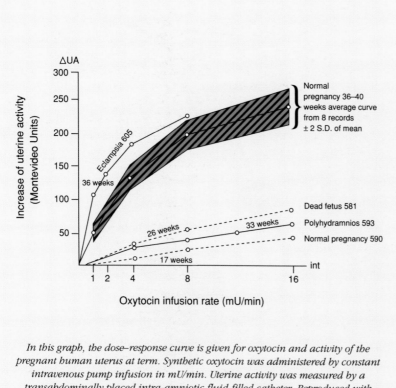

In this graph, the dose–response curve is given for oxytocin and activity of the pregnant human uterus at term. Synthetic oxytocin was administered by constant intravenous pump infusion in mU/min. Uterine activity was measured by a transabdominally placed intra-amniotic fluid-filled catheter. Reproduced with permission from Caldeyro-Barcia et al. (1957)[8]. Copyright Am. Soc. Pharm. & Exp. Ther. Note: The exponential relationship between the dose of oxytocin and uterine activity

Fetal participation in parturition

The onset of labor had attracted the attention of Hippocrates (460–397 BC) and Aristoteles (384–322 BC), both of whom expressed strong views on fetal participation in the process.

Working with sheep, G.C. Liggins from Auckland, New Zealand, made considerable progress towards understanding the role of the fetus[9]. He found that the fetal pituitary produces ACTH which stimulates the adrenal gland and, through glucocorticoids, the placenta. This stimulus produces an estrogen increase, a progesterone decrease and the release of prostaglandin $F_{2\alpha}$ which stimulates the uterus (see figure overleaf).

9. Liggins, G.C. (1973). Foetal participation in the physiological mechanisms of parturition. Foetal and neonatal physiology. In Comline, K.S., Cross, K.W., Dawes, G.S. and Nathanielsz P.W. (eds.) *Proceedings of the Sir Joseph Barcroft Symposium.* (Cambridge: Cambridge University Press)

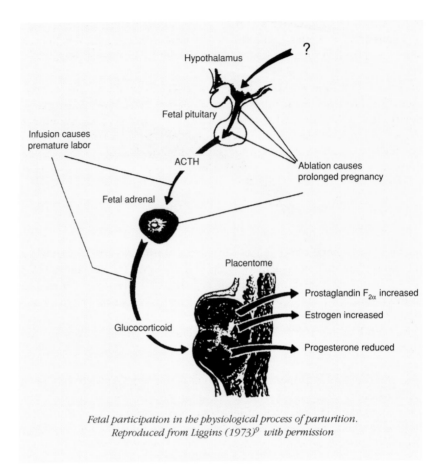

Fetal participation in the physiological process of parturition.
Reproduced from Liggins (1973)[9] with permission

10. Novy, M.J. (1977).
Endocrine and pharmaco-
logic factors which modify
the onset of labour in rhe-
sus monkeys. In Knight, J.
and O'Donnor, M. (eds.)
Fetus and Birth. Ciba
Foundation Symposium,
Vol 47, pp. 259.
(Amsterdam: Elsevier)

11. Honnebier, W.J. and
Swaab, D.F. (1973). The
influence of anencephaly
upon intra-uterine growth of
fetus and placenta and
upon gestation length.
*J. Obstet. Gynaecol. Br.
Commonw.,* **80**, 577

12. Harbert, G.M. and
Spisso, K.R. (1980).
Biorhythms of the primate
uterus (*Macaca mulatta*)
during labor and delivery.
Am. J. Obstet. Gynecol.,
138, 686

Further evidence that the fetal brain is involved in the initiation of labor was found in monkeys in which anencephaly was produced experimentally[10] and in humans in clinical anencephaly without polyhydramnios[11]. In both monkeys and man, anencephaly has been shown to result in labor occurring 'at random' instead of as a sharp occurrence at term.

Maternal participation in parturition

Working with non-medicated rhesus monkeys, Harbert and Spisso[12] found a 24-hour circadian rhythm of uterine activity, with a shift from contractures to contractions being most pronounced in those animals that delivered in the night. From their studies they concluded that, in the non-human primate, specific, directly related prodromal events occur within the maternal organism hours before parturition.

In humans, it has been demonstrated that the oxytocin sensitivity of the uterus gradually increases from early pregnancy until term. These observations possibly reflect the increasing concentration of oxytocin receptors in the myometrium and decidua which occurs during pregnancy. In a study by Fuchs and colleagues[13], the concentration of oxytocin receptors in both tissues was found to rise up to 80–100-fold during the course of pregnancy.

In natural, non-induced labor, birth is precipitated by the release of oxytocin from the posterior lobe of the pituitary. Fuchs and colleagues[14] demonstrated that this endogenous oxytocin is released in spurts and not as a continuous 'infusion'. The number of spurts increase, with a pulse frequency from 1.2 before labor to 6.7 per 30 minutes during the second and third stages.

Activity at night

As shown by Harbert and Spisso[12] in monkeys, uterine activity exhibits a diurnal rhythm with peak activity at night. In humans, the time distribution for spontaneous human birth exhibits a peak at between 3 and 4 o'clock in the morning [14]. This was demonstrated both in America by Kaiser and Halberg[15] and in Prague by the work of Málek and Maly[16]. These observations correlate both with levels of endogenous oxytocin as well as oxytocin sensitivity.

The importance of nocturnal elevations in plasma oxytocin has been demonstrated in monkeys having nocturnal contractions and peak oxytocin values around the time of increased myometrial activity. Honnebier and colleagues demonstrated that these nocturnal contractions could be abolished by an oxytocin antagonist[17].

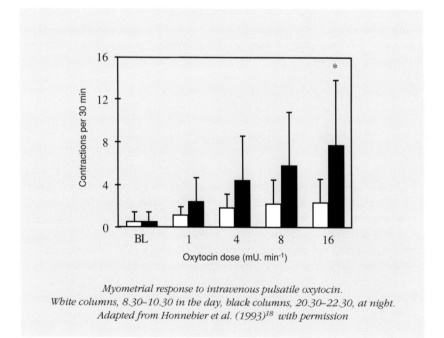

Myometrial response to intravenous pulsatile oxytocin.
White columns, 8.30–10.30 in the day, black columns, 20.30–22.30, at night.
Adapted from Honnebier et al. (1993)[18] with permission

13. Fuchs, A.R., Fuchs, F., Husslein, P., Soloff, M.S. and Fernström, M.J. (1982). Oxytocin receptors and human parturition: a dual role for oxytocin in the initiation of labor. *Science*, **215**, 1396

14. Fuchs, A.R., Romero, R., Keefe, D., Parra, M., Oyarzun, E. and Behnke, E. (1991). Oxytocin secretion and human parturition: pulse frequency and duration increase during spontaneous labor in women. *Am. J. Obstet. Gynecol.*, **165**, 1515

15. Kaiser, I.H. and Halberg, F. (1962). Circadian periodic aspects of births. *Ann. NY Acad. Sci.*, **98**, 1056

16. Málek, J. and Maly ,V. (1962). Characteristics of the daily rhythm of menstruation and labor. *NY Acad. Sci.*, **98**, 1042

17. Honnebier, M.B.O.M., Figueroa, J.P., Rivier, J., Vale, W. and Nathanielsz, P.W. (1989). Studies on the role of oxytocin in late pregnancy in the pregnant rhesus monkey: plasma concentrations of oxytocin in the maternal circulation throughout the 24-h day and the effect of the synthetic oxytocin antagonist [1-ß-Mpa(ß-(CH₂)₅)₁, (Me(Tyr², Orn⁸) oxytocin on spontaneous nocturnal myometrial contractions. *J. Dev. Physiol.*, **12**, 225

18. Honnebier, M.B.O.M.,
Regenstein, A.C.,
Nathanielsz, P.W. and
Main, D.M. (1993). The
myometrial response to a
pulsatile intravenous oxytocin challenge test varies
at different times of the
day in pregnant women. In
Honnebier, M.B.O.M. (ed.)
*The role of the circadian
system during pregnancy
and labour in monkey and
man.* Thesis, University of
Amsterdam

19. Bishop, E.H. (1964).
Pelvic scoring for elective
induction.
Obstet. Gynecol., **24**, 266

Myometrial sensitivity to oxytocin is also highest at night. Again, Honnebier and colleagues[18] (see figure above) have shown that myometrial response to intravenous pulsatile oxytocin in pregnant women is highest during a post meridian challenge (20:30–22:30), than in morning hours (08:30–10:30).

The final maternal role in parturition resides with the cervix. Bishop[19] recognized the importance of the human cervix, and the need for it to be favorable for the success of induction of labor. In his studies, he devised a scoring system which took into account dilatation, effacement, station, consistency and position and results, confirming the importance of cervical status. He stressed, however, that these factors are not independent of each other, for instance an engaged head in a primiparous woman will favor rapid changes in effacement and dilatation of the cervix.

Epilogue

The original observations of Sir Henry Dale have led, through a series of elegant studies, to a more complete understanding of the role of oxytocin and, today, synthetic oxytocin is widely used to induce labor. Basic clinical research and physiological/biochemical studies have indicated that the mother and the fetus should be judged as the 'pilot' and 'co-pilot' in the process of parturition.

Of particular importance has been the finding that the evening and night hours are associated with a higher incidence of childbirth and that this is linked with peak levels of endogenous oxytocin and peak myometrial sensitivity. All this work underlines the conclusion of Honnebier[18], '*A chronopharmacological attitude towards the prevention of premature labor and the induction or augmentation of labor at term may yield new therapeutic strategies.*'

Summary of references

1. Dale, H.H. (1909). The action of extracts of the pituitary body. *Biochem. J.,* **4**, 427
2. Kamm, O., Aldrich, T.B., Grote, I.W., Rowe, L.W. and Bugbee, E.P. (1928). The active principles of the posterior lobe of the pituitary gland. I. The demonstration of the presence of two active principles. II. The separation of the two principles and their concentration in the form of potent solid preparations. *J. Am. Chem. Soc.,* **50**, 573
3. Vigneaud, V. Du., Ressler, C., Swan, J.M., Roberts, C.W., Katsoyannis, P.G. and Gordon, S. (1954). The synthesis of an octapeptide amide with the hormonal activity of oxytocin. *J. Am. Chem. Soc.,* **75**, 4879
4. Berde, B. (1959). *Recent Progress in Oxytocin Research.* (Springfield, Illinois: Charles C. Thomas)

5. Stein, A. (1917). Geburtshilfliche Tagesfragen uber die Anwendung minimaler Dosen von Pituitrin zur Einleitung der Geburt am Ende der Schwangerschaft. *Zentralbl. Gynäkol.,* **41**, 1152

6. Theobald, G.W., Graham, A., Campbell, J., Gange, P.D. and Driscoll, W.J. (1948). The use of post-pituitary extract in physiological amounts in obstetrics. *Br. Med. J.,* **2**, 123

7. Theobald, G.W., Kelsey, H.A. and Muirhead, J.M.B. (1956). The pitocin drip. *J. Obstet. Gynaecol. Br. Emp.,* **63**, 641

8. Caldeyro-Barcia, R., Sica-Blanco, Y., Poseiro, J.J., Gonzalez-Panizza, V., Mendez-Bauer, C., Fielits, C., Alvarez, H., Pose, S.V. and Hendricks, C.H. (1957). A quantitative study of the action of synthetic oxytocin on the pregnant human uterus. *J. Pharmacol. Exp. Ther.,* **121**, 18

9. Liggins, G.C. (1973). Foetal participation in the physiological mechanisms of parturition. Foetal and neonatal physiology. In Comline, K.S., Cross, K.W., Dawes, G.S. and Nathanielsz P.W. (eds.) *Proceedings of the Sir Joseph Barcroft Symposium.* (Cambridge: Cambridge University Press)

10. Novy, M.J. (1977). Endocrine and pharmacologic factors which modify the onset of labour in rhesus monkeys. In Knight, J. and O'Donner, M. (eds.) *Fetus and Birth.* Ciba Foundation Symposium, Vol 47, pp. 259. (Amsterdam: Elsevier)

11. Honnebier, W.J. and Swaab, D.F. (1973). The influence of anencephaly upon intra-uterine growth of fetus and placenta and upon gestation length. *J. Obstet. Gynaecol. Br. Commonw.,* **80**, 577

12. Harbert, G.M. and Spisso, K.R. (1980). Biorhythms of the primate uterus (*Macaca mulatta*) during labor and delivery. *Am. J. Obstet. Gynecol.,* **138**, 686

13. Fuchs, A.R., Fuchs, F., Husslein, P., Soloff, M.S. and Fernström, M.J. (1982). Oxytocin receptors and human parturition: a dual role for oxytocin in the initiation of labor. *Science,* **215**, 1396

14. Fuchs, A.R., Romero, R., Keefe, D., Parra, M., Oyarzun, E. and Behnke, E. (1991). Oxytocin secretion and human parturition: pulse frequency and duration increase during spontaneous labor in women. *Am. J. Obstet. Gynecol.,* **165**, 1515

15. Kaiser, I.H. and Halberg, F. (1962). Circadian periodic aspects of births. *Ann. NY Acad. Sci.,* **98**, 1056

16. Málek, J. and Maly, V. (1962). Characteristics of the daily rhythm of menstruation and labor. *Ann. NY Acad. Sci.,* **98**, 1042

17. Honnebier, M.B.O.M., Figueroa, J.P., Rivier, J., Vale, W. and Nathanielsz, P.W. (1989). Studies on the role of oxytocin in late pregnancy in the pregnant rhesus monkey: plasma concentrations of oxytocin in the maternal circulation throughout the 24th day and the effect of the synthetic oxytocin antagonist [1-ß-Mpa(ß-$(CH_2)_5)_1$, (Me(Tyr^2, Orn^8] oxytocin on spontaneous nocturnal myometrial contractions. *J. Dev. Physiol.,* **12**, 225

18. Honnebier, M.B.O.M., Regenstein, A.C., Nathanielsz, P.W. and Main, D.M. (1993). The myometrial response to a pulsatile intravenous oxytocin challenge test varies at different times of the day in pregnant women. In Honnebier, M.B.O.M. (ed.) *The role of the circadian systems during pregnancy and labour in monkey and man.* Thesis, University of Amsterdam

19. Bishop, E.H. (1964). Pelvic scoring for elective induction. *Obstet. Gynecol.,* **24**, 266

ERYTHROBLASTOSIS FETALIS

Classic Paper No.5

The antenatal prediction of hemolytic disease of the newborn

D.C.A. BEVIS

Senior Registrar, Saint Mary's Hospitals, Manchester

1. Bevis, D.C.A. (1952). The antenatal prediction of haemolytic disease of the newborn.
Lancet, **1**, 395

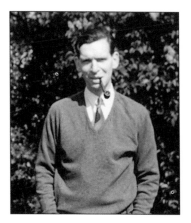

The work of Bevis in the 1950s introduced the clinical possibility of diagnosing hemolytic disease in the fetus, by analyzing blood pigments in amniotic fluid. Earlier, in 1939, a new blood group called Rhesus had been discovered and work with this new group, as well as with the newly discovered CDE/cde alleles, led to the suggestion that erythroblastosis fetalis might be an isoimmune disorder. It became evident from later work that transplacental leakage can occur and that this could result in immunization of the mother. Finally, prophylaxis with anti-D gamma globulin was developed and proved to be of value. The history of erythroblastosis fetalis represents an example of a disease where the pathogenesis, treatment and prophylaxis have been elucidated over a period of 30–40 years as a result of good basic research and a little serendipity.

THE ANTENATAL PREDICTION OF HÆMOLYTIC DISEASE OF THE NEWBORN

D. C. A. BEVIS

M.B. Manc., M.R.C.O.G.

SENIOR REGISTRAR, SAINT MARY'S HOSPITALS, MANCHESTER

ALTHOUGH serological evidence of sensitisation in a rhesus-negative woman indicates the possibility of hæmolytic disease in her child, the probability of this event is difficult to assess. Changes in titre of the maternal antibodies are unreliable evidence (Diamond et al. 1950), and biochemical changes in the mother's serum are equivocal.

A preliminary survey of the help obtained from analysis of the liquor amnii obtained at artificial rupture of the membranes indicated that further investigation was warranted (Bevis 1950), but that specimens should be obtained earlier in pregnancy. In the present investigation amniotic fluid was obtained by abdominal paracentesis starting at the 28th week and repeated at fortnightly intervals until delivery. The specimens were extensively investigated chemically, but only the non-hæmatin iron and the urobilinogen concentrations proved of prognostic value.

METHODS

Paracentesis.—A point midway between the umbilicus and the symphysis pubis is infiltrated with 1% procaine, care being taken to avoid large skin vessels. Uterine paracentesis is then done with a spinal needle (gauge 20), and the liquor amnii is aspirated into an all-glass syringe, about 3 ml. being withdrawn. The puncture is then sealed with plastic. The technique is the same as that used in spinal puncture, but the syringe must be chemically clean as well as sterile.

Analysis.—Specimens were examined as soon after collection as possible but storage overnight at a temperature of 5°C does not affect the results.

Urobilinogen.—The method used is that of Watson (King 1951), 1 ml. of liquo₁ amnii being used and the volume of reagents being reduced proportionally. The standard used was Terwen's. Readings were taken on a single-cell photo-electric absorptiometer (Gallenkamp no. 3615) using an Ilford filter no. 625 (yellow-green) and a Chance ON 20 filter to remove the infra-red rays.

Non-hæmatin Iron.—Many methods of estimation have been tried; but as the amount of iron present is small compared with the amount of serum, and the liquor

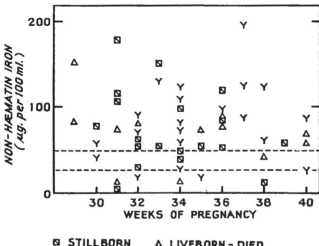

STILLBORN   △ LIVEBORN - DIED
○ NORMAL   Y AFFECTED - LIVED

Fig. I—Non-hæmatin iron in liquor amnii at different stages of pregnancy. Interrupted lines show mean and upper limit of normal (26·7 ± 10·4 μg. per 100 ml.) calculated from controls and unaffected cases.

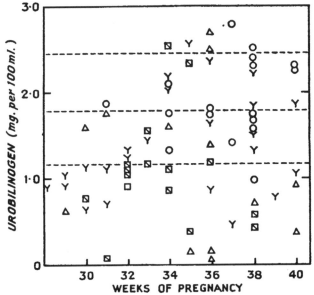

Fig. 2—Urobilinogen in liquor amnii at different stages of pregnancy. Interrupted lines show mean and limits of normal (1·79 ± 0·32 mg. per 100 ml.) calculated from normal cases. Key as in fig. I.

amnii is sometimes stained with meconium, and the proteins are difficult to precipitate completely, the most effective method is one modified from those described by Kitzes et al. (1944) and Thompson (Sandell 1950).

1 ml. of liquor amnii is heated in a bath of boiling water for five minutes to denature the proteins, and 0·2 ml. of 50% trichloroacetic acid is added and the heating continued for a further five minutes. The tube is then cooled and centrifuged at 4000 r.p.m. for five minutes. 1 ml. of the supernatant fluid is transferred to a stoppered tube or volumetric flask (5 ml.), and 1 drop of 10% potassium permanganate solution is added. 2 ml. of iso-butyl alcohol and 1 ml. of 10% potassium thiocyanate are now added, and the tube is shaken for one minute and the alcohol allowed to separate. The coloured layer is next transferred to a cuvette, and water droplets are removed by adding a few milligrammes of anhydrous sodium sulphate. The absorption is then measured with an Ilford filter no. 623 (blue-green). A standard and a blank are run through at each determination.

The colour in butyl alcohol is stable, and the extraction is recommended as a routine (the alcohol can be recovered

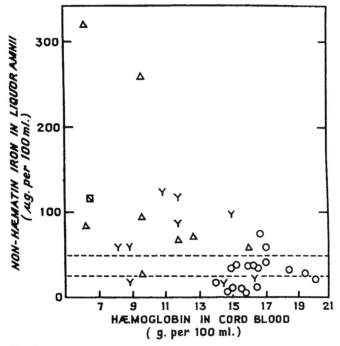

Fig. 3—Non-hæmatin iron in liquor amnii shortly before delivery.
Key as in fig. 1.

by distillation); but, if time is of great importance, the extraction may be omitted and the colour stabilised by the addition of 1·5 ml. of acetone. It must be emphasised, however, that the slightest turbidity in the solution will cause appreciable error in the results.

All reagents must be of analytical grade, and water used for cleaning and the preparation of solutions is glass-distilled.

Glassware (including syringes, specimen tubes, and cuvettes) can be effectively cleaned by immersion in a hot 5% solution of ' Lissapol ' in 5% hydrochloric acid for five to ten minutes followed by six washes with glass-distilled water. This seems to be more effective than the usual dichromate cleaning.

RESULTS

158 specimens of liquor amnii from 69 patients were examined. 54 of the patients were sensitised rhesus-negative women and, of these, 30 gave birth to children with hæmolytic disease of the newborn.

In spite of repeated paracentesis no ill effects were noted in the mothers apart from slight abdominal discomfort for four to six hours, which was never severe enough to stop the patient from doing her normal house-work. Great attention was paid to possible effects of aspiration on the fœtus, but no case of premature

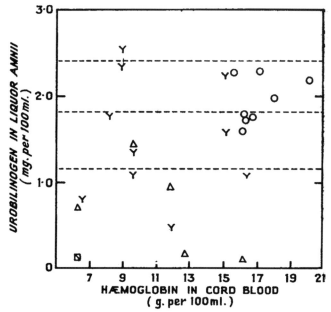

Fig. 4—Urobilinogen in liquor amnii shortly before delivery. Key as in fig. 1.

labour or stillbirth could be ascribed to the procedure, and there was no evidence of skin trauma in the infants.

The results of the estimations of non-hæmatin iron and urobilinogen are shown in figs. 1 and 2, which show that the hæmolytic process produces well-marked changes in the concentrations of these substances. Figs. 3 and 4 show that these concentrations offer some guide to the severity of the disease. The ultimate fate of the children has been difficult to assess because most of the affected babies were treated in the Medical Research Council trial of methods of treatment in hæmolytic disease of the newborn, and minor degrees of kernicterus in surviving children may have been masked by routine blood-transfusions.

Mollison and Cutbush (1951) have shown that the degree of severity of the disease can be expressed as a sigmoid curve capable of probit analysis. As this curve is that found in dose/mortality experiments, the results for iron and urobilinogen have been expressed similarly. The concentration of iron in the liquor amnii proved to be fairly constant throughout the period of pregnancy covered by this investigation (all the constituents of the liquor amnii varied from week to week); and, although the concentration found just before delivery does not fit the curve, the highest concentration in the period under review agrees closely with the curve (fig. 5). As this curve is linear when plotted on a logarithmic scale (fig. 6), the estimation of iron appears to be of great value in assessing the result for the fœtus.

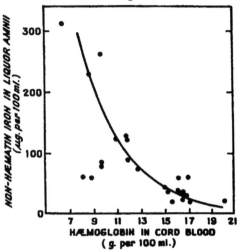

Fig. 5—Highest concentration of non-hæmatin iron in liquor amnii recorded for each case.

The urobilinogen concentration does not behave in the same way, but considerable help is given by the fact that disease of the fœtus was always accompanied by a sudden, although often transitory, decrease in the concentration. This decrease in concentration does not indicate clearly the degree of the hæmolytic process, but a large decrease is of very grave significance.

The concentrations of bilirubin and biliverdin in the liquor amnii do not give any idea of the severity of the disease, nor do they bear any definite relation to the colour of the liquor. The relation of the "icteric index" of the liquor to the severity of the disease is shown in fig. 7. The pigment responsible for the yellow colour has now been identified as mesobilifuscin.

DISCUSSION

It is now known that the liquor amnii is not a static fluid, but that its water-content is changed hourly (Flexner and Gellhorn 1942), although other constituents remain for a longer period. Also, since iron reaches the liquor within forty minutes of administration to the mother (Pommerenke et al. 1942), the liquor is apparently produced by an active secretory process rather than by dialysis. The secretion is probably from the placenta, but it is likely that the amnion plays some part in the process (Kropp 1940). The rôle of fœtal metabolites in the production of the fluid is obscure, but probably some reach the liquor through the skin and lungs, and some possibly through the kidneys.

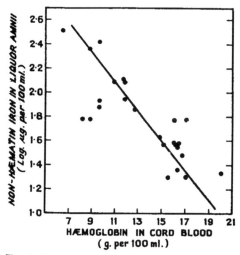

Fig. 6—Points of fig. 5 on logarithmic scale. Regression line is calculated from recorded values. The hæmoglobin in the cord-blood = 28·4 minus 8·4 log Fe.

The concentration of some of the constituents of the liquor are shown in the accompanying table, and the variation in these amounts suggests that an active process is in operation rather than a purely physical transfer across a membrane.

So far as hæmolytic disease of the newborn is concerned, the only definite trends observed are those of non-hæmatin iron and urobilinogen, and these have been indicated in the results.

Winternitz (1926) studied the concentration of urobilin

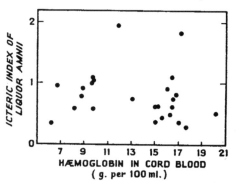

Fig. 7—" Icteric index " of liquor amnii. There is no correlation between this value and the hæmoglobin content of the cord-blood.

in the fœtus and concluded that there was no evidence of a parenteral source, and that the major part found in the fœtus was absorbed from the maternal blood-stream. More recent work on this subject is lacking, but it seems likely that fœtal erythrocytes disintegrate before term, and that therefore some degradation of hæmoglobin does take place in the fœtus. The work of London et al. (1950) has shown that the output of bile pigments in adults is not entirely accounted for by the destruction of mature erythrocytes, and there is some evidence that the reticulo-endothelial system plays an obscure part in this.

Knowledge of iron metabolism has increased rapidly over the past few years, but here again there are wide

COMPOSITION OF LIQUOR AMNII

Constituent	Reference					
	Shrewsbury 1933	Tankard et al. 1934	Makepeace et al. 1931	Cantarow et al. 1933	Uranga Imaz and Gascon 1950	Bevis
Chloride ..	540–670	660	622	—	350	508
Sugar ..	0–91	—	33	0–59	40	27
Protein ..	25–600	350	233	530	210	446
Cholesterol..	Nil	—	—	—	19	8–58
Urea ..	10–73	190	—	—	30	12–37
Bile pigment	Nil	—	—	—	—	0–2·5
Icteric index	—	—	—	—	—	0·2–7·0
Urobilinogen	—	—	—	—	—	1·79
Lævulose ..	—	—	—	—	—	0–11
Iron..	—	—	—	—	—	26 (µg.)
Copper ..	—	—	—	—	—	1·4–120 (µg.)

All values are mg. per 100 ml. except where stated, and refer to mean values at term except where the range is given.

gaps in our knowledge. These gaps are particularly obvious in iron excretion, although there is evidence that large proportions are excreted through the skin (Vanotti and Delachaux 1949). It is therefore clear that, although knowledge of the production of the amniotic fluid is still incomplete, these findings offer an explanation for the results in the present investigation.

The findings for 8 stillbirths where reliable hæmo-globin estimations could not be done were :

Urobilinogen 0·55 ± 0·47 mg. per 100 ml.
Non-hæmatin iron 192 ± 142 µg. per 100 ml.

Both these means are significantly different from the normals.

SUMMARY

The results of analysis of the liquor amnii taken at various times in pregnancy indicate that the concentrations of non-hæmatin iron and urobilinogen offer a reliable guide to the outcome for the fœtus.

Methods of analysis and for obtaining specimens are described, and it is shown that the iron concentration tends to follow a sigmoid curve. The implications of this are briefly discussed.

Thanks are due to the trustees of the Leverhulme Research Fund and the Royal College of Obstetricians and Gynæcologists for a grant to perform this work; to the consultant staff at Saint Mary's Hospitals for referring cases to the clinic and to all members of the medical and nursing staff for their coöperation.

REFERENCES

Bevis, D. C. A. (1950) *Lancet*, ii, 443.
Cantarow, A., Stuckert, H., Davis, R. C. (1933) *Surg. Gynec. Obstet.* 57, 63.
Diamond, L. K., Vaughan, V. C., Allen, F. H. jun. (1950) *Pediatrics*, 6, 630.
Flexner, L. B., Gellhorn, A. (1942) *Amer. J. Physiol.* 136, 757.
King, E. J. (1951) Microanalysis in Medical Biochemistry. 2nd ed., London.
Kitzes, G., Elvehjem, C. A., Schuette, H. A. (1944) *J. biol. Chem.* 155, 653.
Kropp, B. (1940) *Anat. Rec.* 77, 407.
London, I. M., West, R., Shemin, D., Rittenberg, D. (1950) *J. biol. Chem.* 184, 351.
Makepeace, A. W., Fremont-Smith, F., Dailey, M. E., Carroll, M. P. (1931) *Surg. Gynec. Obstet*, 53, 635.
Mollison, P. L.. Cutbush, M. (1951) *Blood*, 6, 777.
Pommerenke, W. T., Hahn, P. F., Bale, W. F., Balfour, W. M. (1942) *Amer. J. Physiol.* 137, 164.
Sandell, E. B. (1950) Colorimetric Determination of Traces of Metals. 2nd ed., New York.
Shrewsbury, J. F. D. (1933) *Lancet*, i, 415.
Tankard, A. R., Bagnall, D. J. T., Morris, F. (1934) *Analyst*, 59, 806.
Uranga Imaz, F. A., Gascon, A. (1950) *Obstet. Ginec. lat.-amer.* 8, 237.
Vanotti, A., Delachaux, A. (1949) Iron Metabolism and Its Clinical Significance. London.
Winternitz, M. (1926) *Klin. Wschr.* 5, 988.

Commentary on Classic Paper No.5

Amniotic fluid has long been recognized as one of the essential products of conception. Thoughts on this fluid pool were probably centered around protection of the fetus, with meconium staining as a possible sign of fetal distress. Deviations of normal quantity, as in poly- (oligo-) hydramnios, were also clinically recognized as pathologic.

An example of how the possibility of using amniotic fluid as a predictor for fetal distress was developed is the work of Bevis on the composition of liquor amnii in hemolytic disease of the newborn. Bevis was Senior Registrar in Obstetrics and Gynecology at St. Mary's Hospitals in Manchester, England.

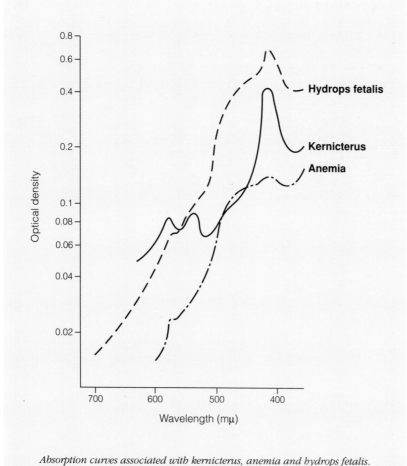

Absorption curves associated with kernicterus, anemia and hydrops fetalis. Adapted from Bevis (1956)[2] with permission

1. Bevis, D.C.A. (1952).
The antenatal prediction of
haemolytic disease of the
newborn.
Lancet, **1**, 395

2. Bevis, D.C.A. (1956).
Blood pigments in
haemolytic disease of the
newborn.
J. Obstet. Gynaecol., **63**,
68

In his paper published in 1952[1], Bevis reported on studies using amniotic fluid obtained at 2-weekly intervals from week 28 through to delivery. His studies indicated that the concentrations of non-hematin and urobilinogen offer a reliable guide to the outcome for the fetus. Later, in 1956, Bevis[2] recognized blood pigments in amniotic fluid, met-hemalbumin at a wavelength of 620 millimicron, and oxyhemoglobin and bilirubin at 460 millimicron.

Bevis wrote 'Amniotic fluid biopsy appears to be a safe procedure and provides suitable material for the prediction of disease in the fetus.' In the same publication he noted that a high concentration of oxyhemoglobin and bilirubin is followed by kernicterus, while a normal concentration of oxyhemoglobin and a high concentration of bilirubin indicated hemolytic anemia (see previous figure). Finally, using spectrophotometric scanning of amniotic fluids, Bevis focused on the increased absorbance which peaked at 450 micron: bilirubin.

3. Liley, A.W. (1961).
Liquor amnii analysis in the
management of the preg-
nancy complicated by rhe-
sus sensitization.
Am. J. Obstet. Gynecol.,
82, 1359

These important early findings of Bevis led to the work of Liley[3] in 1961, which indicated that three zones can be identified (see figure below), based on the optical density of amniotic fluid at 450 millimicron. Each zone represents a degree of severity of disease in the neonate. These zones took into account maturity on the horizontal axis (weeks of pregnancy) and the final, end result, neonatal hemoglobin concentration.

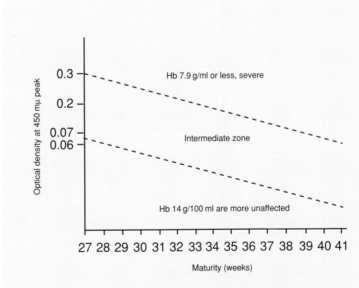

The significance of the 450 mμ peaks recorded
at different maturities.
Adapted from Liley (1961)[3] with permission

Fetal therapy

Improved diagnosis of fetal hemolytic anemia was followed in 1963, by an advance in the treatment of fetal hemolytic anemia, when the first successful intrauterine transfusion was reported by Liley[4]. A new therapy was launched, avoiding preterm delivery and introducing the beginning of fetal treatment.

Originally, intrauterine transfusions were done by the intraperitoneal route, but ultrasound guidance of a transfusion needle directly into the umbilical vein is now the most common method[5].

A new blood group

In 1939, Levine and Stetson[6] described a severe transfusion reaction in a woman with postpartum hemorrhage. They found not only agglutination with the husband's cells (both having group O) but also with 80% of other group O bloods. This suggested a new blood group system, probably in line with the anti-Rh agglutinine of Landsteiner and Wiener[7]. These workers, from the Rockefeller Institute in New York (USA), had found that, when rabbits were injected with the blood of Rhesus monkeys, they formed antibodies, which they called Rh (Rhesus). These antibodies not only agglutinated the monkey's red cells, but also 80% of human red blood cells. The observations of Levine and colleagues[8] represented the first suggestion that erythroblastosis fetalis could be an isoimmune disorder.

Rhesus alleles

Since their original discovery, several types of Rh antigens have been found and Prof. Dr J.J. van Loghem[9], former head of the Blood Transfusion Service at Amsterdam, wrote:

'After the discovery of the Rh factor (1939–1940) it was soon realized that the Rh groups were far more complicated than they seemed at first. By 1943, the American investigator Dr A.S. Wiener had three antisera and had defined six alleles, while the British investigators R.R. Race et al. had four antisera and had defined seven alleles.

Sir Ronald Fisher, a British geneticist and a friend of Dr Race and Dr Ruth Sanger, studying the results of the British work with the four antisera, observed that the reactions of two of them were antithetical, and he supposed that the antigens and the genes recognized by these two antibodies were allelic, and called them C and c. As the reactions of the two remaining antisera were not antithetical, Fisher called them D and E, and he postulated that they also had allelic antigens (and genes), which he called d and e. Furthermore, Fisher assumed that the three pairs of genes must be closely

4. Liley, A.W. (1963). Intra-uterine transfusion of foetus in haemolytic disease. *Br. Med. J.*, **2**, 1107

5. Berkowitz, R.L. and Hobbins, J.C. (1981). Intra-uterine transfusion utilizing ultrasound. *Obstet. Gynecol.*, **57**, 33

6. Levine, P. and Stetson, R. E. (1939). An unusual case of intra-group agglutination. *J. Am. Med. Assoc.*, **113**, 126

7. Landsteiner, K. and Wiener, A.S. (1940). An agglutinable factor in human blood recognized by immune sera for Rhesus blood. *Soc. Exp. Biol.*, **42**, 223

8. Levine, P., Katrin, E.M. and Burnham, L. (1941). Isoimmunization in pregnancy. *J. Am. Med. Assoc.*, **116**, 825

9. Loghem, J.J. van (1983). Classic illustration. *Eur. J. Obstet. Gynecol. Reprod. Biol.*, **16**, 147

linked, as no crossing-over would occur at all and the frequencies would differ very much from those observed.

According to Fisher's theory of three pairs of closely linked genes, an Rh complex could be assembled in eight different ways: CDe, cDE, cde, cDe, Cde, CDE; the eighth combination, CdE, was found in 1948. In 1945, the antiserum anti-e, predicted by Fisher, was discovered by Dr A.E. Mourant; however, the postulated anti-d has never been identified. Fisher's brilliant concept has been of great value in unravelling the genetics of the Rh system.

In 1959, I received from Drs Race and Sanger, on a special occasion, the piece of paper on which Fisher formulated his concept for the first time, followed by the explanatory remarks of Race and Sanger.'

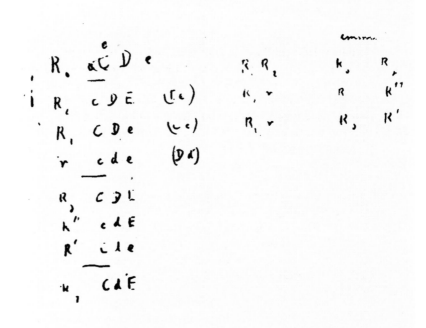

10. Race, R.R. and
Sanger, R. (1975). *Blood
Groups in Man*, 6th edn.
(Oxford: Blackwell
Scientific Publications)

*This was the first writing down by Professor Sir Ronald Fisher of his idea that the less frequent Rh chromosomes might have arisen by crossing-over in heterozygotes for the more frequent chromosomes. He wrote it in 'The Bun Shop', a 'pub' in Cambridge, on the 22nd of June 1944. The Professor is very short-sighted and was not aware of a good deal of beer on the table – the cause of the marks on the lower part of the paper.
Reproduced from Loghem (1983)[9] with permission*

Evidence for transplacental leakage

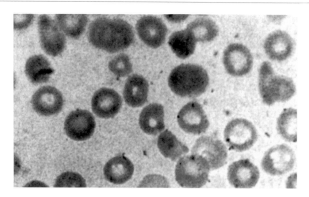

In Alkohol fixierter Blutausstrich, bei pH 3.5 in Citronensäure-Phosphat-Buffer extrahiert und nach May-Grünwald-Giesma gefärbt. Blut eines jungen Säuglings mit 7.5% fetalem Hämoglobin. Gut Hämoglobingefüllte Zellen neben einzelnen mehr oder weniger schwächer gefärbten.
Reproduced from Kleihauer et al. (1957)[11] with permission

Enno Kleihauer, Hildegard Braun and Klaus Betke published their article[11] entitled 'Demonstration von fetalem Hämoglobin in den Erythrozyten eines Blutausstrichs' in 1957. This publication introduced a procedure for detecting HbF cells, which today is known as the Kleihauer–Betke technique[12] and is used widely where a fetomaternal hemorrhage is suspected. Rh transfusion reactions were predominantly associated with pregnancy, the explanation being that the Rh-negative mother had previously been sensitized by an earlier Rh-positive fetus through a 'placental leak'.

That the placental membrane between the fetal and maternal circulations can leak erythrocytes was demonstrated by Kleihauer and colleagues[11]. They made use of the fact that fetal and adult hemoglobins react differently when digested with trypsin and pepsin. In an acid buffer solution, adult Hb is washed out of the erythrocytes so that they appear as ghosts, whereas the fetal Hb remains within the cell and can be made visible by staining (see above figure).

Serendipity of phototherapy

Sister J. Ward, shown in the picture, was the nurse in charge of the Premature Unit at Rochford General Hospital, Essex, England. She was a keen fresh air, outdoor fan and on warm summer days wheeled the more delicate infants out into the courtyard, sincerely convinced that the combination of fresh air and warm sunshine would do them much more good than the stuffy, overheated atmosphere of an incubator. As Dobbs and Cremer wrote[13]: '*One particular fine summer's day in 1956, during a ward round, Sister Ward diffidently showed us a premature baby, carefully*

11. Kleihauer, E., Braun, H. and Betke, K. (1957). Demonstration von fetalem Hämoglobin in den Erthrozyten eines Blutausstrichs. *Klin. Wochenschr.*, **35**, 637

12. Knörr, K. (1985). Classic illustration. *Eur. J. Obstet. Gynecol. Reprod. Biol.*, **19**, 333

13. Dobbs, R.H. and Cremer, R.J. (1975). Phototherapy. *Arch. Dis. Child.*, **50**, 833

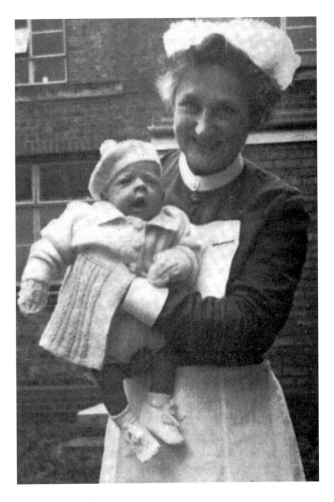

Figure reproduced with permission from Dobbs, R. H. and Cremer, R. J. (1975)[13].
Also published as classic illustration in Eur. J. Obstet. Gynecol. Reprod. Biol.,
13, *59–60, 1982*

undressed and with fully exposed abdomen. The infant was pale yellow except for a strongly demarcated triangle of skin, very much yellower than the rest of the body.'

Sister Ward explained that jaundice was more intense where a corner of the sheet had covered the skin area. Subsequent observations thereafter by the biochemists P.W. Perryman and D.H. Richards revealed that sunlight had an action on blood samples *'behaving like traffic lights as they turned from red to yellow and then green'*.

Confirmation of a photo-oxidative action was given by a simultaneous increase in oxidation–reduction potential measured electrically. An apparatus was constructed to illuminate jaundiced babies, care being taken to protect the baby's eyes by a simple plastic shield. The clinical and biochemical findings[14] were published in 1958. Ten years were then to pass before phototherapy was virtually rediscovered in America, after which it quickly gained a measure of recognition and respectability. However, the major contribution made by Sister J. Ward and the biochemists P.W. Perryman and D.H. Richards should not be forgotten.

Prophylaxis with anti-D

In immunology, it was well known that passively administered antibodies could prevent active immunization by its specific antigen.

Freda *et al.*[15] in the United States and Clarke *et al.*[16] in Great Britain achieved a high degree of protection from isoimmunization by administering anti-D immunoglobulin to Rh-negative male volunteers who had been infused with Rh-positive erythrocytes.

Early trials administering Rh-immune globulin within 72 hours of delivery were excitingly successful[17–19] and this form of treatment is now common practice. Today, the only reasons for women 'escaping prophylaxis' are either neglect in cases of bleeding during pregnancy or inadequate doses of anti-D.

Epilogue

We now know that erythroblastosis fetalis is a hemolytic anemia of the fetus and newborn, which occurs when the blood of the infant contains an antigen lacking in the mother's blood. This stimulates maternal antibody formation against the infant's erythrocytes, leading to hemolysis and anemia. The history of this condition is an interesting example of where the pathogenesis, treatment and prophylaxis of a disease have been solved over a 30–40-year period.

Beginning with the observations described in the original paper of Bevis, the efforts of biochemists, clinicians, geneticists and immunologists, not to mention the timely observations of Sister J. Ward, have not only unravelled the cause of this disease, but have introduced the possibility of 'fetal therapy' bringing a better outlook for mother and child.

14. Cremer, R.J., Perryman, P.W. and Richards, D.H. (1958). Influence of light on the hyperbilirubinaemia of infants. *Lancet*, **1**, 1094

15. Freda, V.J., Gorman, J.G. and Pollack, W. (1964). Successful prevention of experimental Rh sensitization in man with anti Rh gamma 2-globulin antibody preparation. *Transfusion*, **4**, 26

16. Clarke, C.A., Donohoe, W.T.A., McConnel, R.B. *et al.* (1963). Further experimental studies on the prevention of Rh haemolytic disease. *Br. Med. J.*, **1**, 979

17. Hamilton, E.G. (1967). Prevention of Rh iso immunization by injection of anti-D antibody. *Obstet. Gynecol.*, **30**, 812

18. Pollack, W., Singer, H.D., Gorman J.G. *et al.* (1968). The prevention of isoimmunisation to the Rh factor by passive immunisation with Rh D immune globulin. *Haematology*, **2**, 1

19. Chown, B., Duff, A.M., James, J. *et al.* (1969). Prevention of primary Rh immunization: first report of the Western Canadian Trial. *Can. Med. Assoc. J.*, **100**, 1021

Summary of references

1. Bevis, D.C.A. (1952). The antenatal prediction of haemolytic disease of the newborn. *Lancet,* **1**, 395
2. Bevis, D.C.A. (1956). Blood pigments in haemolytic disease of the new born. *J. Obstet. Gynaecol.,* **63**, 68
3. Liley, A.W. (1961). Liquor amnii analysis in the management of the pregnancy complicated by rhesus sensitization. *Am. J. Obstet. Gynecol.,* **82**, 1359
4. Liley, A.W. (1963). Intra-uterine transfusion of foetus in haemolytic disease. *Br. Med. J.,* **2,** 1107
5. Berkowitz, R.L. and Hobbins, J.C. (1981). Intra-uterine transfusion utilising ultrasound. *Obstet. Gynecol.,* **57**, 33
6. Levine, P. and Stetson, R.E. (1939). An unusual case of intra-group agglutination. *J. Am. Med. Assoc.,* **113**, 126
7. Landsteiner, K. and Wiener, A.S. (1940). An agglutinable factor in human blood recognized by immune sera for Rhesus blood. *Soc. Exp. Biol.,* **42,** 223
8. Levine, P., Katrin E.M. and Burnham, L. (1941). Isoimmunization in pregnancy. *J. Am. Med. Assoc.,* **116**, 825
9. Loghem, J.J. van (1983). Classic illustration. *Eur. J. Obstet. Gynecol. Reprod. Biol.,* **16,** 147
10. Race, R.R. and Sanger, R. (1975). *Blood Groups in Man*, 6th edn. (Oxford: Blackwell Scientific Publications)
11. Kleihauer, E., Braun, H. and Betke, K. (1957). Demonstration von fetalem Hämoglobin in den Erthrozyten eines Blutausstrichs. *Klin. Wochenschr.,* **35**, 637
12. Knörr, K. (1985). Classic illustration. *Eur. J. Obstet. Gynecol. Reprod. Biol.,* **19**, 333
13. Dobbs, R.H. and Cremer, R.J. (1975). Phototherapy. *Arch. Dis. Child.,* **50**, 833
14. Cremer, R.J., Perryman, P.W. and Richards, D.H. (1958). Influence of light on the hyperbilirubinemia of infants. *Lancet,* **1**, 1094
15. Freda, V.J., Gorman, J.G. and Pollack, W. (1964). Successful prevention of experimental Rh sensitization in man with anti Rh gamma 2-globulin antibody preparation. *Transfusion,* **4,** 26
16. Clarke, C.A., Donohoe W.T.A., McConnel, R.B. *et al.* (1963). Further experimental studies on the prevention of Rh haemolytic disease. *Br. Med. J.,* **1**, 979
17. Hamilton, E.G. (1967). Prevention of Rh iso immunization by injection of anti-D antibody. *Obstet. Gynecol.,* **30,** 812
18. Pollack, W., Singer, H.D., Gorman, J.G. *et al.* (1968). The prevention of isoimmunisation to the Rh factor by passive immunisation with Rh D immune globulin. *Haematology,* **2**, 1
19. Chown, B., Duff, A.M., James, J. *et al.* (1969). Prevention of primary Rh immunization: first report of the Western Canadian Trial. *Can. Med. Assoc. J.,* **100**, 1021

EARLY PREGNANCY LOSS

Signs and symptoms of early pregnancy

ALFRED HEGAR

Gynäkologischen Universitätsklinik, Freiburg i. B.

1. Hegar, A. (1895).
Diagnose der frühesten
Schwangerschaftsperiode.
Dtsch. Med.
Wochenschr., **35**, 564

Alfred Hegar's paper, published in 1895, is an example of the meticulous clinical observer describing the signs, symptoms and findings during vaginal examination in early pregnancy. This early publication represents the beginning of our scientific understanding of pregnancy and sets the standard for research in the future. The subsequent discovery of the pregnancy hormone (human chorionic gonadotropin), the accurate anatomical descriptions of the human embryo (Carnegie stages) and the observations of the products of conception, have contributed much to our current understanding.

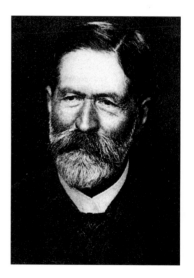

Donnerstag № 35. 29. August 1895.

DEUTSCHE
MEDICINISCHE WOCHENSCHRIFT.

Mit Berücksichtigung des deutschen Medicinalwesens nach amtlichen Mittheilungen, der öffentlichen Gesundheitspflege und der Interessen des ärztlichen Standes.

Begründet von Dr. Paul Börner.

Einundzwanzigster Jahrgang.

Verantwortlicher Redacteur: **Prof. Dr. A. Eulenburg,** Berlin. — Verlag: **Georg Thieme,** Leipzig-Berlin.
Lichtensteinallee 3. Postadresse: Leipzig, Seeburgstr. 31.

I. Aus der gynäkologischen Universitätsklinik in Freiburg i. B.
Diagnose der frühesten Schwangerschaftsperiode.

Von Geheimrath Prof. Dr. **Hegar.**

Man unterscheidet zwischen sicheren und unsicheren Zeichen der Schwangerschaft. Als ein sicheres Zeichen gilt das, welches, auch allein vorhanden, die Schwangerschaft ausser Zweifel lässt. Die Erscheinungen gehören hierher, welche direkt durch das Ei und die Frucht hervorgerufen werden, wie Fötalherztöne, Kindesbewegungen.

Eine Täuschung ist hier möglich durch eine falsche Wahrnehmung unserer Sinne und durch falsche Deutung einer richtigen Wahrnehmung. Wir hören Herztöne, welche aber nicht der Frucht, sondern der Mutter entstammen.

Ein unsicheres Zeichen macht die Schwangerschaft nur mehr oder weniger wahrscheinlich. In diese Kategorie fallen die Veränderungen, welchen die Sexualorgane infolge der Befruchtung unterliegen, ferner die correlativen Veränderungen im Bau und in der Function anderweitiger Organe und Systeme und endlich die consensuell-nervösen Symptome.

Zu den oben erwähnten Quellen des Irrthums kommt noch hinzu, dass wir bei richtiger Wahrnehmung und Deutung der Erscheinung deren Ursache falsch bestimmen. Wir finden eine Geschwulst im Unterleibe, deuten sie ganz richtig als eine Vergrösserung des Uterus, beziehen sie aber auf Schwangerschaft, während sie einem Tumor angehört.

Der Werth der unsicheren Zeichen ist ein sehr verschiedener. Selbstverständlich sind die Veränderungen in den Sexualorganen selbst von hervorragender Bedeutung; die correlativen Erscheinungen, welche wir an den Brüsten wahrnehmen, können jedoch ebenfalls grossen Werth erlangen. Man hat auch correlative Modificationen des Keislaufes, des Stoffwechsels, der Harnsecretion diagnostisch zu verwerthen gesucht, bis jetzt jedoch ohne Erfolg, da unsere Kenntnisse darüber noch mangelhaft sind. Nur die Pigmentirungen werden noch als freilich wenig wichtige Indicien in den Lehrbüchern aufgeführt. Caeteris paribus haben solche Erscheinungen, welche, wie die blaue Verfärbung der Vaginalschleimhaut, dem Auge zugänglich sind, gewisse Vorzüge vor den lediglich durch das leichter zu täuschende Tastorgan erkennbaren Symptomen.

Je schärfer sich der Contrast zwischem dem veränderten und dem gewöhnlichen Zustand eines Körpertheiles ausprägt, desto werthvoller wird das Zeichen.

Die bekannten Symptome an den Brüsten, Entwickelung der Venen, der Montgomery'schen Drüsen, Schwellung des glandulären Gewebes, Colostrum, haben bei einer Person, welche, wie wir sicher wissen, vorher nie schwanger war, eine sehr grosse Bedeutung, dagegen eine sehr geringe bei einer Frau, welche schon mehrere Schwangerschaften vor nicht zu langer Zeit durchgemacht hat. Die Fortpflanzung hinterlässt immer Spuren, und eine vollständige Rückbildung der durch sie bedingten Veränderungen findet nicht mehr statt.

Zuweilen gewinnen sonst sehr wenig geschätzte Zeichen mehr Werth, wenn sie schon früher regelmässig in den vorhergehenden Schwangerschaften, jedoch nie ausserhalb dieser, beobachtet wurden. So erkennen manche Frauen ihren Zustand sofort an dem sogleich eingetretenen Vomitus matutinus. Auch Speichelfluss oder eine Neuralgie des Trigeminus sollen so als Omina gedient haben.

Ein Zeichen ist um so höher zu schätzen, je weniger es durch andere Ursachen hervorgerufen werden kann und je leichter diese anderen Ursachen zu erkennen sind. Diese günstigen Umstände erleichtern uns sehr die Methode der Exclusion, welche wir bei der Diagnose der Schwangerschaft zur Vermeidung von Irrthümern häufig anwenden müssen.

Gewöhnlich trifft man mehrere, selbst zahlreiche Zeichen, und selbstverständlich können solche Combinationen die Schwangerschaft viel wahrscheinlicher machen, selbst ausser Zweifel setzen. Auch bei der Combination tritt die Methode der Exclusion ein. Endlich können zeitliche Verhältnisse und Beziehungen uns bei Aufstellung unserer Diagnose grosse Hülfe gewähren, wie z. B. Vergleich zwischen Grösse des Uterus und dem Termin der zuletzt dagewesenen Menstruation, oder Beobachtungen, nach welchen eine Geschwulst allmählich so aus dem Becken herauswächst, wie dies der Uterus in der Schwangerschaft thut.

Man kann so mit Hülfe der sogenannten unsicheren Zeichen nicht selten zu einer allen Irrthum ausschliessenden Diagnose gelangen, auch in früheren Perioden des Zustandes. Eine Person, welche noch nie schwanger war, verliert ihre vorher ganz regelmässige Periode, zeigt die bekannten Veränderungen an den Brüsten sehr deutlich, ebenso eine bläuliche Färbung der Vagina, einen runden Muttermund mit Schleimpfropf, eine weich anzufühlende Vergrösserung des Uteruskörpers, deren Grad dem seit der zuletzt beobachteten Periode verflossenen Zeitraum entspricht. Ohne Zweifel besteht Schwangerschaft.

Freilich ist die Sachlage recht häufig viel weniger günstig, und die gewöhnliche Ansicht, nach welcher die Diagnose der Schwangerschaft wohl in den späteren Monaten, jedoch nicht in früheren Perioden vollständig sicher zu stellen sei, hat daher eine gewisse Berechtigung. Glücklicherweise sind wir jetzt im Besitz von Hülfsmitteln, durch welche wir die Schwangerschaft auch in ihren ersten Stadien, selbst bei Complicationen, bestimmt zu erkennen vermögen.

Ehe ich darauf eingehe, will ich nur kurz die wichtigsten Erscheinungen besprechen, welche bis jetzt zur Diagnose der frühesten Schwangerschaftszeit verwendet wurden.

Die an verschiedenen Körperstellen auftretenden Pigmentirungen können wohl nur einen gewissen Verdacht wecken, obgleich bei Blondinen die Lentigines und das Chloasma oft überaus scharf gegenüber dem sonst hellen Teint hervortreten.

Der Vomitus matutinus muss schon höher taxirt werden. Magenkrankheiten, Nierenleiden, consensuell nervöse Reizungen, welche ja vorzugsweise in pathologischen Processen der Sexualorgane ihre Quelle haben, lassen sich meist ausschliessen.

Das Ausbleiben der Periode hat um so mehr Werth, je regelmässiger diese vorher eingetreten war. Depascirende Krankheiten, wie besonders Chlorose, Tuberkulose, acute Krankheiten und ihre Folgen, Vergiftungen, wie die mit Morphin, lassen sich oft leicht als Ursachen ausschliessen; ebenso Wechsel des Wohnorts. Schwieriger ist dies mit den Gemüthsaffecten, da gerade die Furcht oder in selteneren Fällen der Wunsch, schwanger zu sein, hier eine grosse Rolle spielen.

Die blaue Färbung der Vulva, der Scheidenschleimhaut und des Portio vaginalis haben mit Recht eine ganz besondere Beachtung erfahren; doch viele andere Ursachen jener venösen Hyperämie sind vorhanden, wie Herzfehler, Lebercirrhose, comprimirende Geschwülste; vor allem aber jene neuerdings viel besprochenen Zustände der Erschlaffung und Atrophie in der Musculatur, den Fascien, dem Bindegewebe der Bauchwände und des Beckens, sowie in dem Bauchfell und seinen Bändern. Die Gefässe büssen ihre Stütze bei dem Schwund und der Relaxation des umgebenden Gewebes ein; die Circulation wird durch Muskelthätigkeit nicht mehr gefördert. Die Gefässwände nehmen wohl auch an der Ernährungsstörung Antheil. Wir wissen, dass Chlorose, Anämie, Erschöpfung durch chronische oder acute Krankheiten, eine durch unpassende Kleidung, schwere körperliche Arbeit anhaltend gesteigerter Druck an jenen Zuständen die Schuld tragen. Häufiger fällt diese auf vorausgegangene Schwangerschaften, bei welchen die Bauchwände oft bis zum Verlust ihrer Elasticität gedehnt werden, während bei der Geburt Dehnungen, Quetschungen, selbst Zerreissungen der Fascien und der Musculatur im Becken eine grosse Rolle spielen.

Wenn das Auftreten der blauen Farbe im Genitalschlauch einen diagnostischen Werth für die Schwangerschaft haben soll, so müssen die erwähnten anderen Ursachen ausgeschlossen werden können. Freilich wird die venöse Hyperämie ungemein stark, wenn zu jenen Zuständen Schwangerschaft hinzutritt. Bei Mehrschwangeren sehen wir daher die blaue Farbe im allgemeinen viel intensiver ausgebildet, als bei Erstschwangeren. Aber auch bei diesen ist sie unter abnormen Verhältnissen zuweilen äusserst intensiv. Ich fand bei jungen Personen, welche zurückgebliebene Körperentwickelung, schlecht ausgebildete Musculatur, überhaupt mangelhafte Ernährung und Anämie zeigten, zuweilen einen so starken Blutreichthum der Venen, dass die Schleimhaut des Scheidenausgangs blauschwarz erschien und selbst die unteren Extremitäten zahlreiche varicöse Gefässe zeigten.

Bei Erstschwangeren haben wir in den Veränderungen des Scheidentheils noch wichtige Hülfszeichen. Die Portio vaginalis verliert ihre ausgesprochen abgeplattete, conische Form oder zeigt diese wenigstens in geringerem Grade. Der Muttermund erhält eine runde Gestalt, und in ihm befindet sich ein grauweisser, festanhaftender Schleimpfropf, welcher sich von dem normalen glasigen Secret des Cervicalcanals scharf unterscheidet. Freilich können Krankheitszustände, wie insbesondere Endometritis colli, verbunden mit consecutiver Schwellung des tiefer liegenden Gewebes derartige Erscheinungen ebenfalls hervorrufen. Bei Personen, welche geboren haben, hat die Vaginalportion für gewöhnlich schon eine cylindrische Form, und der Muttermund ist so verschieden gestaltet, das Secret so oft ungewöhnlich oder geradezu abnorm, dass man kaum Anhaltspunkte hat, um eine etwaige Veränderung durch die Schwangerschaft als solche zu erkennen.

Die diagnostisch werthvollsten Zeichen bietet uns der Uteruskörper. Sein Breitendurchmesser ist sehr bald vergrössert. Noch mehr fällt aber, gegenüber der früheren platten Form, die Zunahme des Sagittaldurchmessers auf. Während früher an der Vorderfläche des Organs der Hals gewöhnlich in einen mehr oder weniger flachen Bogen übergeht, springt dieser winklig vom Hals ab und bietet eine bauchige Vorwölbung dar. Dies kann nun freilich auch durch pathologische Processe bedingt sein. Allein zu dieser eigenthümlichen Form tritt nun noch die weich-elastische Consistenz, welche bei jenen Erkrankungen sonst nie beobachtet wird.

Selten, wenigstens in den ersten Monaten, sind Wechsel in der Consistenz vorhanden, so dass das Organ abwechelnd hart oder weich gefühlt wird.

Um das Verzeichniss der bis jetzt bekannten Schwangerschaftszeichen der früheren Perioden zu vervollständigen, wäre endlich noch das Circulationsgeräusch zu nennen, zu welchem verschiedene pathologische Processe, wie Fibrome, Tumoren des Eierstockes ebenfalls Anlass geben können. Wir sind, wie schon erwähnt wurde, bei richtiger Verwerthung dieser angegebenen, schon lange bekannten Zeichen und ihrer stets vorhandenen Combinationen vielfach in Stand gesetzt, die Schwangerschaft der ersten Monate mit Gewissheit oder wenigstens mit grösster Wahrscheinlichkeit zu diagnosticiren. Freilich werden wir auch zuweilen, besonders bei Complicationen, im Stich gelassen.

Glücklicherweise haben wir nun noch ein weiteres Hülfsmittel, welches auf der Compressibilität des unteren Körperabschnittes beruht. Ich bin darauf geführt worden, als ich einen Aufsatz von A. Martin[1]) las, worin dieser eine Hypertrophie des Gebärmutterhalses beschreibt, bei welcher während eingetretener Schwangerschaft sich der Zusammenhang des weichen unteren Körperabschnittes und des Halses nur schwer nachweisen lässt.

Da der Hals beträchtliche Dimensionen annehmen kann, so kann man ihn leicht für einen etwa normal grossen Uteruskörper halten, während man diesen in seinem vergrösserten und erweichten Zustand für einen Tumor ansieht und so einen leicht verhängnissvollen Irrthum begeht.

Ich zweifelte sogleich an der Deutung, nach welcher das Alles auf einen pathologischen Zustand zurückzuführen sei, und stellte daher eine grössere Reihe von Untersuchungen in den verschiedensten Zeiten der Schwangerschaft an. Hierbei zeigte sich die Zusammendrückbarkeit als eine physiologische Eigenschaft des unteren Körperabschnittes, welche sich schon in sehr frühem Stadium der Schwangerschaft, selbst zuweilen schon in der vierten Woche, nachweisen lässt.

Ich habe den Zustand als Zusammendrückbarkeit, Compressibilität bezeichnet und glaube, dass dies der richtige Ausdruck dafür ist, da die Bezeichnung Erweichung leicht zu irrigen Anschauungen, insbesondere zu der Ansicht führen kann, als wenn die schon lange bekannte Erweichung der Uteruswand der einzige oder wichtigste Factor bei der Entstehung des Phänomens sei.

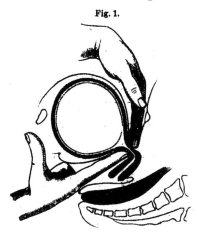

Fig. 1.

Der Nachweis der Zusammendrückbarkeit wird dadurch geliefert, dass bei dem ja gewöhnlich nach vorn gelagerten Uteruskörper der Zeigefinger der einen Hand in das vordere Scheidengewölbe eingeführt wird, während die Finger der anderen Hand über den Fundus herüber gegen den unteren Theil der hinteren Wand vordringen. Die Finger suchen sich nun einander entgegenzukommen (Fig. 1). Ist der Uterus retrovertirt, so geht der eine Finger ins hintere Scheidengewölbe, die andere Hand dringt zum unteren Theil der vorderen Wand.

---

[1]) Zur Kenntniss der Hypertrophia colli uteri supravaginalis. Zeitschrift für Geburtshülfe und Gynäkologie Bd. VI, S. 101.

Am besten gelingt der Nachweis, wenn der Finger der einen Hand in den Mastdarm eingeführt wird, doch muss er nicht in der Ampulle bleiben, da er sonst nur durch die Falten des Sphincter ani tertius den unteren Körperabschnitt erreicht. Er muss durch den Schlupf des Sphincters hindurchgehen, wo er dann unmittelbar an die Stelle gelangt. Der mediale Theil des Uterus ist am meisten zusammendrückbar, während die beiden Seitengegenden mehr Widerstand leisten. Zuweilen glaubt man eine nur kartenblattdicke Gewebsschicht zwischen den Fingern zu haben, ein andermal erscheint diese 4—5 mm dick. Sehr auffallend ist der Unterschied zwischen dem sich wie eine feste Walze anzufühlenden Hals gegenüber dem oberhalb des Isthmus beginnenden nachgiebigen Gewebe, welches, wenn zusammengedrückt, sich in die Breite legt, wie ein entfalteter Fächer.

Was nun die Entstehung des Phänomens betrifft, so hielt man es seit Erscheinen der ersten durch meine Schüler [2][3] erfolgten Publicationen und selbst noch später nach Erscheinen der Sonntag'schen Arbeit [1] für eine Folge der Erweichung, welche sich sehr bald nach der Befruchtung in der Uteruswand ausbildet. Man betrachtete es so höchstens als einen neuen Nachweis der schon längst bekannten Gewebseigenschaft.

Neuerdings noch hat ein Redner auf dem gynäkologischen Congress in Wien diese Zusammendrückbarkeit davon abgeleitet, dass das Ei nicht zum Orificium internum herabreiche, die Finger daher oberhalb dieses nur die Wände der Gebärmutter zwischen sich haben, welche dann bei ihrer Weichheit leicht comprimirt werden könnten. In dem ersten Monat reicht allerdings der untere Eipol nicht ganz bis zum inneren Muttermund. Allein die Entfernung ist doch so wenig gross, dass die beiden Hände nothwendig noch ein Segment des Eies zwischen sich haben müssen.

Mit Ablauf der ersten fünf bis sechs Wochen nach der letzten Menstruation geht das Ei aber tiefer herab, und vom vierten Monat an liegt es fast unmittelbar über dem Orificium internum. Solche Verhältnisse fand ich wenigstens an den Präparaten des hiesigen anatomischen Museums und an den Abbildungen (Coste, Hunter), welche mir zu Gebote standen. Zeichnungen, bei welchen die Eihöhle eröffnet ist, sind nicht maassgebend, da hier durch Entleerung des Fruchtwassers die Durchmesser verkürzt sein können.

Die Compressibilität lässt sich auch in der Gegend der Tuben nachweisen, wie dies Landau [2] richtig bemerkt; und nicht nur da, sondern in grösserem oder geringerem Grade überall, selbst in der Mitte des Corpus uteri. Darüber kann kein Zweifel bestehen, dass hier das Ei sei und von dem Druck der Finger getroffen werde, während man dies an den erwähnten anderen Stellen, wenn auch nur mit scheinbarer Berechtigung, in Abrede stellen kann. Trifft nun der Druck nicht nur die Uteruswand, sondern auch das

[2] Reinl, Prager med. Wochenschrift 1884, No. 26, Bd. IX.
[3] Compes, Berliner klin. Wochenschrift 1885, No. 38.
[1] Das Hegar'sche Schwangerschaftszeichen. Sammlung klinischer Vorträge, Neue Folge No. 58.
[2] Landau, Zur Diagnose der Schwangerschaft in den ersten Monaten. Deutsche med. Wochenschrift 1893, No. 52.

Ei, so muss dieses bei Anstellung des Versuches oberhalb des Isthmus oder in der Nähe der Tubarostien entweder in toto zurückweichen, oder das Fruchtwasser in der Eiblase muss nach einer anderen Region des Uterus gedrängt werden. Bei Compression der mittleren Körpergegend ist nur letzteres möglich.

Bei einem solchen Vorgang muss die durch den Druck bedingte Raumverminderung, welche die Höhle des Corpus uteri in der comprimirten Gegend erleidet, durch Dehnung der Wand an anderen, der Compression nicht ausgesetzten Stellen wieder ausgeglichen werden (Fig. 2).

Der Versuch giebt uns, was physiologisch von Interesse ist, Aufschluss über die physikalische Beschaffenheit der Uteruswand. Diese kann nicht starr sein; sie kann sich aber auch nicht in einem hohen Grade der Spannung befinden, weil sie sonst grösseren Widerstand leistete oder zerrisse.

Fig. 2.   Fig. 3.

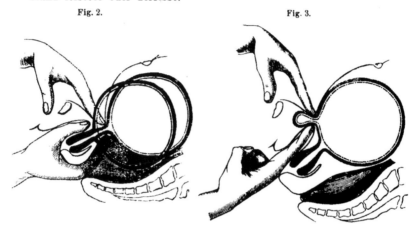

Ein von mir erst seit kurzem aufgefundenes neues Phänomen, welches für die Diagnose der Schwangerschaft vielleicht von gleich grossem Werth sein dürfte, setzt dieselben physikalischen Bedingungen voraus und bestätigt das eben Gesagte. Der Amerikaner Dickinson[3]) spricht von einer Falte, welche er in früher Zeit der Schwangerschaft an der vorderen Uteruswand vorgefunden habe. Sie soll durch Contractionen zustande kommen. Ich habe mich vergeblich bemüht, sie aufzufinden. Allein es gelingt leicht, eine künstliche Falte zu bilden, wenn der im Scheidengewölbe befindliche Finger dem von den Bauchdecken aus herabgeführten Finger der anderen Hand mit Druck auf den Uterus entgegengedrängt wird (Fig. 3).

[3]) The diagnosis of pregnancy between the second and eigth week by bimanual examination. American Journ. of Obst. 1892, Vol. 25, S. 384.

Man bildet so eine Falte aus Uteruswand, wie man eine Falte aus Darmwand formirt, wenn man in einer Hernie die Darmschlinge nachweisen will.

Ich habe übrigens diese Faltenbildung erst in etwas späterer Zeit, wenigstens noch nicht in den ersten zwei Monaten, nachzuweisen Gelegenheit gehabt, daher ich noch nicht genau sagen kann, ob und wie oft sie in letzterer Periode aufzufinden sei.

Ich kann auch nicht sagen, ob bei dieser Faltenbildung das Ei in toto verschoben oder ob auch die Eihäute in die Falte hineingelangen und dann nur das Fruchtwasser verdrängt werde (Fig. 3 und Fig. 4).

Vielleicht existiren hier Verschiedenheiten, je nach dem Elasticitätsgrad der Eihäute. Man sieht ja zuweilen bei der Geburt die Fruchtblase wurstförmig aus der Scheide hervorragen; ein andermal wölbt sich der untere Pol nur in flacher Wölbung durch den geöffneten Muttermund, und die Häute reissen eher, als dass sie weiter vortreten. Die Sache ist nicht ganz ohne Belang; verdränge ich das Ei in toto, so verschiebe ich die Uteruswände an den Eihäuten, und Anlass zu Gefässzerreissungen ist gegeben. Verdränge ich das Fruchtwasser, so werden zunächst die nicht in die Falte genommenen Abschnitte der Eihäute den verstärkten Druck aushalten und sich dehnen müssen. Sind sie wenig elastisch, so werden sie reissen, und zwar wohl gewöhnlich über dem Orificium internum, woselbst sie am wenigsten Stütze durch die Uteruswand haben, und der Abort wird ganz sicher erfolgen; aber Gefahr wird auch im ersteren Fall durch die Blutungen an der Eiperipherie eintreten.

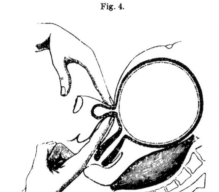

Fig. 4.

Bei Compression in der Mitte des Uteruskörpers ist wohl am leichtesten Fehlgeburt zu erwarten. Man verzichtet deshalb am besten darauf.

Dies führt mich zu der Schattenseite unseres diagnostischen Hülfsmittels. Wenn die Experimente gewaltthätig und wiederholt angestellt werden, läuft man das Wagniss, eine Fehlgeburt herbeizuführen, man mag diese oder jene Stelle, diese oder jene Modification des Versuchs zur Feststellung der physikalischen Beschaffenheit der Uteruswand benützen. Es giebt wohl kein sichereres und weniger gefährliches Mittel zur Herbeiführung des künstlichen Aborts. Ein Missbrauch zu verbrecherischer Abtreibung ist sehr nahe gelegt, da auch die Entdeckung und der Nachweis einer dolosen Handlung nur sehr schwer möglich ist.

Leider sind auch bei unserer Diagnose, wie überall, Quellen des Irrthums vorhanden. Bei Rückwärtslagerungen findet man nicht ganz selten den Uteruskörper etwas weich, wohl auch zusammen drückbar, jedoch nur in geringem Grade und nie so ausgesprochen, wie bei Schwangerschaft. Reponirt man das Organ, so erlangt es seine gewöhnliche Festigkeit meist sehr rasch, da die geringe Consistenz wohl nur durch Stauung und leichte ödematöse Infiltration entstanden zu sein scheint.

Geschwülste, wie erweichte Fibromyome, Echinococcus können ebenfalls zu einer Täuschung Anlass geben. Ich sah einmal ein Angiofibrom von der Grösse einer Wallnuss, welches in der hinteren Wand gerade oberhalb des Isthmus sass. Dabei fanden sich aber noch andere Fasergeschwülste von der gewöhnlichen Beschaffenheit an anderen Stellen. Die differentielle Diagnose wird bei diesen Zuständen keine grosse Schwierigkeiten bereiten.

Ebensowenig bei Hämatometra oder Hydrometra infolge angeborener oder erworbener Atresie des Halscanals. Hier giebt die Geschichte des Falles oft Auskunft. Die Menstruation ist bei der angeborenen Form überhaupt nie dagewesen. Cauterisation, Operationen am Gebärmutterhals, schwere Geburt, gangränescirende Entzündungen sind bei der erworbenen Form vorhergegangen. Auch der Befund gestaltet sich verschieden.

Die neuen Zeichen sind, wie man sieht, äusserst zuverlässig. Sie sind als sichere, in dem althergebrachten Sinne dieses Ausdrucks, zu bezeichnen, insofern sie direkt durch das Ei bedingt werden. Sie haben aber auch noch den Vorzug, dass die Zustände, welche etwas Aehnliches vorzutäuschen vermögen, wenig zahlreich und dabei leicht zu erkennen sind.

Commentary on Classic Paper No.6

Hegar[1] described one of the earliest objective signs of human pregnancy. He noted during vaginal examination that there was a selective softening of the lower part of the uterus, resulting in increased compressibility between the cervix and the pregnant corpus uteri. The discovery of this sign was of particular value at that time period, because it could differentiate between pregnancy and uterine tumors. The sign was first noted by his assistant, C. Meinl, in 1884[2].

Human chorionic gonadotropin (hCG)

In 1927 and 1928, Aschheim and Zondek[3,4] demonstrated that the urine of pregnant women contained a gonad-stimulating substance which, when injected subcutaneously into intact immature female mice, induced follicular maturation. Aschheim and Zondek believed that this gonadotropic substance was produced by the anterior pituitary, but subsequent work by other investigators demonstrated that the placenta and not the pituitary was responsible for the production of the hormone and consequently it was given the name human chorionic gonadotropin (hCG).

1. Hegar, A. (1895). Diagnose der frühesten Schwangerschaftsperiode. *Dtsch. Med. Wochenschr.*, **35**, 564

2. Meinl, C. (1884). *Präque Med. Wochenschr.*, **9**, 157

3. Aschheim, S. and Zondek, B. (1927). Hypophysenworderlappen hormon und ovarialhormon im Harn von Schangeren. *Klin. Wochenschr.*, **6**, 1322

4. Aschheim, S. and Zondek, B. (1928). Die Schwangerschafts-diagnose aus dem Harn durch Nachweis des Hypophysen vorderlappen-hormons. I. Grundlagen und Technik der Methode (B. Zondek). *Klin. Wochenschr.*, **7**, 1404. II. Praktische und theoretische Ergebnisse aus den Harnuntersuchungen. (S. Aschheim). *Klin. Wochenschr.*, **7**, 1453

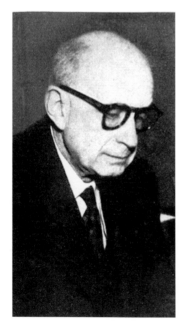 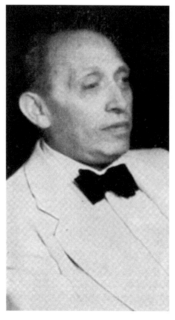

Selmar Aschheim   *Bernhard Zondek*
Reprinted with permission of Macmillan Publishing Company
from Obstetric and Gynecologic Milestones by Harold Speert, MD.
Copyright © 1958 Harold Speert, MD.

Human embryonic development

5. Mall, F.P. (1899–1908). *Contributions to the Study of the Pathology of Early Human Embryos.* (Baltimore)

Our understanding of the details of early human development began with the work of Franklin P. Mall in the 1890s at the Johns Hopkins University[5,6] and his founding of the Carnegie Department of Embryology in 1914, as well as the collection of very early specimens by Hertig and Rock in the 1940s and 1950s.

6. Keibel, F.K.J. and Mall, F.P. (1910–12). *Manual of Human Embryology*, 2 vols. (Philadelphia: J.B. Lippincott)

In 1944, Hertig and Rock[7] at Harvard University in Boston, Massachusetts (USA), studied 12 fertilized ova discovered in surgically removed uteri. The ages of the ova were recorded as mean values on the basis of coital dates.

Hertig and Rock were able to demonstrate implantation of the human blastocyst at day six or seven of its development. The solid syncytiotrophoblast developed lacunae on the eighth day and was observed to begin receiving maternal blood at day eleven.

7. Hertig, A.T. and Rock, J. (1944). On the development of the early human ovum, with special reference to the trophoblast of the previllous stage: a description of 7 normal and 5 pathologic human ova. *Am. J. Obstet. Gynecol.*, **47**, 149

In contrast to the monkey (*Macaca mulatta*), which has a superficial type of implantation, the human ovum was observed to have an interstitial type of implantation in which the blastocyst becomes completely embedded within the endometrium.

Ultrasound

The introduction of ultrasound into Obstetrics[8] represented a major advance, allowing the developing embryo to be studied repeatedly throughout its development.

Robinson[9] studied 80 pregnant women, all of whom were certain of the dates of their last menstrual periods and cycle variation. In this study, Robinson recognized uncertainties as to the normal variation of the timing of ovulation (plus or minus two days) as well as the inaccuracy of fetal crown–rump length (plus or minus 2 mm) and the biological variation in growth. Notwithstanding these factors, the crown–rump length curve that Robinson published is now widely used to estimate the age of the embryo to within three days.

8. Donald, I. (1963). Use of ultrasonics in diagnosis of abdominal swellings. *Br. Med. J.*, **2**, 1154

9. Robinson, H.P. (1973). Sonar measurement of fetal crown–rump length as a means of assessing maturity in the first trimester of pregnancy. *Br. Med. J.*, **4**, 28

Using ultrasound, the embryonic heart action can be documented as early as 35 days after the beginning of the last menstrual period and after 25 days in patients where the embryo has been transferred after *in vitro* fertilization. From 6 to 9 weeks of gestation there is a rapid increase in the mean heart rate from 113 to 167 beats per minute.

10. Vries, J.I.P. de, Visser, G.H.A. and Prechtl, H.F.R. (1982). The emergence of fetal behaviour. I. Qualitative aspects. *Early Human Dev.*, **7**, 301

The first discernible movements of the fetus, apart from heart action, occur at 7 weeks postmenstruum. In a study of 11 fetuses by De Vries *et al.* in 1982[10], a specific sequence of developmental events was observed, including startles, general movements, hiccups, isolated arm and leg, head and hand movements and breathing movements.

Early pregnancy loss

The study of spontaneous abortion or recurrent abortion is not simple, because of the fact that reproduction is associated with a tremendous loss of gametes and conceptions. This was illustrated by the theoretical calculations of Roberts and Lowe (see table below)[11], published in 1975, which postulated a 78% failure of all human conceptions.

11. Roberts, C.J. and Lowe, C.R. (1975). Where have all the conceptions gone? Lancet, 1, 498

—	No. in millions
Married women aged 20–29	2·437
Annual acts of coitus (assuming a mean of twice a week)	253·448
Annual acts of unprotected coitus (assuming one in four is unprotected)	63·362
Unprotected acts occurring within 48-hour period around ovulation (i.e., 1/14)	4·526
Assume one in two of these results in fertilisation ..	2·263
Actual number of infants (live and stillborn) born to these women	0·505
Estimated loss (2·263 − 0·505)	1·758
Percentage loss $\left(\frac{1\cdot758}{2\cdot263}\times100\right)$	78%

Estimated fetal loss (married women aged 20–29 in England and Wales, 1971). Reproduced from C.J. Roberts and C.R. Lowe [11] with permission

Earlier, in 1956, Hertig *et al.*[12] had published a paper studying biologic wastage in early human pregnancy, in which they examined the Fallopian tubes, uterine cavities and endometria of women with planned elective hysterectomies. Ovulation dates were calculated on the basis of basal body temperature charts and coital times were recorded. All women were of proven fertility with a mean age of 33 years.

12. Hertig, A.T., Rock, J., Adams, E.C. and Menkin, M.C. (1956). Thirty-four fertilised human ova, good, bad and indifferent, recovered from 210 women with known fertility. A study of biologic wastage in early human pregnancy. *Paediatrics*, **23**, 202

Four of eight pre-implanted embryos were found to be morphologically abnormal in comparison to other embryos of a comparable age. Nine out of 26 implanted embryos were so morphologically abnormal that further embryonic development seemed unlikely.

13. Miller, J.F., Williamson, E., Glue, J., Gordon, Y.B., Grudzinskas, J.G. and Sykes, A. (1980). Fetal loss after implantation. A prospective study. *Lancet*, **2**, 554

Later, in 1980, Miller *et al.*[13] observed a 43% pregnancy loss rate out of 152 conceptions in 623 cycles of volunteer women. In the majority of cases the sole evidence of pregnancy was an increased concentration of urinary hCG. Judging this 43% against the 78% of Roberts and Lowe, it would appear that most conceptional losses must occur before implantation. Exalto[14] summarized the literature on early pregnancy loss and showed that the earlier the study period, the higher the rate of loss, up to 80–90% just after conception.

14. Exalto, N. (1984). The nature of pregnancy wastage. In Rolland, R., Heineman, M.J., Hillier, S.J. and Vemer, H. (eds.) *Gamete Quality and Fertility Regulation*. (Amsterdam: Excerpta Medica)

Chromosomal aberrations

15. Boué, J. and Boué, A. (1968). Chromosomal aberrations in human spontaneous abortion. *Mammalian Chromosome Newsletter*, **9**, 246

In a study by Boué and Boué[15], the frequency of chromosomal anomalies in spontaneous abortions was found to be around 50%, compared to 0.6% among liveborn children. The anomalies found were mostly trisomy, monosomy and polyploidy. Spontaneous abortion in these cases points to a highly effective form of natural selection, eliminating malformed products of conception.

16. Poland, B.J. and Yuen, B.H. (1978). Embryonic development in consecutive specimens from recurrent spontaneous abortions. *Am. J. Obstet. Gynecol.*, **130**, 512

In 1978, Poland and Yuen[16] reported on a comprehensive study of embryos and fetuses over a period of 10 years. In a group of women with repeated failure of pregnancy, the chromosomal anomalies were found to be the same as those found in sporadic cases of spontaneous abortion, namely trisomies and triploids.

Trisomy is associated with increased maternal age in both liveborn infants and aborted fetuses. The activation of the process of meiosis is triggered by the midcycle luteinizing hormone and may be associated, or causally linked, to a faulty division of chromosomes during fertilization. Unlike trisomy, triploidy is not an age-related phenomenon but is considered to be a fault of fertilization. Chromosomal translocations are also known to be linked with repeated spontaneous abortion.

17. Houwert-Jong, M.H. de, Eskes, T.K.A.B., Termijtelen, A. and Bruinse, H.W. (1989). Habitual abortion: a review. *Eur. J. Obstet. Gynecol. Reprod. Biol.*, **30**, 39

Genetic factors are now reported in the literature in 9.5–13.2% of couples with three or more recurrent abortions. Abnormalities found are translocations (44%), mosaicism (48%) and deletions or inversions (8%)[17].

Hydatidiform mole

The discovery of the origin of the hydatidiform mole provides a beautiful example of the contribution of clinical science to embryology. Its androgenic origin was described long before animal studies were performed. Also, genomic imprinting found its first example in the 'mole-syndrome'.

18. Park, W.W. (1957). The occurrence of sex chromatin in chorionepitheliomas and hydatiform moles. *J. Pathol. Bacteriol.*, **74**, 197

In studying hydatidiform moles, Park (1957)[18] found a preponderance of Barr bodies. When the number of chromosomes in man was shown to be 46, a comparison with earlier studies of hydatidiform moles showed that the majority was 46(XX). This deviation from the 'normal' sex ratio in human concepti was an early impetus to further research.

19. Vassilakos, P. and Kajii, T. (1976). Hydatidiform mole: two entities. *Lancet*, **1**, 259

In 1976 Vassilakos and Kajii[19] suggested that hydatidiform moles were two entities: the complete form being 46(XX) and the partial hydatidiform mole being triploid or aneuploid, showing trisomy for one chromosome.

20. Kajii, T. and Ohama, K. (1977). Androgenetic origin of hydatiform mole. *Nature*, **268**, 633

21. Wake, N., Takagi, N. and Sasaki, M. (1978). Androgenesis as a cause of hydatidiform mole. *J. Natl. Cancer Inst.*, **60**, 51

Two Japanese research groups made the interesting observation that, in complete hydatidiform moles, all pairs of chromosomes were paternally derived. No maternal chromosomes were present and therefore the conceptus was called androgenetic[20,21]. This finding was possible because of the development of staining techniques for banding human chromosomes.

Pathology of villi

Three types of villi have been described[22] in cases of spontaneous abortion.

type I   in which the majority of villi showed hydatidiform change. This type show the highest correlation with chromosomal abnormalities

type II   in which the majority of villi showed postmortem changes of fibrosis

type III in which the majority of villi showed a normal aspect including fetal vessels containing normoblasts.

In 1990, Houwert-De Jong *et al.*[23] found abnormal villi in 62% of 44 women with unexplained recurrent miscarriage. There was, however, no statistically significant difference between this and 58% of 105 women with sporadic miscarriage. From these results, the authors question whether or not recurrent abortion is an entity from a morphologic point of view.

Hypersecretion of luteinizing hormone

Lesley Regan and colleagues[24] from the Department of Obstetrics and Gynaecology, St. Mary's Hospital Medical School, London (UK) found that levels of luteinizing hormone (LH) exceeding 10 IU/l in the early follicular phase of the menstrual cycle were associated with an increased risk of spontaneous miscarriage. In the high LH group, 65% of the pregnancies ended in miscarriage, whereas there were only 15 (12%) miscarriages in the group with normal levels of LH. These authors concluded that hypersecretion of LH before conception plays an important role in miscarriage and they postulated that an abnormal secretion of LH can interfere with the completion of the first meiotic division in the pre-ovulatory follicle. Importantly, this finding offers the possibility of a simple predictive test for women before pregnancy, that could be used to identify patients with an endocrine abnormality that can be remedied.

Immunology

In 1953, Medawar[25] described an immunological conundrum associated with pregnancy. He asked, 'How does the pregnant mother contrive to nourish within itself, for many weeks or months, a fetus that is an antigenically foreign body?' Medawar noted that the mother does not always contrive to do so and, as an example, he pointed to the immunization against the fetus in cases of hemolytic Rhesus disease.

Since then, immunological techniques have been used to elucidate the role of the fetus as an allograft. A depressed maternal immunity during preg-

22. Rushton, D. (1981). Examination of products of conception from previable human pregnancies. *J. Clin. Pathol.*, **34**, 819

23. Houwert-Jong, M.H. de, Bruinse, H.W., Eskes, T.K.A.B., Mantingh, A., Termijtelen, A. and Kooijman, C.D. (1990). Early recurrent miscarriage: histology of conception products. *Br. J. Obstet. Gynaecol.*, **97**, 533

24. Regan, L., Owen, E.J. and Jacobs, H.S. (1990). Hypersecretion of luteinising hormone, infertility and miscarriage. *Lancet*, **1**, 1141

25. Medawar, P.B. (1953). Some immunological and endocrinological problems raised by the evolution of viviparity in vertebrates. *Symp. of the Soc. for Exp. Biol.*, **7**, 320

26. Branch, D.W., Scott, J.R., Kochenour, N.K. *et al.* (1985). Obstetric complications associated with the lupus anticoagulant. *N. Engl. J. Med.*, **313**, 1322

27. Carp, J.H.A., Toder, V., Mashiach, S., Nebel, L. and Serr, D.M. (1990). Recurrent miscarriage: a review of current concepts, immune mechanisms and results of treatment. *Obstet. Gynecol. Surv.*, **45**, 657

28. Hibbard, B.M. (1964). The role of folic acid in pregnancy with particular reference to anaemia, abruption and abortion. *Br. J. Obstet. Gynaecol.*, **71**, 529

29. Steegers-Theunissen, R.P.M., Boers, G.H.J., Blom, J.H., Trijbels, J.M.F. and Eskes, T.K.A.B. (1992). Hyperhomocysteinaemia and recurrent spontaneous abortion or abruptio placentae. *Lancet*, **1**, 1122

30. Aerts, L.A.G.J.M. van, Klaasboer, H.H., Postma, N.S., Pertijs, J.C.L.M., Copius Peereboom, J.H.J., Eskes, T.K.A.B. and Noordhoek, J. (1993). Stereospecific *in vitro* embryotoxicity of homocysteine in pre- and post-implantation rodent embryos. *Toxicol. in vitro*, in press

nancy with respect to humoral and cellular immunity has been reported, especially at the fetal/maternal interface. A number of possible mechanisms that may be involved in the non-rejection of the allogenic fetal-placental unit are currently being studied. These include placental histocompatibility antigens, immune suppressive factors like progesterone, hCG, human placental lactogen, alkaline phosphatase, early pregnancy factor, alpha-fetoprotein, maternal interphase and maternal and fetal blocking antibodies.

Antiphospholipid antibodies have been widely reported to cause fetal loss (up to 89%)[26]. However, the prevalence of these antibodies, including lupus anticoagulant and cardiolipin antibodies, in a population of habitual aborters is reported to be low[27].

So far, intensive work in reproductive immunology has failed to give clear-cut answers to the precise mechanisms involved in early or even late pregnancy loss.

Occupational hazards

Reproductive epidemiology also takes its share of research into spontaneous abortion. Using case referent or cohort designs, odds ratios and relative risks, the contribution of the environment and toxic influences on human reproduction become more and more evident. Agents and environments implicated include anesthetic agents, laboratory work, copper smelting, soldering and chemical sterilization using ethylene oxide and glutaraldehyde.

Folates

In 1964, Hibbard[28] used the excretion of formimino-glutamic acid (FIGLU) to assess the folic status of 700 patients suffering from (recurrent) spontaneous abortion. He found evidence for a defect in folate metabolism in 31–48% of patients (low levels of serum and red cell folate).

This 'defect' has more recently been explained by studying methionine–homocysteine metabolism. In 1992, Steegers-Theunissen and colleagues[29] found evidence for hyperhomocystinemia as a possible risk factor for women with unexplained recurrent early pregnancy loss. Using a standardized methionine loading test, hyperhomocystinemia was found in 22% of these women.

Methionine is an essential amino acid for methyl donation in DNA synthesis and homocysteine is a toxic intermediate product. In the rat embryo *in vitro* model, homocysteine has been shown to interfere with embryonic growth and development[30]. The folates, pyridoxine (vitamin B6) and vitamin B12, are essential co-factors in methionine metabolism and for the functioning of the enzymes involved in the various steps in transsulfuration and remethylation of homocysteine.

It seems likely that Hibbard's suggestion of folate supplementation could solve at least a part of the clinical problem. However, this suggestion awaits a proper clinical placebo-randomized trial. Rather than talking about vitamin deficiency, as in Hibbard's original work, it seems now that we can also introduce the words vitamin-dependency. Hyperhomocystinemia might be a marker for a defect in methionine metabolism, a defect related to the involved enzymes and vitamin co-factors.

Uterine malformations

In 1953, Howard W. Jones and Georgeanna Seegar Jones[31] drew attention to the association between the double uterus and repeated abortion. They observed that one in four women would have serious reproductive problems and made a plea for surgical unification.

Later studies confirmed that uterine anomalies are found more frequently in patients exhibiting second-trimester abortions or premature delivery, varying from 15 to 33%. The poorest reproductive performance is found in women with an unicornuate uterus or complete bicornuate uterus. However, before performing constructive surgery, it is necessary to realize that, in the case of a double uterus, one or both uteri may be dysfunctional.

Cervical insufficiency

In 1955, Shirodkar[32] published a method 'closing the cervix with a fascia lata strip'. It took many years, however, to realize that not every woman benefited from this procedure.

The Medical Research Council and the Royal College of Obstetricians and Gynaecologists organized a multicenter randomized trial[33]. Results suggested that the operation had an important beneficial effect in only one in 25 cases. The basis for the low success rate of this form of treatment of the cervix is the insufficient knowledge we have on uterine behavior during pregnancy. This can be illustrated in the beautiful drawing of the non-pregnant uterus as done by Aschoff in 1906[34]. In most textbooks the human uterus is illustrated as having a cavity; however, as shown in his drawing, Aschoff recognized that the uterine cavity is a space that has to unfold during pregnancy.

31. Jones, H.W. and Seegar Jones, G.E. (1953). Double uterus as an etiological factor in repeated abortion: indications for surgical repair. *Am. J. Obstet. Gynecol.*, **65**, 325

32. Shirodkar, V.N. (1955). A new method of operative treatment for habitual abortions in the second trimester of pregnancy. *Antiseptic*, **52**, 299

33. MRC/RCOG Working Party on Cervical Cerclage (1993). Final report of the Medical Research Council / Royal College of Obstetricians and Gynaecologists Multicentre Randomised Trial of cervical cerclage. *Br. J. Obstet. Gynaecol.*, **100**, 516

34. Aschoff, L. (1906). Das untere Uterinsegment. *Zeitschrift für Geburtshilfe und Gynäkologie*, **58**, 328

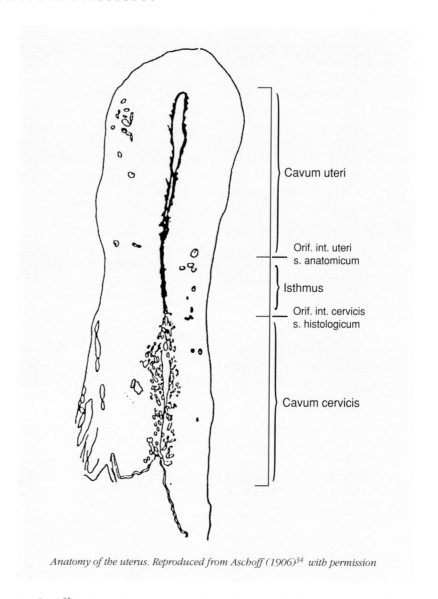

Cavum uteri

Orif. int. uteri
s. anatomicum

Isthmus

Orif. int. cervicis
s. histologicum

Cavum cervicis

Anatomy of the uterus. Reproduced from Aschoff (1906)[34] with permission

35. Danforth, D.N. (1947). The fibrous nature of the human cervix, and its relation to the isthmic segment in gravid and nongravid uterus. *Am. J. Obstet. Gynecol.*, **53**, 541

Danforth[35] took up this message and carefully studied the cervical and isthmic compartment of 12 pregnant and 46 non-pregnant uteri. In the non-pregnant uterus Aschoff had recognized two internal uterine ostia: the histological internal os marked the microscopic point of transition from endocervical mucosa to isthmic mucosa and the anatomical internal os some 6–10 mm superior to this. The structure lying in between these two ostia was designated as the isthmus uteri.

Danforth fixed and sectioned the specimens directly from the operating table and studied the intrinsic structure of the cervix and the isthmic segment, especially concentrating on the fibrous or muscle concentrations in the various areas.

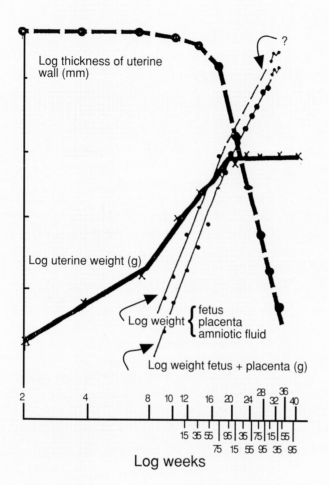

Double logarithmic presentation of the thickness of the uterine wall, the weight of the uterus and the weight of the uterine content during pregnancy. A clear point of intersection is seen at the 24th week of amenorrhea after which distension starts. Adapted from Stolte and Eskes (1967)[36] with permission

Danforth's summary and conclusions are clear: there is no such thing as a separate distinct entity, the isthmus (or lower uterine segment), but just a muscular (corpus) and fibrous part (cervix) of the uterus. The complex nature of the unfolding of the pregnant uterus can be illustrated by the thickness of the uterine wall, the weight of the uterus and the contents during human pregnancy, as shown in the previous figure[36]. From these data, it is clear that distension occurs after the 24th week especially after a growth period of uterus and contents.

The previous studies are in line with the current tendency to be very restrictive in the indication for cervical cerclage and, in preference, to perform abdominal cerclage after organogenesis in the well-developed uterus (in selected cases).

36. Stolte, L.A.M. and Eskes, T.K.A.B. (1967). Cervical insufficiency. In Wood, C. and Walters, W.A.W. (eds.) Proceedings of Fifth World Congress of Gynaecology and Obstetrics, p. 729. (London, Sydney: Butterworths)

Epilogue

Almost every two years a new therapy is published for the treatment of habitual abortion. The clinician, when making his or her choice, is confronted with a number of considerations:

a) The intake criteria for the various studies which may vary from 0 to 28 weeks.
b) The lack of a scientific basis for a certain treatment.
c) The virtual lack of placebo-randomized studies and the fact that often too few patients are included.
d) The possible teratologic effects of medication.
e) The possible disadvantages of immunotherapy.
f) The fact that, in cases of idiopathic recurrent abortion, 60% of women do reach a viable pregnancy by observation and tender loving care only.

A possible approach to this problem is first of all to have more basic information on all the processes of fertilization, implantation, growth and development of the conceptus. This information is also essential for diagnosis with couples confronted with the problem of early pregnancy loss. Necessary data would include knowledge as to the correct medical-obstetrical history identifying the period of pregnancy where the loss occurred, a study of the previous conceptus (pathology of villi), chromosomal translocations, the quality of the menstrual cycle (hormones and endometrium), immunologic aspects, including anti-phospholipids, occupational hazards, the role of folates (homocysteine), and the form and function of uterus and cervix.

In his or her choice of therapy, the clinician is hampered by the fact that not many placebo-randomized trials are performed with a sufficient number of patients to demonstrate the efficacy of a certain treatment. This means that the same clinician has tended to correct the specific deviation from normal that is found in a specific clinical situation. For the time being, there seems to be no other choice. However, it is worth remembering that 'in dubio abstine' is also a modality of treatment, especially knowing that in cases of unexplained loss the outlook for a subsequent pregnancy is reasonable.

For the time being approaches to improve the outlook for a subsequent pregnancy have to focus on the quality of oocytes in menstrual cycles during which conception takes place (improving LH levels), genetic composition and uterine environment, metabolism and immunological processes.

Summary of references

1. Hegar, A. (1895). Diagnose der frühesten Schwangerschaftsperiode. *Dtsch. Med. Wochenschr.*, **35**, 564
2. Meinl, C. (1884). *Prägue Med. Wochenschr.*, **9**, 157

3. Aschheim, S. and Zondek, B. (1927). Hypophysenvorderlappen hormon und ovarialhormon im Harn von Schwangeren. *Klin. Wochenschr.*, **6**, 1322

4. Aschheim, S. and Zondek, B. (1928). Die Schwangerschaftsdiagnose aus dem Harn durch Nachweis des Hypophysenvorderlappenhormons. I. Grundlagen und Technik der Methode (B. Zondek). *Klin. Wochenschr., 7*, 1404. II. Praktische und theoretische Ergebnisse aus den Harnuntersuchungen (S. Aschheim). *Klin. Wochenschr., 7*, 1453

5. Mall, F.P. (1899–1908). *Contributions to the Study of the Pathology of Early Human Embryos.* (Baltimore)

6. Keibel, F.K.J. and Mall, F.P. (1910–12). *Manual of Human Embryology,* 2 vols. (Philadelphia: J.B. Lippincott)

7. Hertig, A.T. and Rock, J. (1944). On the development of the early human ovum, with special reference to the trophoblast of the previllous stage: a description of 7 normal and 5 pathologic human ova. *Am. J. Obstet. Gynecol.*, **47**, 149,

8. Donald, I. (1963). Use of ultrasonics in diagnosis of abdominal swellings. *Br. Med. J.,* **2**, 1154

9. Robinson, H.P. (1973). Sonar measurement of fetal crown–rump length as a means of assessing maturity in the first trimester of pregnancy. *Br. Med. J.,* **4**, 28

10. Vries, J.I.P. de, Visser, G.H.A. and Prechtl, H.F.R. (1982). The emergence of fetal behaviour. I. Qualitative aspects. *Early Human Dev.,* **7**, 301

11. Roberts, C.J. and Lowe, C.R. (1975). Where have all the conceptions gone? *Lancet,* **1**, 498

12. Hertig, A.T., Rock, J., Adams, E.C. and Menkin, M.C. (1956). Thirty-four fertilised human ova, good, bad and indifferent, recovered from 210 women with known fertility. A study of biologic wastage in early human pregnancy. *Paediatrics,* **23**, 202

13. Miller, J.F., Williamson, E., Glue, J., Gordon, Y.B., Grudzinskas, J.G. and Sykes, A. (1980). Fetal loss after implantation. A prospective study. *Lancet,* **2**, 554

14. Exalto, N. (1984). The nature of pregnancy wastage. In Rolland, R., Heineman, M.J., Hillier, S.J. and Vemer, H. (eds.) *Gamete Quality and Fertility Regulation.* (Amsterdam: Excerpta Medica)

15. Boué, J. and Boué, A. (1968). Chromosomal aberrations in human spontaneous abortion. *Mammalian Chromosome Newsletter,* **9**, 246

16. Poland, B.J. and Yuen, B.H. (1978). Embryonic development in consecutive specimens from recurrent spontaneous abortions. *Am. J. Obstet. Gynecol.*, **130**, 512

17. Houwert-Jong, M.H. de, Eskes, T.K.A.B., Termijtelen, A. and Bruinse, H.W. (1989). Habitual abortion: a review. *Eur. J. Obstet. Gynecol. Reprod. Biol.*, **30**, 39

18. Park, W.W. (1957). The occurrence of sex chromatin in chorion-epitheliomas and hydatiform moles. *J. Pathol. Bacteriol.,* **74**, 197

19. Vassilakos, P. and Kajii, T. (1976). Hydatidiform mole: two entities. *Lancet,* **1**, 259

20. Kajii, T. and Ohama, K. (1977). Androgenetic origin of hydatiform mole. *Nature,* **268**, 633

21. Wake, N., Takagi, N. and Sasaki, M. (1978). Androgenesis as a cause of hydatidiform mole. *J. Natl. Cancer Inst.,* **60**, 51

22. Rushton, D. (1981). Examination of products of conception from previable human pregnancies. *J. Clin. Pathol.,* **34**, 819

23. Houwert-Jong, M.H. de, Bruinse, H.W., Eskes, T.K.A.B., Mantingh, A., Termijtelen, A. and Kooijman, C.D. (1990). Early recurrent miscarriage: histology of conception products. *Br. J. Obstet. Gynaecol.,* **97**, 533

24. Regan, L., Owen, E.J. and Jacobs, H.S. (1990). Hypersecretion of luteinising hormone, infertility and miscarriage. *Lancet,* **1**, 1141

25. Medawar, P.B. (1953). Some immunological and endocrinological problems raised by the evolution of viviparity in vertebrates. *Symp. of the Soc. for Exp. Biol.,* **7**, 320

26. Branch, D.W., Scott, J.R., Kochenour, N.K. *et al.* (1985). Obstetric complications associated with the lupus anticoagulant. *N. Engl. J. Med.,* **313**, 1322

27. Carp, J.H.A., Toder, V., Mashiach, S., Nebel, L. and Serr, D.M. (1990). Recurrent miscarriage: a review of current concepts, immune mechanisms and results of treatment. *Obstet. Gynecol. Surv.,* **45**, 657

28. Hibbard, B.M. (1964). The role of folic acid in pregnancy with particular reference to anaemia, abruption and abortion. *Br. J. Obstet. Gynaecol.,* **71**, 529

29. Steegers-Theunissen, R.P.M., Boers, G.H.J., Blom, J.H., Trijbels, J.M.F. and Eskes, T.K.A.B. (1992). Hyperhomocysteinaemia and recurrent spontaneous abortion or abruptio placentae. *Lancet,* **1**, 1122

30. Aerts, L.A.G.J.M. van, Klaasboer, H.H., Postma, N.S., Pertijs, J.C.L.M., Copius Peereboom, J.H.J., Eskes, T.K.A.B. and Noordhoek, J. (1993). Stereospecific *in vitro* embryotoxicity of homocysteine in pre- and post-implantation rodent embryos. *Toxicol. in vitro,* in press

31. Jones, H.W. and Seegar Jones, G.E. (1953). Double uterus as an etiological factor in repeated abortion: indications for surgical repair. *Am. J. Obstet. Gynecol.,* **65**, 325

32. Shirodkar, V.N. (1955). A new method of operative treatment for habitual abortions in the second trimester of pregnancy. *Antiseptic,* **52**, 299

33. MRC/RCOG Working Party on Cervical Cerclage (1993). Final report of the Medical Research Council / Royal College of Obstetricians and Gynaecologists Multicentre Randomized Trial of cervical cerclage. *Br. J. Obstet. Gynaecol.,* **100**, 516

34. Aschoff, L. (1906). Das untere Uterinsegment. *Zeitschrift für Geburtshilfe und Gynäkologie,* **58**, 328

35. Danforth, D.N. (1947). The fibrous nature of the human cervix and its relation to the isthmic segment in gravid and nongravid uterus. *Am. J. Obstet. Gynecol.,* **53**, 541

36. Stolte, L.A.M. and Eskes, T.K.A.B. (1967). Cervical insufficiency. In Wood, C. and Walters, W.A.W. (eds.) *Proceedings of Fifth World Congress of Gynaecology and Obstetrics*, p. 729. (London: Butterworths)

TERATOLOGY

Classic
Paper
No.7

Does the administration of diethylstilbestrol during pregnancy have therapeutic value?

WILLIAM J. DIECKMANN

Department of Obstetrics and Gynecology of the University of Chicago and the Chicago Lying-in Hospital

1. Dieckmann, W.J., Davis, M.E., Rynkiewicz, L.M. and Pottinger, R.E. (1953). Does the administration of diethylstilbestrol during pregnancy have therapeutic value? *Am. J. Obstet. Gynecol.,* **66**, 1062

This paper of Dieckmann and colleagues (1953)[1] has been chosen because it contains all the 'ingredients' for a prospective study into the effect of medication during pregnancy. The choice was also made in memory of all those clinicians who were involved in the two dramas, DES and thalidomide. Considerably more information is now available from human embryology, including the importance of timing and in particular the development of the fetal brain. However, although the pathogenesis of congenital malformations remains largely unknown, progress towards prevention is being made.

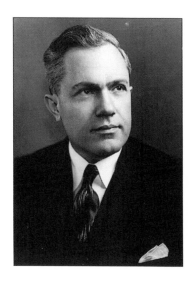

DOES THE ADMINISTRATION OF DIETHYLSTILBESTROL DURING PREGNANCY HAVE THERAPEUTIC VALUE?*†

W. J. Dieckmann, M.D., M. E. Davis, M.D., L. M. Rynkiewicz, S.M., and
R. E. Pottinger, S.M., Chicago, Ill.

(From the Department of Obstetrics and Gynecology of the University of Chicago and the Chicago Lying-in Hospital)

IN 1946 Smith and Smith[1] suggested that increasing amounts of diethylstilbestrol should be administered to all women during pregnancy to prevent or decrease the hazards of the late complications of pregnancy for mothers and babies. The basis for such prophylactic therapy as well as the active therapy of these pregnancy complications stems from a series of experiments by the Smiths on the steroid hormones in normal and abnormal pregnancy.[2] These laboratory observations and their theoretical implications were supported by clinical observations, part of which were made under the supervision of the Smiths and part were the collected reports of other clinical observers.

The use of diethylstilbestrol to prevent and to treat pregnancy complications is based on the supposition that there develops a deficiency in the production of progesterone and other steroids by the placenta which predisposes to or causes these pregnancy complications. The secretion of these steroids can be stimulated by diethylstilbestrol. The increased amounts of steroids made available by the placenta postpone, reduce the severity of, or prevent some of the late complications of pregnancy.

The laboratory experiments which provided the background for this interesting concept of the Smiths have lacked confirmation by other investigators. Davis and Fugo[3, 4] in two reports noted that the administration of diethylstilbestrol to patients during pregnancy did not result in an increased output of urinary pregnanediol, a measure of progesterone metabolism. Sommerville, Marrian and Clayton[5] confirmed these observations and noted a drop in urinary pregnanediol and no gross change in endogenous estrogen. Although many additional experimental data will be necessary to determine the role of diethylstilbestrol in placental steroid metabolism, this paper will confine itself to the clinical implications of the Smith concept.

Smith and Smith in 1949[6] reported on the influence of diethylstilbestrol on the progress and outcome of pregnancy in a series of primigravidas. As

*This investigation was supported in part by a research grant, PHS RG2570, from the National Institutes of Health, Public Health Service.
†Presented at the Seventy-sixth Annual Meeting of the American Gynecological Society, Lake Placid, N. Y., June 15 to 17, 1953.

controls they used a series of primigravidas who received no special treatment. They recorded the following conclusions: (1) It decreased the incidence of the late toxemias of pregnancy. (2) The premature infants born were unusually large for their gestational age. (3) The incidence of postmaturity was decreased. (4) The incidence of unexplained stillbirths was apparently decreased. (5) The neonatal death rate was decreased.

The most serious criticism of this study is the lack of adequate controls. Patients to whom trial medication is administered inevitably receive more meticulous study and medical care than other patients cared for simultaneously. In two nutrition studies conducted by Dieckmann and associates[7] patients who were cooperative and sufficiently intelligent to follow the dietary instructions, keep good records, and attend clinic regularly had a lower incidence of abortion, premature delivery, pre-eclampsia and eclampsia, as well as a lower perinatal death rate, when compared with those of similar groups of women delivered concurrently at this hospital. However, when these figures were compared with those obtained in a control group in which the women received identical treatment with those on the nutrition study there were no significant differences.

The prophylactic administration of diethylstilbestrol and its therapeutic use in pregnancy complications have created widespread interest. To prevent, to postpone, or to ameliorate some of the common hazards of childbirth for mothers and babies is certainly a worthy goal. That all this can be accomplished by the daily consumption of a few tablets is indeed enticing. However, a careful perusal of the literature reveals that most of the clinical data are not supported by adequate controls.[8, 9]

The properly conducted clinical trial demands (1) that patients and staff should have no knowledge of the medication on trial; (2) that a similar group of patients should receive placebo medication which is not discernible from the medication on trial; and (3) that the two groups of patients must be treated simultaneously and as nearly alike as possible. In only one study recently reported by Ferguson[10] have these criteria been met. He concluded that diethylstilbestrol had no effect on the incidence of pre-eclampsia, prematurity, perinatal mortality, fetal weight, and size of the placenta.

We felt that it was timely to conduct a strictly scientifically controlled clinical experiment to determine the value of diethylstilbestrol in our obstetric practice. The first patient was admitted to this study on Sept. 29, 1950. The study terminated Nov. 20, 1952.

The following criteria were used: The sampling was to be sufficiently large so that the results would be statistically significant. A control group of patients who were managed similarly and simultaneously was necessary. It was decided that 2,000 patients registered consecutively in our prenatal clinics prior to the twentieth week of gestation would provide an adequate number. Every other patient would serve as a control. In order to eliminate the personal element, each patient was assigned a code number known only to one individual who was not a clinician. The identity of the two groups was not available until after the data were tabulated by the statistician. A study sheet in duplicate containing pertinent information and the dosage schedule was kept for each patient. One copy was retained in the prenatal record and the other was in the patient's possession so that she could record the daily dosage of tablets.

Four different tablets were designed for this experiment, tablets containing 5 and 25 mg. of diethylstilbestrol and similar tablets containing a placebo. Incorporated in all the tablets was 3 mg. of phenol red, an easy tracer substance. This dye is eliminated in the urine and each urine sample was checked for its presence in order to ascertain if the patient was taking her tablets. She was not aware of this check and some women were eliminated from the study because their urine samples consistently contained no dye.

The following schedule for the administration of tablets was followed: The initial dose varied from 5 to 37.5 mg., depending on the period in the gestation when the patient registered in our clinic. The maximum daily dose of 150 mg. was administered during the thirty-fourth and thirty-fifth weeks of the pregnancy. The duration of the pregnancy was calculated from the menstrual data. The 25 mg. tablets containing stilbestrol or the placebo were scored so that they could easily be broken in half and only one-half consumed.

Each patient was instructed as to the beginning dose and the continuing amounts to be taken. She was asked to note each daily dose on the printed schedule, thereby providing her with a constant reminder to take her medication. At each prenatal visit this schedule was reviewed with her and a notation made as to the degree of patient cooperation. When she completed her medication at the end of the thirty-fifth week, she returned the remaining tablets and her medication chart.

Every patient on registering in our prenatal clinics who was thought to be pregnant between 6 to 20 weeks, inclusive, was offered a box of tablets without charge. Included were women who were known to have complications such as chronic hypertensive vascular disease, diabetes mellitus, or repeated abortions. Each patient was told that previous reports indicated that the tablets were of value in preventing some of the complications of pregnancy and that they would cause no harm to her or the fetus. No coercion was used but she was asked to return the tablets if she did not wish to cooperate. No special clinics or procedures were instituted.

She was instructed to save the urine from bedtime to the next morning on the day of her routine clinic visit and bring in a small specimen. It was tested for phenol red by alkalinizing with 10 per cent sodium hydroxide. A red color merely indicated that the patient had taken one or more of the stilbestrol or placebo tablets. We could not determine how many tablets she took per day or week because of the individual differences in absorption and excretion of phenol red. The amount of this dye was such that a few patients tested negative in periods when they were taking only one pill; all tested positive with two or more tablets. In the patient who was taking the pills regularly whose urine was tested at fairly frequent clinic visits starting at 7 weeks, the sequence of expected test reports was negative-positive, positive, negative-positive when the switch to 25 mg. pills was made, and then positive until administration was discontinued. In general, the reports based on testing for phenol red correlated well with those based on the patient's statements to the clinic staff.

Each set of boxes of pills carried a label with the number which was to be assigned to the patient taking that particular batch of pills. The numbers ran consecutively. Approximately equal numbers of stilbestrol and placebo pills were given out during the period of the study. When the pills were given out to the patient, the number on the boxes was assigned to her and recorded in the record and on the two medication sheets. The patient's name, unit number, and study number were listed in a book kept by the clinic staff.

R. E. P. packaged all the tablets, kept records of the number of boxes sent out, and was the only person who knew the code numbers which he placed in a sealed envelope. At the completion of the study, the sealed envelope containing the code was opened in the presence of three people, the numbers checked with R. E. P., and found to be correct. Because there was a difference in our results from those reported by the Smiths, we wished to determine if there had been a mix-up in the stilbestrol and placebo tablets, which were identical. A representative from Eli Lilly and Company selected tablets from each of the containers and sent them to his company for analysis. Their report states that the tablets marked "stilbestrol" contained the substance in the proper amounts. A colorimetric test for stilbestrol in our laboratory was positive for the same batch of tablets designated "stilbestrol."

The statistician, who had considerable experience with medical charts in our specialty, coded all the pertinent data from the patient's record on IBM cards. W. J. D. served as her consultant when any question arose concerning the interpretation of factual data in the record. He did not know which tablets had been taken by the patient.

A large number of data were accumulated in this study. They concern the reproductive histories of 1,646 mothers and their babies cared for in a teaching institution and the beneficiaries of present-day obstetrical care. This report will concern itself only with some of the questions that have been raised by the ever-increasing use of diethylstilbestrol in obstetrics.

A total of 2,162 patients were entered in this study, evenly divided between those who received stilbestrol and those who received placebos. When the final data were tabulated there remained 1,646 suitable records. Thus 22 per cent of women to whom tablets were given were dropped from the study.

In brief, women were dropped from our study for the following reasons: (a) 125 women cancelled their reservations because they moved or delivered elsewhere; (b) 198 women did not take the tablets regularly according to schedule; (c) 52 women aborted prior to the end of 21 days of medication; (d) the remainder were dropped because of such reasons as not pregnant, husband objected to medication, nausea, etc.

The data presented in the following discussion and tables concern 840 patients who took graduated amounts of diethylstilbestrol according to the schedule in Table I suggested by the Smiths, beginning prior to the twentieth week and continuing uninterruptedly for at least 5 weeks. Serving as controls were 806 women who took similar tablets according to the same schedule containing only a placebo and the dye and cared for simultaneously by the same medical staff under similar conditions. The statistician and the clinicians are in agreement that these two groups of patients are comparable and can be treated as such.

TABLE I.　DAILY DOSAGE OF DIETHYLSTILBESTROL

WEEKS PREGNANT	DIETHYLSTILBESTROL
7-8	5 mg.
9-10	10 mg.
11-12	15 mg.
13-14	20 mg.
15-16	25 mg.
17, 18 and 19	37.5 mg.
20-21	50 mg.
22-23	67.5 mg.
24-25	75 mg.
26-27	87.5 mg.
28-29	100 mg.
30-31	112.5 mg.
32-33	125 mg.
34-35	150 mg.

The distribution of patients in the two groups can be noted in Table II. It is entirely accidental that the several categories of patients are so evenly divided between those who received diethylstilbestrol and those in the control group to whom a placebo was administered. The term primigravida is used in our data to indicate the first pregnancy. If the patient has had one or more additional pregnancies which terminated prior to viability she is considered a primipara in the current pregnancy studied. If she has had one or more viable babies prior to the current pregnancy she is classified as a multipara.

TABLE II.　DISTRIBUTION OF CASES BY HISTORY

	STILBESTROL		CONTROL	
	NO.	%	NO.	%
Primigravidas	314	37.4	316	39.2
Gravida ii (1 abortion)	103	12.3	91	12.8
Gravida iii (2 abortions)	19	2.3	18	2.2
Gravida iv (3 abortions)	9	1.1	8	1.0
Gravida v (4 abortions)	1	.1	0	–
Multiparas, normal	287	34.1	284	35.2
Multiparas with abortion and other abnormalities	36	4.3	25	4.5
Multiparas, abnormal, no abortion	71	8.5	64	7.9
Total	840		806	
All primiparas	446		433	
All multiparas	394		373	

Fig. 1 is a graphic distribution of the period in gestation when the patients in this study began to take tablets. Forty-one per cent of the women began to take stilbestrol prior to the eleventh week compared to 43 per cent of the controls; 43 per cent of each group started medication prior to the fifteenth week of the gestation; 14.4 per cent of the stilbestrol group and 11.8 per cent of the controls began prior to the nineteenth week. The average time of the patient's entry into the study was 11.5 weeks for the primiparas and 12.5 weeks for the multiparas.

In the experimental statistical approach to a clinical problem it is important to compare similar groups of patients in so far as human material will allow. Table III records the mean figures for age, height, and weight increment during pregnancy of the stilbestrol-treated group and the control group. It is surprising how closely these groups compare with each other. The multiparas averaged about three years older than the primiparas. The initial mean weights of the two groups were almost similar. The total weight gain during pregnancy in the primiparas was 9.8 kilograms, compared with 9.5 kilograms in the controls; 9.3 kilograms in the multiparas, compared with 8.7 kilograms for the controls. There was very little difference in their weight loss by the tenth postpartum day.

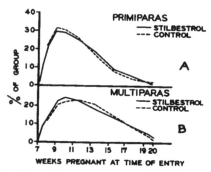

Fig. 1.—Shows the distribution of times of entry to study.

The duration of pregnancy is the most important factor in prematurity. The several criteria for calculating the length of gestation have wide limits of error. It is usually agreed that the menstrual data provide the most simple and probably the most accurate means of calculating the due date. Using the first day of the last normal menstrual period to determine the expected delivery date, the mean length of pregnancy was 38.7 weeks in the primiparas on stilbestrol medication and 39.3 weeks in the controls; 38.6 weeks in the multiparas on stilbestrol and 39.4 weeks in their controls. Analysis of the length of pregnancy for all cases shows a statistically significant longer duration of pregnancy for both control primiparas and multiparas, at the $P = 0.01$ level. Statistical analysis of the uncorrected data shows that stilbestrol did shorten the duration of the pregnancy before the thirty-seventh week, as shown in Table IV. It is obvious that there is a marked increase in the number of primiparas and multiparas in the stilbestrol group over that of the control group up to 37 weeks. These data seem to indicate that stilbestrol favors premature labor. It may be due to an excess amount of hormone. If the patient reaches 37 or more weeks of gestation, the previous administration of stilbestrol has no further effect, but before that time it appears to change the balance in that more patients deliver prematurely. Data corrected to compare with the Smiths' are shown in Fig. 4.

TABLE III. AGE, HEIGHT, WEIGHT, AND DURATION OF PREGNANCY
(MEAN FIGURES)

	STILBESTROL GROUP		CONTROL GROUP	
	PRIMIPARAS	MULTIPARAS	PRIMIPARAS	MULTIPARAS
Age (years)	26.7	29.5	26.4	29.0
Height (cm.)	162.2	162.0	162.2	161.5
Weight (kilograms, minimum)	57.9	59.8	58.5	59.5
Weight gain	9.8	9.3	9.5	8.7
Weight loss in puerperium	7.4	7.2	7.7	7.5
Length of gestation (weeks) (Term 40 weeks)	38.7	38.6	39.3	39.4

TABLE IV. TIME OF DELIVERY BASED ON DATE OF LAST MENSTRUATION

WEEKS' GESTATION	PRIMIPARAS		MULTIPARAS	
	STILBESTROL	CONTROL	STILBESTROL	CONTROL
29-36	5.1%	3.6%	8.4%	4.9%
37-42	89.8%	92.2%	88.3%	88.5%
43 and over	5.1%	4.2%	3.3%	6.6%

TABLE V. TOXEMIAS OF PREGNANCY

	PRIMIPARAS				MULTIPARAS			
	STILBESTROL		CONTROL		STILBESTROL		CONTROL	
	NO.	%*	NO.	%*	NO.	%*	NO.	%*
Pre-eclampsia-eclampsia	16	3.5	13	3.0	1	0.3	3	0.8
Essential hypertension	11	2.5	6	1.4	11	2.8	10	2.7
Chronic glomerulo-nephritis	2	0.4	1	0.2	3	0.8	0	--
Pyelonephritis	0	--	0	--	1	0.3	0	--
Abruptio placentae	3	0.7	2	0.5	2	0.5	3	0.8
Total	446		433		394		373	
		(840)				(806)		

*Percentage of group.

TABLE VI. WEIGHT OF BABIES

	PRIMIPARAS				MULTIPARAS			
	STILBESTROL		CONTROL		STILBESTROL		CONTROL	
WEIGHT IN GRAMS	NO.	%	NO.	%	NO.	%	NO.	%
1,000-1,299	3	0.7	1	0.2	4	1.1	2	0.6
1,300-2,499	29	6.8	16	3.8	23	6.1	17	4.8
2,500-4,499	387	91.7	400	95.5	342	90.9	332	93.2
4,500 and over	3	0.7	2	0.5	7	1.9	5	1.4
Total cases	422		419		376		356	
Average weight all babies	3,200		3,300		3,300		3,300	
Average weight of babies 2,500 grams and over	3,300		3,360		3,407		3,395	

Abortion.—During the last five years the incidence of abortion (1 to 999 grams or before the twenty-eighth week) was 8.3 per cent. The data in Fig. 2 exhibit the incidence of abortion among the several groups of patients studied. Abortions occurred in 4.7 per cent of primiparas on stilbestrol, compared with 2.5 per cent of the controls; in 3.3 per cent of the multiparas on stilbestrol, compared with 1.6 per cent of the controls. Although the abortion rate in the stilbestrol group was higher than in the control group, the total number of patients was too small to be statistically significant. Since most abortions occur before the seventeenth week, and since patients were omitted if they had less than 5 weeks of treatment, it is obvious why the abortion rate was lower than the hospital incidence.

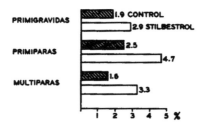

Fig. 2.—Depicts the incidence of abortion (fetuses weighing 1 to 999 grams).

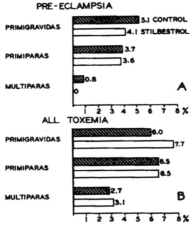

Fig. 3.—A, The incidence of pre-eclampsia. B, The incidence of pre-eclampsia and hypertensive disease in the various groups of patients.

Toxemias of Pregnancy.—In Table V are listed all of the patients who exhibited clinical findings which warranted the diagnosis of toxemia of pregnancy. It will be noted that the incidence of pre-eclampsia was 3.5 per cent in the primiparas on stilbestrol compared to 3 per cent in the control group; 0.3 per cent in the multiparas compared with 0.8 per cent in the controls. The incidence of essential hypertension was 2.5 per cent in the primiparas on stilbestrol in contrast to 1.4 per cent in the controls; it was 2.8 per cent in the multiparas compared with 2.7 per cent in the controls.

Fig. 3 presents a graphic distribution of the toxemia patients after the histories were carefully reviewed by Dieckmann and corrected to conform

Am. J. Obst. & Gynec.
November, 1953

TABLE VII. INCIDENCE OF PREMATURES BY WEIGHT
(PERCENTAGE OF CASES)

WEIGHT OF BABY	UNDER 1,500 GRAMS		1,500-1,999 GRAMS		2,000-2,499 GRAMS		TOTALS	
	STILBESTROL	CONTROL	STILBESTROL	CONTROL	STILBESTROL	CONTROL	STILBESTROL	CONTROL
Primigravidas	1.9	.6	2.2	1.9	4.1	2.5	8.3	5.1
Other primiparas	2.3	--	.8	--	5.3	4.3	8.3	4.3
Multiparas, normal	3.8	1.8	.3	.4	3.5	2.8	7.7	4.9
Multiparas with abortion and other abnormalities	5.5	4.0	2.8	8.0	5.5	16.0	13.9	28.0
Multiparas, abnormal, no abortions	8.4	1.6	2.8	--	2.8	7.8	14.1	9.4
All primiparas	2.0	.5	1.8	1.4	4.5	3.0	8.3	4.8
All multiparas	4.8	1.9	1.0	.8	3.6	4.6	9.4	7.2
All cases	3.3	1.1	1.4	1.1	4.0	3.7	8.8	6.0

to the data presented by the Smiths. These corrected results differ very little from the uncorrected data in Table V. The several groups were too small to treat statistically. However, not only did the administration of diethylstilbestrol fail to decrease the incidence of toxemias but there was no difference in the time of onset of this complication nor in its severity in the two groups of patients studied. One must conclude that the prophylactic administration of stilbestrol has no therapeutic value in decreasing the hazards of late pregnancy toxemias.

Birth Weights of Babies.—In Table VI are listed all of the babies according to their birth weights. It is obvious that in the various weight categories there was a slightly greater percentage of babies that weighed less in the stilbestrol group as compared with those in the control group in both primiparas and multiparas. The average weight of all babies of primiparas on stilbestrol was 3,200 grams compared with 3,300 grams for the controls; the babies of multiparas on stilbestrol, as well as those on placebos, averaged 3,300 grams.

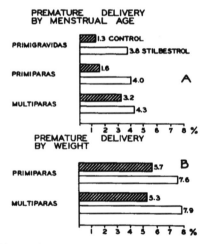

Fig. 4.—*A*, The incidence of premature babies by menstrual age. *B*, By weight of the babies.

Prematurity.—The diagnosis of prematurity is based on the weight, length of the gestation, and physical findings of the baby. The duration of pregnancy is not easy to determine accurately, for it is subject to wide variation. The physical signs of prematurity, including x-ray study of ossification centers, are not reliable indices, nor do they provide sharp end points. Weight is the most reliable criterion for prematurity. During the past five years the over-all incidence of premature delivery based on babies weighing 1,000 to 2,499 grams was 6.6 per cent. Table VII lists the incidence of prematurity by weight. In the group of women on stilbestrol, 8.8 per cent of the babies weighed less than 2,500 grams compared with 6 per cent in the control group. In the stilbestrol group 3.3 per cent weighed under 1,500 grams, 1.4 per cent weighed 1,500 to 1,999 grams, and 4 per cent weighed 2,000 to 2,499 grams. This compares with 1.1 per cent, 1.1 per cent, and 3.7 per cent in the control group.

Fig. 4 is a graphic presentation of the data on premature babies corrected to conform to the data presented by the Smiths by omitting women with known hypertension, diabetes mellitus, chronic nephritis, twins, etc. In A the premature babies are classified by menstrual age and in B by weight. It is obvious that using either criterion for prematurity, a greater number of premature babies were delivered to women to whom stilbestrol was administered as compared with the control group.

Premature infants of mothers who took stilbestrol did not appear to differ from those of the control mothers at the same gestational age. If prematurity was defined in terms of weight of the baby, the incidence was higher, but not significantly so, for all stilbestrol groups. On the basis of week of delivery, there was a real difference between stilbestrol and control cases. Both primiparas and multiparas tended, with fair statistical significance, to deliver earlier in the stilbestrol groups, and the primiparas who took stilbestrol delivered a significantly larger number of infants before the thirty-eighth week.

Postmaturity.—This is exceedingly difficult to define. The menstrual data are so unreliable that they are of little value in determining postmaturity. Undoubtedly, the size of the baby need not bear a direct relationship to his maturity. In our data, Table IV, delivery occurred at an estimated 43 weeks or longer in 5.1 per cent of the primiparas on stilbestrol compared to 4.2 per cent of the controls. The figures for multiparas were 3.3 per cent and 6.6 per cent, respectively. In Table VI the number of babies that weighed more than 4,500 grams is comparable in the several groups of patients. The administration of stilbestrol did not prevent postmaturity.

TABLE VIII. PERINATAL MORTALITY
(ALL DEATHS OF FETUSES 1,000 GRAMS AND OVER)

	PRIMIPARAS		MULTIPARAS	
	STILBESTROL	CONTROL	STILBESTROL	CONTROL
Stillbirths:				
Antepartum, under 24 hours	0	2	0	1
Antepartum, more than 24 hours	4	0	2	1
Intrapartum	1	2	0	2
Total stillbirths	5 (1.1%)	4 (0.9%)	2 (0.5%)	4 (1.1%)
Neonatal:				
Under 24 hours	2	0	5	2
1-10 days	5	0	4	1
Over 10 days	0	1	0	0
Total neonatal	7 (1.6%)	1 (0.2%)	9 (2.3%)	3 (0.8%)
Perinatal	12 (2.7%)	5 (1.1%)	11 (2.8%)	7 (1.9%)

The pediatricians who studied our babies could find no differences in the strength, vigor, nursing ability, weight loss, and other criteria of growth and development in babies born of mothers who had received stilbestrol and those who had taken placebos. There were no statistically significant differences in the length of babies in these two groups. It must be concluded that the prophylactic administration of diethylstilbestrol to mothers did not decrease the incidence of prematurity based on fetal weight nor did it result in larger babies for their gestational age.

Perinatal mortality includes all stillbirths and neonatal deaths of babies weighing 1,000 grams or more. From 1946 to 1952 the incidence of stillbirths was 0.95 per cent and of neonatal deaths was 1.06 per cent. Data for this study are given in Table VIII. The stillbirth rate in primiparas on stilbestrol was 1.1 per cent compared with 0.9 per cent in the control group; in multiparas it was 0.5 per cent compared to 1.1 per cent. The neonatal death rate of infants born to primiparas on stilbestrol was 1.6 per cent compared to 0.2 per cent in the control group; in multiparas it was 2.3 per cent compared to 0.8 per cent in the controls. The perinatal mortality was 2.7 per cent in all the women who were taking stilbestrol compared to 1.5 per cent in the women in the control group.

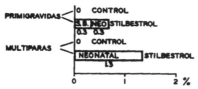

Fig. 5.—Shows the stillbirth and neonatal death rates (1,000 or more grams) for the various groups of patients.

Fig. 5 is a graphic presentation of perinatal mortality after the data were corrected by the deletion of patients with known essential hypertension, diabetes mellitus, chronic glomerular nephritis, etc., to conform to the data presented by the Smiths. Although the sizes of the groups are too small to have statistical significance it is apparent that all the fetal deaths occurred in infants of the women who received stilbestrol.

Our data on perinatal mortality do not indicate that the prophylactic administration of diethylstilbestrol influenced favorably the fetal salvage.

Congenital Anomalies.—All anomalies present in the babies at birth are listed in Table IX. It will be noted that most of these are minor and of no great importance. However, it is obvious that there are no differences between the two groups of patients. It can be concluded that diethylstilbestrol did not increase or decrease the occurrence of fetal anomalies.

Nausea and Vomiting.—The ability of the pregnant patient to consume huge amounts of diethylstilbestrol without nausea or vomiting is an old observation. In our data, 15 women (1.4 per cent of the original group) discontinued stilbestrol because of nausea or vomiting. However, 16 women (1.5 per cent of the original group) who were taking placebos stopped the tablets for the same reason. All of those dropping out because of nausea specifically reported that the pills made them sick, and many stated that the nausea decreased sharply as soon as they stopped. Yet half of these women were actually taking placebos.

Since our data were at variance with those of the Smiths, they were all rechecked. The charts of patients with toxemia of pregnancy, premature delivery, stillbirths and neonatal deaths, and any other complication or abnormality, were examined again by one of the senior authors with no knowledge of the kind of medication. There was no significant change in any of the results.

TABLE IX. CONGENITAL ANOMALIES

TYPE OF ANOMALY	PRIMIPARAS		MULTIPARAS	
	STILBESTROL	CONTROL	STILBESTROL	CONTROL
Minor	7	7	9	4
Skin, as papilloma	7	12	7	6
Cystocele, hydrocele	4	3	3	2
Harelip, cleft palate, etc.	1	0	0	1
Clubfeet, multiple digits	2	5	6	2
Mongolism	0	0	0	1
Brain and spinal cord	1	0	0	0
Cardiac, etc.	2	1	1	2
Gastrointestinal	1	0	0	0
Genitourinary	0	2	0	3
Multiple major	2	2	1	3
Total anomalies	27	32	27	24
Total infants	426	415	376	361

Conclusions

A strictly controlled clinical trial of the therapeutic value of diethylstilbestrol administered to patients during pregnancy in reducing the hazards of some of the late complications of pregnancy for mothers and babies has been reported.

The various complications were studied in the total unselected group of patients divided into primigravidas, primiparas, and multiparas. Then the groups were again studied after all groups were corrected to compare with the Smiths'.

The results of the administration of diethylstilbestrol in graduated amounts to 840 patients according to a schedule suggested by the Smiths were compared with the results of an identical placebo tablet given to 806 patients. Stilbestrol did not reduce the incidence of abortion, prematurity, or postmaturity. Premature babies of stilbestrol-treated mothers were no longer nor more mature for their gestational ages than comparable prematures in the control group of placebo-treated mothers. It did not decrease the incidence of perinatal mortality. It did not decrease the frequency of the toxemias of pregnancy.

Acknowledgment is made to Eli Lilly and Company for aid in making the stilbestrol and placebo tablets with the dye and for the final determination of the stilbestrol; to Lillian Natusko for the examination of the urines for phenol red; to the staff and residents for their cooperation.

References

1. Smith, O. W., and Smith, G. van S.: AM. J. OBST. & GYNEC. 51: 411, 1946.
2. Smith, G. van S., and Smith, O. W.: Physiol. Rev. 28: 1, 1948.
3. Davis, M. Edward, and Fugo, N. W.: Proc. Soc. Exper. Biol. & Med. 65: 283, and 66: 391, 1947.

4. Davis, M. Edward, and Fugo, N. W.: Proc. Soc. Exper. Biol. & Med. 69: 436, 1948.
5. Sommerville, I. F., Marrian, G. F., and Clayton, B. E.: Lancet 1: 680, 1949.
6. Smith, O. W., and Smith, G. van S.: Am. J. Obst. & Gynec. 58: 994, 1949.
7. Dieckmann, W. J., Turner, D. F., Meiller, E. J., Savage, L. J., Hill, A. J., Straube,
   M. T., Pottinger, R. E., and Rynkiewicz, L. M.: J. Am. Dietet. A. 27: 1046, 1951.
8. Gitman, L., and Koplowitz, A.: New York State J. Med. 50: 2823, 1950.
9. Smith, O. W., and Smith, G. van S.: New England J. Med. 241: 562, 1949.
10. Ferguson, J. H.: Am. J. Obst. & Gynec. 65: 592, 1953.
11. Canario, E. M., Houston, G., and Smith, C.: Am. J. Obst. & Gynec. 65: 1298, 1953.

Commentary on Classic Paper No.7

This paper of Dieckmann and colleagues (1953)[1] can be regarded as the first important clinical study on the effect of medication on the outcome of pregnancy. Dieckmann's interest in this area of research was triggered by a paper by Smith and Smith[2] in 1949, who suggested that increasing amounts of diethylstilbestrol (DES) should be administered to all women during pregnancy to prevent complications.

DES is a non-steroidal benzene-like substance with the ability to produce estrogenic effects when taken orally. The hypothesis of Smith and Smith, that DES could have a clinically beneficial effect, was based on the fact that estrogens could promote uterine circulation, could stimulate progesterone production of the placenta and finally could bring a large percentage of normal primigravidas to term. Dieckmann and his group considered that a properly conducted clinical trial was the only way to investigate this hypothesis. In this paper, Dieckmann and colleagues introduced the basic principles of a good clinical trial, much as would be expected in a trial today. They specified that patients and staff should have no knowledge of the medication on trial, that a similar group of patients should have placebo medication and that the two groups of patients should be treated simultaneously and as nearly alike as possible.

In Dieckmann's study, a total of 2162 patients were investigated. Because of a drop out of 22%, a total of 1646 suitable records remained for evaluation. From the results, the authors concluded that the administration of DES in graduated amounts did not reduce the incidence of abortion, prematurity, postmaturity, the frequency of toxemias, or perinatal mortality. Clinical evidence failed to support the hypothesis of Smith and Smith, despite the good theoretical reasoning.

The theory behind the hypothesis

When examining the paper of Dieckmann, the first question that comes to mind is, 'What was the evidence that DES would have been of benefit anyway?'

In 1946, Smith and colleagues[3] published the results of a study into the effect of DES. Their results demonstrated that *the urinary excretion of pregnanediol rose steadily while diethylstilbestrol was being taken and dropped precipitously each time it was omitted'*. Thoughts on possible variation of pregnanediol excretion or the inclusion of a placebo are, however, lacking in this paper.

1. Dieckmann, W.J., Davis, M.E., Rynkiewicz, L.M. and Pottinger, R.E. (1953). Does the administration of diethylstilbestrol during pregnancy have therapeutic value? *Am. J. Obstet. Gynecol.*, **66**, 1062

2. Smith, O.W. and Smith, G.V.S. (1949). Use of diethylstilbestrol to prevent fetal loss from complications of late pregnancy. *N. Engl. J. Med.*, **241**, 562

3. Smith, O.W., Smith, G.V.S. and Hurwitz, D. (1946). Increased excretion of pregnanediol in pregnancy from diethylstilbestrol with special reference to the prevention of late pregnancy accidents. *Am. J. Obstet. Gynecol.*, **51**, 411

4. Smith, O.W. (1948). Diethylstilbestrol in the prevention and treatment of complications of pregnancy. *Am. J. Obstet. Gynecol.*, **56**, 821

In a later publication, Smith[4] reported on 632 pregnant women receiving stilbestrol for reasons such as to prevent threatened abortion, prophylactically for complications of pregnancy or premature delivery and for women with hypertension or diabetes. The author noted success rates, in terms of living and well babies, of 77–78% and 'toxic reactions' were only seen in 1.4%.

One year later, Smith and Smith[2] reported on further results in 180 women. In their evaluation of the results they relied on:

a) the past history of the patients,
b) a comparison with results in the literature.

From this time onwards, this treatment became known as the 'Smith and Smith regimen', and was adopted in various countries. For many years, the results of the placebo-randomized controlled trial of Dieckmann and colleagues[1] failed to influence clinicians, who believed at that time that a reduction of fetal loss from 77% in past obstetric histories to 20% on stilbestrol was sufficient evidence of its efficacy.

Complications of DES therapy

5. Herbst, A.L., Ulfelder, H. and Poskanzer, D.C. (1971). Adenocarcinoma of the vagina: association of maternal stilbestrol therapy with tumor appearance in young women. *N. Engl. J. Med.*, **284**, 878

It took 23 years from the first publication of the clinical use of DES to recognize that the low incidence of toxic reactions noted by Smith in 1948 [4] was not always true. In 1971, Herbst and colleagues published a striking observation of adenocarcinoma of the vagina in young women exposed *in utero* to DES[5]. The DES drama was not restricted to adenocarcinoma of the vagina. Anatomical anomalies of the uterus (T-shaped) were also found, as well as reproductive failure in DES-exposed women[6].

6. Kaufman, R., Adam, E., Binder, G.L. and Gerthoffer, E. (1980). Upper genital tract changes and pregnancy outcome in offspring exposed *in utero* to diethylstilbestrol. *Am. J. Obstet. Gynecol.*, **37**, 299

In 1980, Barnes and colleagues[7] compared 618 subjects who had prenatal exposure to DES with 618 controls. As in previous studies, they also found an increased risk of an unfavorable outcome of pregnancy associated with DES exposure, but gave a more optimistic view, stating that at least 81% had one full-term live birth.

7. Barnes, A.B., Colton, Th., Gundersen, J., Noller, K.L., Titley, B.C., Strama, Th., Townsend, D.E., Hatab, P. and O'Brien, P.C. (1980). Fertility and outcome of pregnancy in women exposed *in utero* to diethylstilbestrol. *N. Engl. J. Med.*, **302**, 609

All this led to a project called the National Cooperative Diethylstilbestrol Adenosis Project (DESAD), which looked at complications associated with DES treatment in pregnancy. This example was followed in more countries where DES was being prescribed by too many doctors and used by too many women. An increased risk of an unfavorable outcome of pregnancy associated with DES exposure was published in 1980[7] in the same Journal that originally accepted the paper of Smith and Smith in 1949 which advocated the use of DES!

Interference with first meiotic cell division?

A hitherto unexpected finding associated with DES treatment, that might have implications for spontaneous abortion, is the observation by Eskes and Scheres[8] of a karyogram in abortion tissue demonstrating a trisomy in the 11th pair of chromosomes, a rare finding in all trisomic patterns published so far. The suggestion given is that DES can interfere with the first meiotic division occurring *in utero*.

8. Eskes, T.K.A.B. and Scheres, J.M.J.C. (1984). Does diethylstilbestrol influence the fetal ovary? (in Dutch). *Ned. Tijdschr. Geneesk.*, **128**, 1601

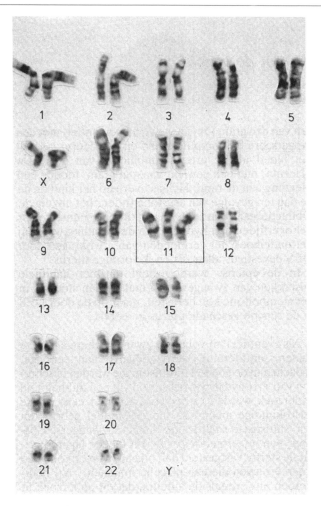

Karyogram of a spontaneous abortion in the 6th week (empty sac with chorionic villi) in a DES-exposed woman. Reproduced from Eskes and Scheres (1984)[8] with permission

The thalidomide drama

9. Lenz, W. and Knapp, K. (1962). Thalidomide embryopathy. *Arch. Environ. Health*, 5, 100

In 1962, Lenz and Knapp[9] described a drug-related syndrome similar to a natural condition, originally identified in 1917 in a doctoral thesis from Dr Hélène Socin at Basel. This condition, namely phocomelia, had a rare spontaneous occurrence in nature, but was now duplicated by the ingestion of the sedative thalidomide.

Lenz and Knapp[9] observed that, in every country where thalidomide had been introduced on a large scale, typical malformations were observed after its introduction. Retrospective histories on 112 mothers of malformed infants brought to light acceptable evidence of thalidomide intake in early pregnancy in 90 cases. Lenz and Knapp concluded: *'The exact time relation between intake of thalidomide and development of the affected organs seems to be conclusive proof of a causal connection. We can conceive of no other acceptable explanation.'*

10. Lenz, W. (1965). Discussion in symposium on *Embryopathic Activity of Drugs*, edited by Robson, J.M., Sullivan, F.M. and Smith, R.L.J. (London: Churchill)

In a later publication, Lenz[10] presented a figure (see below) showing the relationship between malformations of the thalidomide type and sales of the drug. He commented that, 'There is an approximate parallelism between the two curves suggesting that they could be causally related. The time separation between the two curves, i.e. about 9 months, is as one would expect on biological grounds.'

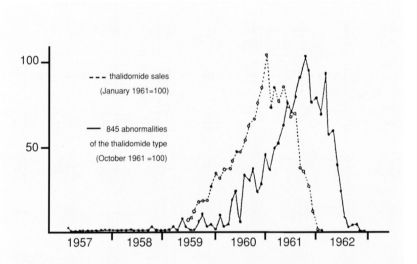

The relationship between malformations of the thalidomide type and the sales of thalidomide (figures for F.R.G., excluding Hamburg).
Note that the distance between the curves is ± 9 months. Adapted from W. Lenz (1965)[10] with permission

The Carnegie Stages

An important landmark for human embryology was the publication of the *Manual of Human Embryology* by Keibel and Mall[11] based on measurements and staging made by Mall[12,13]. Further studies on the detail of the human embryo had to await the founding of the Carnegie Department of Embryology by Franklin P. Mall in 1914, as well as the collection of very early specimens by Hertig and Rock in the 1940s.

The Carnegie collection was transferred from Baltimore to Davis (California) in 1973 and serves as a Bureau of Standards for primate embryology[14]. Twenty-three embryonic stages are now meticulously described from age 1 day till 60 days, postovulatory. Today, the possibility of measuring crown–rump length by ultrasound, even from the third week onwards, greatly facilitates insight into early human development.

The importance of timing

In practice, the type of malformations observed in a fetus can be related to the critical or sensitive period of development. For instance, the closure of the neural tube and the early development of the heart take place in the third postconceptional week while the development of the genital system occurs around 6–9 weeks postconception. Importantly, the central nervous system remains sensitive to noxious influences throughout pregnancy.

The fetal brain

The work of Dominick P. Purpura at the Albert Einstein College of Medicine, New York, USA, has done much to advance our knowledge of the development of the fetal brain and its sensitivity to noxious influences[15].

The methods of study used have a direct bearing on the developmental pathobiology of the neuron. Employed were the rapid Golgi method, evoked potentials and camera lucida drawings, allowing a stereometric insight into the brain.

There are several messages from this type of research:

- The development of appropriate and sufficient synaptic relations between neurons is necessary for normal neuronal operations.

- Significant alterations in somadendritic membrane surfaces of neurons invariably result in brain dysfunction.

11. Keibel, F. and Mall, F.P. (1910 &1912). *Manual of Human Embryology*, 2 volumes. (Philadelphia: Lippincott)

12. Mall, F.P. (1907). On measuring human embryos. *Anat. Rec.*, **1**, 129

13. Mall, F.P. (1914). On stages in the development of human embryos from 2 to 25 mm long. *Anat. Anz.*, **46**, 78

14. O'Rahilly, R. (1973). Developmental stages in human embryos. Including a survey of the Carnegie collection. (Washington DC: Carnegie Institution of Washington)

15. Purpura, D. P. (1977). Developmental pathobiology of cortical neurons in the immature human brain. In Gluck, L. (ed.) *Intrauterine Asphyxia and the Developing Fetal Brain*. (Chicago, London: Year Book Medical Publishers Inc.)

- The normal full-term neonate is most likely equipped with all the cortical neurons it will ever possess. Most of these have acquired their basic dendritic branching patterns, at, or shortly after, birth.

- Much of the development of the dendritic surface area of cortical neurons occurs during the last trimester, making the preterm infant particularly vulnerable to noxious influences.

The etiology and prevention of congenital malformations

16. Kalter, H. and Warkany, J. (1983). Congenital malformations: etiologic factors and their role in prevention. *N. Engl. J. Med.,* Part I, **308**, 424; Part II, **308**, 491

Kalter and Warkany[16] studied etiologic factors and their role in the prevention of congenital malformations. They estimated that monogenic and chromosomal causes of congenital malformations accounted for approximately 13.5% of the total number of defects. Unfortunately, attempts to reduce the frequency of such defects are limited to genetic counselling and induced abortion.

With respect to major environmental causes of congenital malformations, diabetes mellitus, anticonvulsant drugs and infections such as rubella, toxoplasmosis and cytomegalic infection are associated with about 5% of all major congenital malformations. Intensified efforts at metabolic control of diabetes, before and in early pregnancy, the development of non-teratogenic anticonvulsant medication and timely recognition of infections could make important contributions to prevention.

Another important group of malformations consists of those for which environmental and genetic components (ecogenetic) are responsible. These so-called multifactorial defects constitute about 20% of all malformations. Evidence of such multifactorial origins exists for neural tube defects in which dietary compounds, especially folic acid, are involved in etiology and prevention.

17. Hibbard, E.D. and Smithells, R.W. (1965). Folic acid metabolism and human embryopathy. *Lancet,* **1**, 1254

Progress in primary prevention

One of the consequences of failure of the neural tube to close (in the third postconceptional week) is the occurrence or recurrence of anencephaly or spina bifida.

18. Smithells, R.W., Sheppard, S., Schorah, C.J., Seller, M.J., Nevin, N.C., Harris, R., Read, A.P. and Fielding, D.W. (1980). Possible prevention of neural tube defects by periconceptional vitamin supplementation. *Lancet,* **1**, 339

Hibbard and Smithells[17] recognized the importance of folates to cell growth, focusing on megaloblastic anemia, placental abortion, spontaneous abortion and birth defects. Smithells and colleagues[18] suggested that a multi-vitamin supplement in the periconceptional period could reduce the occurrence rate of neural tube defects (NTD). The prospective Medical Research Council vitamin study helped to resolve this issue when, in a placebo-randomized trial, it was demonstrated that 4 mg folic acid in the periconceptional period resulted in a 72% protective effect on the recurrence of NTD[19].

The mechanism behind the action of folic acid is now under investigation, with the answer probably in the metabolism of methionine-homocysteine[20].

International organizations

The International Clearing House is a worldwide organization that reports on the prevalence of major congenital malformations. From its information, areas of high and low prevalence can be readily identified. In the chart for 1974 to 1988 it can be seen that, for neural tube defects, there was a high prevalence in Mexico and Ireland but a low prevalence in Finland and Japan[21].

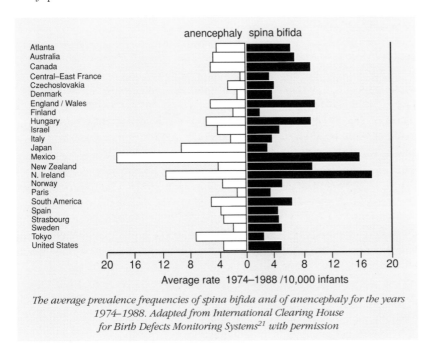

The average prevalence frequencies of spina bifida and of anencephaly for the years 1974–1988. Adapted from International Clearing House for Birth Defects Monitoring Systems[21] with permission

A registry, similar to the International Clearing House, now also exists in Europe (Eurocat), providing the basis for further epidemiological studies in regard to pathogenesis and prevention.

Classification of medication risks

After the thalidomide and DES disasters, it became clear that more demanding measures were necessary than the standard teratological studies required before a drug could be marketed.

19. MRC Vitamin Study Research Group (1991). Prevention of neural tube defects: results of the Medical Research Council vitamin study. *Lancet*, **2**, 131

20. Steegers-Theunissen, R.P.M., Boers, G.H.J., Trijbels, J.M.F. and Eskes, T.K.A.B. (1991). Neural tube defects and derangement of homocysteine metabolism. *N. Engl. J. Med.*, **324**, 199

21. International Clearing House for Birth Defects Monitoring Systems (1991). *Congenital Malformations Worldwide. A Report from the International Clearing House for Birth Defects Monitoring Systems.* (Amsterdam: Elsevier Science)

One of those measures, apart from drug surveillance, is the development of a system in which the teratological risks are classified. Such a system has now been introduced in the USA, Australia and Sweden. The classification system is divided into four categories, A, B, C and D (or X).

Category A	free from teratological risks in man
Category B	not enough information available
category B1	non-teratogenic in animals
category B2	insufficient information in animals
category B3	teratogenic in animals
Category C	reversible damage possible without anatomical defects
Category D (or X)	teratological risks

Epilogue

22. Gregg, N.M. (1941). Congenital cataract following german measles in the mother. *Trans. Ophthalmol. Soc. Aust.*, **3**, 35

Fifty years ago the important observation of Gregg[22], that there is a linkage between congenital cataract and the infection of the mother with rubella during pregnancy, signalled the beginning of our awareness of teratogenic effects.

Since then, not only infections but also medication and environmental influences have been implicated as teratological influences. The classic paper of Dieckmann represented the first real evidence that drug therapy could fail and even had untoward effects on the development of the fetus as was observed by Herbst[5]. This was followed by the disastrous thalidomide episode. With hindsight, we are now aware of the susceptibility of the fetus and are able to take precautions that will hopefully prevent such disasters occurring in the future.

23. Czeizel, A.E., Intödy, Z. and Modell, B. (1993). What proportion of congenital abnormalities can be prevented? *Br. Med. J.*, **306**, 499

The effect of rubella infection can be solved by vaccination programs for young girls and the drug-related problem can be tackled by a more accurate prescribing behavior, judging medication risks during the various periods of pregnancy. Finally, more insight into environmental influences should lead to preventive actions as already suggested by Czeizel and colleagues[23].

Nevertheless, the cause of more than 50% of teratological abnormalities is still not known and urgently requires more and new initiatives for research.

Summary of references

1. Dieckmann, W.J., Davis, M.E., Rynkiewicz, L.M. and Pottinger, R.E. (1953). Does the administration of diethylstilbestrol during pregnancy have therapeutic value? *Am. J. Obstet. Gynecol.,* **66**, 1062

2. Smith, O.W. and Smith, G.V.S. (1949). Use of diethylstilbestrol to prevent fetal loss from complications of late pregnancy. *N. Engl. J. Med.,* **241**, 562

3. Smith, O.W., Smith, G.V.S. and Hurwitz, D. (1946). Increased excretion of pregnanediol in pregnancy from diethylstilbestrol with special reference to the prevention of late pregnancy accidents. *Am. J. Obstet. Gynecol.,* **51**, 411

4. Smith, O.W. (1948). Diethylstilbestrol in the prevention and treatment of complications of pregnancy. *Am. J. Obstet. Gynecol.,* **56**, 821

5. Herbst, A.L., Ulfelder, H. and Poskanzer, D.C. (1971). Adenocarcinoma of the vagina: association of maternal stilbestrol therapy with tumor appearance in young women. *N. Engl. J. Med.,* **284**, 878

6. Kaufman, R., Adam, E., Binder, G.L. and Gerthoffer, E. (1980). Upper genital tract changes and pregnancy outcome in offspring exposed *in utero* to diethylstilbestrol. *Am. J. Obstet. Gynecol.,* **37**, 299

7. Barnes, A.B., Colton, Th., Gundersen, J., Noller, K.L., Titley, B.C., Strama, Th., Townsend, D.E., Hatab, P. and O'Brien, P.C. (1980). Fertility and outcome of pregnancy in women exposed *in utero* to diethylstilbestrol. *N. Engl. J. Med.,* **302**, 609

8. Eskes, T.K.A.B. and Scheres, J.M.J.C. (1984). Does diethylstilbestrol influence the fetal ovary? (in Dutch). *Ned. Tijdschr. Geneesk.,* **128**, 1601

9. Lenz, W. and Knapp, K. (1962). Thalidomide embryopathy. *Arch. Environ. Health,* **5**, 100

10. Lenz, W. (1965). Discussion in symposium on *Embryopathic Activity of Drugs,* edited by Robson, J.M., Sullivan, F.M. and Smith, R.L.J. (London: Churchill)

11. Keibel, F. and Mall, F.P. (1910 & 1912). *Manual of Human Embryology,* 2 volumes. (Philadelphia: Lippincott)

12. Mall, F.P. (1907). On measuring human embryos. *Anat. Rec.,* **1**, 129

13. Mall, F.P. (1914). On stages in the development of human embryos from 2 to 25 mm long. *Anat. Anz.,* **46**, 78

14. O'Rahilly, R. (1973). Developmental stages in human embryos. Including a survey of the Carnegie collection. (Washington, DC: Carnegie Institution of Washington)

15. Purpura, D. P. (1977). Developmental pathobiology of cortical neurons in the immature human brain. In Gluck, L. (ed.) *Intrauterine Asphyxia and the Developing Fetal Brain.* (Chicago, London: Year Book Medical Publishers Inc.)

16. Kalter, H. and Warkany, J. (1983). Congenital malformations: etiologic factors and their role in prevention. *N. Engl. J. Med.,* Part I, **308**, 424; Part II, **308**, 491

17. Hibbard, E.D. and Smithells, R.W. (1965). Folic acid metabolism and human embryopathy. *Lancet,* **1**, 1254

18. Smithells, R.W., Sheppard, S., Schorah, C.J., Seller, M.J., Nevin, N.C., Harris, R., Read, A.P. and Fielding, D.W. (1980). Possible prevention of neural tube defects by periconceptional vitamin supplementation. *Lancet,* **1**, 339

19. MRC Vitamin Study Research Group (1991). Prevention of neural tube defects: results of the Medical Research Council vitamin study. *Lancet,* **2**, 131

20. Steegers-Theunissen, R.P.M., Boers, G.H.J., Trijbels, J.M.F. and Eskes, T.K.A.B. (1991). Neural tube defects and derangement of homocysteine metabolism. *N. Engl. J. Med.,* **324,** 199

21. International Clearing House for Birth Defects Monitoring Systems (1991). *Congenital Malformations Worldwide. A Report from the International Clearing House for Birth Defects Monitoring Systems.* (Amsterdam: Elsevier Science)

22. Gregg, N.M. (1941). Congenital cataract following german measles in the mother. *Trans. Ophthalmol. Soc. Aust.,* **3**, 35

23. Czeizel, A.E., Intôdy, Z. and Modell, B. (1993). What proportion of congenital abnormalities can be prevented ? *Br. Med. J.,* **306**, 499

THE MENSTRUAL CYCLE

Classic
Paper
No.8

Variation of the human menstrual cycle through reproductive life

ALAN E. TRELOAR *ET AL.*

Chief, Reproductive Anthropometry Section, National Institute of Child Health and Human Development, Bethesda, Maryland, and Research Associate, University of Minnesota, Minneapolis

1. Treloar, A.E., Boynton, R.E., Behn, B.G. and Brown, B.W. (1967). Variation of the human menstrual cycle through reproductive life. *Int. J. Fertil.*, **12**, 77

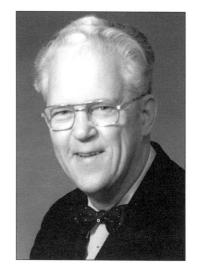

The work of Treloar, carried out before oral contraceptives became widely available, has been chosen because it represents an important publication in the history of our understanding of the menstrual cycle. It was also chosen because it is the result of a long interest by the author in the life events of women, including menarche, the interval length of the menstrual cycle and menopause, the paper being published after 34 years of observations. The following commentary describes the fascinating clinical and scientific history of our understanding of the endocrine mechanisms which govern the ovarian–pituitary–hypothalamic axis, focusing on sex steroids and proteins. It is interesting to note that all this was accomplished around 90 years after the original discovery of ovulation in the human, as characterized by the shift in basal body temperature which occurs half-way through the menstrual cycle.

INTERNATIONAL JOURNAL OF FERTILITY
Jan.-Mar., 1967, Vol. 12, No. 1, Part 2, pp. 77-126
Printed in U.S.A.

Variation of the Human Menstrual Cycle through Reproductive Life

ALAN E. TRELOAR, PH.D.,* RUTH E. BOYNTON, M.D.,† BORGHILD G. BEHN, PH.D.,‡ and BYRON W. BROWN, PH.D.§ (U.S.A.)

The temporal characteristics of human menstrual rhythm are defined in the public mind by conventional thought. Questions concerning this periodicity continue to be accorded commonplace answers, even to the point where repetition seems to have become persuasive of what is supposed to be truth. The inadequacy of fact concerning this phenomenon, established by scientific inquiry involving complete coverage of human menstrual life, is remarkable.

Nominal association of this cyclic human phenomenon with the rhythmic regularity of motions of the moon has no doubt contributed to delusion concerning the interval length and its regularity. A conviction of personal normality in these matters seems characteristic of the majority of women who, in giving medical histories, rather consistently continue to affirm that they menstruate "regularly," and "every 28 days." Only a minority do otherwise without prompting or challenge. Some concede a little to individuality by preferring to claim a 30-day interval, or have another preference for a nearby number, usually even but perhaps an odd multiple of five. Still fewer will go so far in approximation as to define the interval in weeks as three, five, or even a greater number. The inference that this pattern attests to one fact alone, wide variability between persons in the menstrual interval, seems to have had appeal only to those few who were not uncomfortable in being unconventional.

Three decades ago, the statistical concepts of one of the authors were challenged by a conflict, defined in printer's ink, concerning length and variability of the human menstrual cycle. Several extensive compilations of data had been assembled from patient histories recorded in hospital files and in private practice. This information recalled from memory had been augmented by responses to questions presented to large numbers of school girls and student nurses. The collected findings from these sources of information contrasted

* Chief, Reproductive Anthropometry Section, National Institute of Child Health and Human Development, Bethesda, Maryland, and Research Associate, University of Minnesota, Minneapolis.

† Professor and Director Emeritus, University Health Service, University of Minnesota.

‡ Statistician, Reproductive Anthropometry Section, National Institute of Child Health and Human Development.

§ Professor and Chief, Biometry Division, School of Public Health, University of Minnesota.

sharply with the results available from studies of currently made records of successive onsets of menstrual flow. However, the latter series of data were few in number and covered rather short periods of experience; in that sense only they were unimpressive by comparison.

No attempt will be made at this point to assemble the results of that search of the earlier literature. Suffice it to say in summary that the limited but concurrent records of menstruation available at that time were statistically consistent with established patterns of biologic variation.[1-8] On the other hand, the numerically impressively large response to inquiry seemed to reflect a heterogeneity of accommodations to fancied normality.[9-14] It was obvious that much remained to be done in the way of current record keeping before the cyclical characteristics of this fundamental biologic rhythm would be adequately described. It was in this setting that our interest in planning a research foray in this field was matured in 1933.[*]

For present purposes we must also be content with very brief reference to results of closely related activities on the frontiers of human reproductive physiology. In the third and fourth decades of this century the remarkable investigations by Ogino and Knaus abroad, and by Corner, Hartman, Hertig, and Rock in this country, citing only a few in both cases among the better known, led to a hypothesis of ovulation in relation to menstruation which had enormous appeal in its dissipation of mystery. Since then this theory has become so important in obstetrical thinking that recognition of new evidence as challenging to the established view may be difficult to achieve. Experience has repeatedly shown that the elegance of simplicity can be its weak point. The deterministic character of early theories usually yield to probabilistic concepts as fuller comprehension is matured.

ASSEMBLY OF RECORDS CURRENTLY MADE

Through the past 30 years we have been gathering the data we deemed obtainable and necessary to define, as factually as reasonably seemed possible, the temporal characteristics of the human menstrual cycle and some of its associated phenomena. This report presents the first comprehensive statement of the findings of this study concerning the menstrual cycles, age-specific throughout menstrual life.[†]

Initiation of the Program. In the latter part of 1934, Miss Esther Doerr, a graduate student at the University of Minnesota, commenced her research program under the guidance of two of the authors to define quantitatively the rhythm pattern of the human menstrual cycle through current recording of dates of onset and cessation of flow. The experience of a relatively large group of single women was sought for this purpose. The problem and a plan for its solution were presented personally to selected groups by Miss Doerr. Approximately 500 record-keeping collaborators were enrolled, chiefly from women's

---

[*] It is entirely coincidental that the extensive investigations by Vollman involving current recording of menstruation and the signs of ovulation were also started in Switzerland in 1934. Vollman's first report of this work appeared in 1940.[15]

[†] A brief account of some early results was given in 1939 by Treloar.[16]

physical education classes and other selected groups at the University; to a minor extent these were supplemented by sorority members, a somewhat more mature age group from the Minneapolis YWCA, and a few personal friends.

A specially printed card was designed at that time for keeping the records of menstruation of the collaborating women. These cards were collected for analysis at the close of calendar year 1935, at which time a report on any illnesses which might have influenced menstruation was requested. A new card for continuing the record through the next calendar year was issued at the same time, and thus a continuing reporting system was initiated.

Miss Doerr's thesis for the M.A. degree, embracing a statistical study of the data assembled for calendar year 1935, has been on file with the University of Minnesota Graduate School and the University Library since 1936. Those data now form part of the very much larger accumulation through a long coverage in time, and from a broader enrollment of collaborators. The expanded series is defined below.

Augmentation of the Coverage. Success of the initial efforts led promptly to broadening of the program. A presentation of the need for accurate data was made to all female enrollees in the entering classes at the University of Minnesota starting in the fall of 1935; this was continued through four years of class admissions. Each girl in the course of her physical examination, given by physicians at the University Health Service, was informed of the project purpose and procedure, invited to join, and given a form to be used for entering certain identification and impression records in case she decided to become a collaborator. This routine procedure resulted in approximately one half of the girls in each entering class electing to join the study.

Contact with all collaborators has been maintained by mail as far as possible over the succeeding years, principally for an interchange annually of new cards for old and return of report forms. Approximately one half of those who initially accepted the invitation proved their continuing interest by returning their first year record card at the next interchange for the following year's history. The forces of attrition—dropout from college with the collaborator erroneously implying this meant leaving the study, change of address without adequate record for our needs, to some degree no doubt a slackening of interest in this activity, and retirement through hysterectomy or menopause—have led, until recently, to a varying annual reduction in the number of these collaborators.

Menarchial Experience. Records of the beginning of menstrual experience have been secured through two channels of information. All girls joining the study at ages beyond menarche were requested to recall age at menarche and record this on the form which initiated their collaboration. The lapse of time in each case from this biologically memorable event was usually a matter of five to eight years for most students. There was opportunity for conventional ideas to influence the recall from memory and introduce some error in these cases.

After record keeping habits had become well established and the married status had become characteristic, we began soliciting our collaborators to enroll their daughters in this personally useful habit as they entered menstrual life. The response to this invitation has been gratifying. We are now securing an increasing number of current records from menarche onwards from this source, enlarged somewhat by relatives and friends from the same age group. These data, plus complete records of past menstruations maintained by two girls joining the study as university enrollees, constitute the recorded menarche and early years of experience in our study.

Records of Menopause. Special problems arose as the menopausal period was entered and retirement from active collaboration seemed imminent. Our dependence on mailed records meant that menopause must ordinarily be confirmed by filing a return for a calendar year with the information that there was no menstrual flow in that year. As menopausal changes were experienced, collaborators apparently tended to assume that their blank or perhaps only sparsely filled cards were no longer of interest and that they had therefore graduated from this study. Many terminations of collaboration are undoubtedly due to this inference occasioned by the advent of menopause and its increased irregularity. These losses of particularly valuable information were not anticipated; special efforts to offset them were begun in 1952 after the problem was recognized.

The menopausal picture will be presented herein solely with respect to the records of those who have continued as active collaborators for at least one calendar year beyond the last known menstrual period. This is a rather stringent requirement, but only through this definition of confirmed menopause can we be reasonably sure that we are free of the entanglements of arbitrarily truncated histories.

The attrition through confirmed menopause is now being offset by accessions from daughters entering at menarche.

INTERRUPTIONS OF RECORD

A record is not accepted for inclusion in this analysis unless it contains six months or more of uninterrupted menstruation entries. All records of more than one year of collaboration are not necessarily complete in the sense of being continuous, for collaborators were initially urged, and are reminded every year, not to enter any record by recall of an uncertain date, but instead to indicate clearly any break in continuity of the entries. A record so broken is accepted provided the history spans at least two calendar years.

Events normally intervene to bring pause to the usual pattern of menstrual life. Pregnancy terminated by delivery or abortion is the most common of such events. We are reporting elsewhere our study of over 2000 live births for which the date of onset of the last maternal menstrual period was recorded as currently as the date of the birth itself.

NORMAL AND ANORMAL INTERVALS

A record on the card of all surgery, any major illnesses, and use of medications which might be of influence on the menstrual cycle, has been requested of all collaborators. A report form returned with each record card after the year's close gives further opportunity for such notes. The primary purpose of these additional records was to permit designation of those menstrual intervals which were suspect of being abnormal because of disturbing interventions.

There is no difficulty in recognizing surgery and major illnesses as potentially affecting menstrual rhythm. Use of pharmaceuticals presents a very different problem, one which we have learned we cannot resolve satisfactorily. Analgesics are not in the same class as preparations intended to influence endocrinal balances in the body. Add the obscurity provided by trade names, inadequate specification of prescription medicines, the problems of personal shorthand and other brevities, and it frequently becomes impossible to discriminate in the record entries between pharmaceutical preparations intended to control menstrual experience and other drugs which serve only as palliatives. As a result, use of only the more obvious and better known drugs, as recorded, led to designation of an interval as being possibly so influenced.

All intervening surgery and major illnesses, together with drug usage as limited above, led us to designation of an interval between menstruations as anormal in the sense that there was reason to suspect it *might* be so. This determination was made independently of any change, discernible or otherwise, in the length of the interval. Roughly 1 per cent of all menstrual intervals recorded in this study have been coded as anormal in accord with the above designations in our processing of the records. Separation of so small a proportion has a barely detectable influence on the over-all picture. Special study of the anormal menstrual intervals is not appropriate to this paper. It is pertinent to note, however, that to ignore them in most analyses and deal with all recorded intervals is merely to overlook some "needles in a haystack." Limitation of the statistical analyses in this report to years prior to 1962 avoids any serious impact from the use of birth control drugs.

Our use of the words "normal intervals" herein must not be transposed in inference to imply "normal women." In the absence of evidence to the contrary, we consider all collaborators in this study to be menstrually normal; we designate about 1 per cent of all their menstrual intervals as possibly deviant intervals because of potentially disturbing interventions. In many cases there isn't any discernible effect of these interventions on the menstrual interval itself, but this is certainly not true in all cases. The truly anormal intervals must fall well below 1 per cent.

We gave close attention to the individual menstrual history following delivery in distinguishing post partum bleeding episodes from resumption of menstruation. Difficult cases arose so rarely that any effects of such empirical decisions would become imperceptible in the summations.

Age and Calendar Time

Our menstrual data have been assembled in terms of the calendar year as the time unit embraced. The analyses of these data have all been made separately for each year of age from menarche to menopause. This has required the assignment of a single year of age to each collaborator for each complete calendar year of history. The rule we have followed for defining the chronologic age of a collaborator for a given calendar year has been to assign the number of her birthday which occurred in that year. The net effect of this rule is to treat the collaborator's record as if her birthday occurred on the first day of January. Thus this rule tends to overstate age when conventionally given as the number of the last birthday. In terms of "age at nearest birthday" our procedure is devoid of defect.

The year of menstrual experience or age since menarche is also a meaningful biologic time scale of particular usefulness in this study. A rule for calculation of menstrual year has therefore been required, a rule readily adaptable to the records as they were acquired. The rule established for this calculation was as follows: A collaborator's menstrual year is her chronologic age minus her age at menarche as recorded when she entered the study.

The more precise information on actual date of menarche which became available later as daughters joined the study had to conform to the simple rule for menstrual year already established. Thus when menarche occurs within the calendar year and after the birthday, that calendar year is zero on the menstrual year scale. When menarche precedes the birthday within the same calendar year, the menstrual year is not the zero year but the first. All menstrual years have been computed uniformly by application of this rule, and charts of menstrual histories are so scaled in terms of menstrual year. Therefore, when date of menarche is known it may be plotted in year 0 or in year 1 on the menstrual year scale, according to whether the birthday preceded menarche or followed it. This problem is avoidable only when dates of menarche and of birth are both known. We feel fortunate to have many such pairs of dates, or in lieu of this to have secured records of menarche age by recall within a relatively few years from incidence of that event.

The technical discrepancies introduced by these time scales are of small consequence in their bearing on the problems being considered; the other variation patterns are so large by comparison that the time scaling problems become of minor consequence.

THE ORIGINAL RECORDS

Reproductions of the face and reverse of the basic card as printed for the 1965 calendar year form Figures 1 and 2 herein. *Bold face characters* indicate the first day of each week. The arrangement of dates in four-week lines permits immediate recognition of the two principal features of any uncomplicated pattern of menstrual cyclicity. Perfect regularity will always be represented by a straight line pattern of the onset dates. This line is vertical when the periodicity is 28 days. The straight line approaches the left (reading from *top to bottom*) if the periodicity is regular but less than 28 days; it inclines to the right if the period is constant but greater than 28 days. The degree of irregularity in intervals between onset dates is reflected in the amount of departure of the indicated dates from a straight line array.

The interchange of record cards has been initiated usually at year's end. A covering letter seeking to maintain interest as well as to give special instructions and reinforce needed emphases, together with an updating report form,

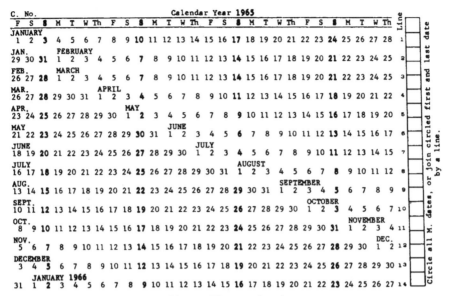

Figure 1. The record card.

accompanied each mailing. Processing information received on the report form accompanied critical survey of the returned card with its recorded flows. Intervals between menstrual onsets for each collaborator's record card were calculated and recorded at this time in the boxes at the right of the card.

Collaborators either circle all days of menstrual flow or circle just the days of onset and cessation for each flow period, joining these two circled dates by a line. Some have indicated the days of "show" (or spotting) by a dot above the date; all are now requested to do this. It was relatively easy to recognize the occasionally recorded single-day indication of midcycle bleeding in these latter entries. Occurrence of spotting symbols just prior to the first circled day of flow sometimes presented a question in fixing the onset of menstrual flow, but this problem was rarely a troublesome one. Usually peculiar to a few histories, spotting tends to become more common in the menopausal years.

Errors of Interpretation. The determination of intervals between onsets of menstruation involves recognition of any difference between "true" menstrual flow and any simulating vaginal discharges. It is only in the presence of easily recognizable definite criteria which will separate menstruation from vaginal bleedings of other origin that those who compile such menstruation records can determine what is a menstrual flow and what is not. The void in criteria of discriminatory value is too easily masked among physicians by speculative assertion originating in hypothesis. No one is entirely free from the influence of such speculations and may yield to their pressures. Our resistance to them has been strong, enough so perhaps to lead us occasionally to accept a very short interval that some physicians would dismiss as involving a "nonmenstrual flow."

NOTATIONS concerning: periods accidentally omitted from the record, any peculiarities of a period, and records of surgery (named), illnesses (diagnoses) and medications, all identified by line number or date.

————————————————————————————————

————————————————————————————————

————————————————————————————————

————————————————————————————————

————————————————————————————————

————————————————————————————————

————————————————————————————————

————————————————————————————————

————————————————————————————————

————————————————————————————————

————————————————————————————————

————————————————————————————————

————————————————————————————————

————————————————————————————————

————————————————————————————————

————————————————————————————————

————————————————————————————————

This card is a research document. Please return it to: Health Service, Study Office W163, University of Minnesota, Minneapolis, Minn. 55455.

Figure 2. Reverse of the record card.

In the absence of any helpful guiding notes from the collaborator, we have treated any indicated flow of approximately the usual length for her menstrual period as being an independent menstrual flow, provided that it is separated by at least two days from an adjacent flow of like kind. The onset dates had therefore to be separated by at least two days *more* than the duration of flow. Fortunately such small separations are rare indeed; an interval of less than 10 days so generated between menstrual onsets is most uncommon in our records. Intervals longer than 10 days grow smoothly in number to the modal value for that age of collaborator.

When the interval between two consecutive menstruations has an intervening nonmenstrual bleeding, not diagnosed as such, the true menstrual interval will be erroneously divided into two intervals. As a consequence, the mean interval for the year would be lowered and the standard deviation would normally be increased. When one or more days of simulating vaginal discharge immediately preceding a menstrual flow are included in error with the true flow period, one menstrual interval is shortened and its successor is lengthened by the same amount. Thus the mean in this case is not affected, but the variability of intervals is increased. The effect of these relatively rare occurrences on the total picture of menstrual interval distribution is small, so small indeed that we feel the effect is trivial.

Scientists must always be alert (1) to detect errors in their basic data, (2) to trace such errors to the originating sources, and (3) to evaluate the impact of those errors on any allocation of effects to causative forces. Experience often sharpens this alertness in statisticians to the point of its engendering a consuming skepticism about the worth of basic data, including the kind which forms the original material in this analysis. It has been with a keen appreciation of the necessity for such alertness, without excess of it, that we have maintained throughout the years of this study a close review of every one of the original record cards.

The Suspect Record. It has been an unexpectedly rare occurrence to receive a record card warranting detailed "follow-through" to evaluate suspicion that it might not be a record of events made correctly and currently. In this connection we wondered from the beginning when we would encounter the false "28-day regular" record, with claims to which medical histories in hospitals are still so replete. Such a card did finally arrive after five years' experience had yielded nearly 3000 person-years of history. By that time, enduring regularity of any length of interval seemed a myth and this record card immediately became suspect. But no detectable sign of faking was evident. Eight years of subsequent review of this collaborator's history simply confirmed her, among all our recorders, as the most regular menstruator by a wide margin, a unique record maker indeed. That her average interval happened also to be very nearly 28 days throughout her 11 years of recorded history is of independent interest. Statistically, in our files her record would warrant challenge as too extreme a deviate, but we lack any supporting evidence of such a proposition.

Another type of interval for which we have watched is that which might validate the claim commonly made by girls that they occasionally "skip" a menstrual period. Are these true failures in an otherwise rhythmic physiologic pattern, or may they simply be misinterpretations of unusually long intervals? With the mean and standard deviation of interval calculated for each person-year of history to help us, we particularly watched all cards for many years to detect substantial evidence of "skipped" periods. It proved to be a fruitless effort; when evidence of that kind appeared it usually proved transient; information available elsewhere indicated failure to record a period at the proper time. It seems to us that long intervals between periods do not approach simple multiples of previous average interval lengths any more than chance itself would seem to prescribe.

We feel we have exercised all the alertness that would be deemed reasonable as well as pertinent. We conclude that the data as accepted testify to the acumen of our collaborators in judging the importance of accuracy in this personal record as a guide to social if not private behavior. What errors are included in these records, and approximations not noted as such must escape us, are surely not of any practical consequence in limiting applicability of the conclusions we reach.

Data Handling Procedures

This project was the recipient of major support for analysis purposes late in 1960 when provision was made by contract with an interested industrial corporation to cover three years of data processing activity. Access to powerful computer facilities at the University of Minnesota was prospective only at that time; accordingly, the design of data input cards was accommodated to limitation of operations to an IBM 101 statistical machine and related facilities. Because of this limitation, a single card per person-year of menstrual experience was designed to receive the coded data. Thus this initial study necessarily became restricted to a few items of top priority from all data available in each person-year of experience. Only the intervals between menstrual onsets and the interrupting events of pregnancy, coded by type as well as length of each interval, could be accommodated on one card for each year. Processing of these cards was initiated 18 months later, using a computer of large capacity. Thus the designed limitation for input to a single card per person-year proved unnecessary. The complications of double punching devices incorporated in those cards were also regretted.

Presentation of Results

Through calendar year 1961 this study had accumulated 25,825 person-years of menstrual experience. Slightly over 2700 collaborators had recorded sufficient history of periodic flow and intervening events to enable calculation of over a quarter of a million intervals between onsets of consecutive menstruations. These intervals exclude those embracing somewhat over 2750 intervening pregnancies.

It is a major concern that the results of analysis of this unusually extensive array of data be presented in a form allowing rapid comprehension of the outcome without loss of significant detail. It is with this in view that we choose to rely chiefly on graphic presentations of changes observed through chosen spans of menstrual experience. For those seeking details in numerical form we assemble those tabulations most likely to be in demand. In Table I the frequency distribution of years of recorded experience per person covered by this analysis is presented.

I. A Pattern of Change in Interval with Age

In its contour lines for a selection of percentile values, Figure 3 portrays the frequency distribution, changing with age, of intervals between menstrual

TABLE I
Frequency Distribution of Years of Recorded Menstrual Experience per Person

Years of Record	No. of Persons		Years of Record	No. of Persons	
	1935 to 1961	1935 to 1962*		1935 to 1961	1935 to 1962*
1	725	725	16	19	19
2	299	299	17	26	26
3	186	186	18	28	28
4	140	140	19	39	37
5	90	90	20	28	29
6	96	96	21	53	54
7	64	64	22	68	68
8	53	53	23	76	72
9	61	61	24	123	125
10	34	34	25	129	128
11	31	31	26	104	103
12	41	41	27	100	101
13	28	28	28	1	4
14	32	32	29	1	1
15	27	27			
Total persons				2,702	2,702
Total person-years				25,825	25,844

* Adds only the final year record (1962) of 19 menopause cases confirmed at the close of 1963.

onsets made available for this study, from menarche* through age 51 years. The outer *broken lines* follow increments of unity in the percentile scales, from 1 to 5 per cent for the shortest intervals and from 95 to 99 for the longest intervals. Between these zones the *solid lines* change by increments of 10 per cent, the median line (50 per cent) being drawn more heavily. The *solid dots* not connected laterally indicate the quartile values (25 and 75 percentiles) at each age. These quartile values demark between them a central span of days at each age within which one half of the menstrual intervals fell, or, alternatively, the two values of menstrual interval at each age outside of which in actual experience of the population of women studied one quarter of the menstrual intervals fell.

The data presented in Figure 3 do not include the records within the span of chronologic ages 52 to 56, the latter being at present the latest age attained by a collaborator at menopause. Data through these last five years are relatively scanty, making percentile line representation very irregular and risking impressions based chiefly on sampling errors. This problem is resolved in a later section. The predominant characteristic of Figure 3 will be recognized as the scope of change in variability of intervals between onsets with advance through the years of menstrual experience. Within this total range of 40 years in age, the two decades from about age 21 to 39 inclusive are notable for their compara-

---

* We omit four intervals for 3 persons who experienced menarche in the calendar year of their 10th birthday and had a second flow (in 1 case a third) in that year.

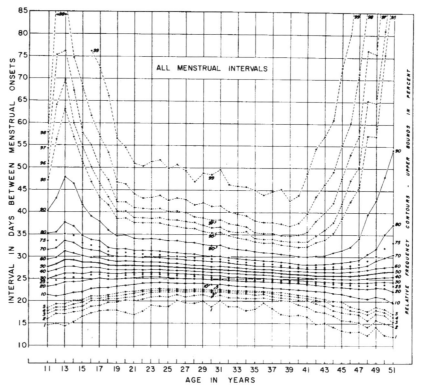

Figure 3. Contours for the frequency distribution of all menstrual intervals changing with age.

tive compactness in variation. But even in this middle zone of menstrual life the range of variation, as defined for the central 98 per cent of all intervals, extends at its minimum (at age 36) over a span of 23 days. While the *lower bound* (1 per cent line) rises from 17 days at age 21 to about 20 days in the middle of the span and then returns to 17 again at age 39, the *upper bound* of 99 per cent falls progressively from 50 days to nearly 42 days through these same years.

Beyond these two central decades of age, the dispersion increases rapidly the further one proceeds below 20 or above 40 years. The changes occur much more rapidly toward longer intervals than toward the short, but they occur in both directions nevertheless.

Table II in its second column gives the total frequencies on which these percentile points at each age are based.

Rejection of Intervals Designated Anormal. The contours of Figure 3 encompass all recorded menstrual intervals within the age span covered including the possibly anormal ones which involve medical experiences and interventions. Table II also gives the distribution by age of the intervals designated as potentially anormal. The proportion that these intervals are of all

TABLE II

Distribution of Menstrual Intervals by Chronologic Age and Normality

Age	Total (2)	Normal (3)	Anormal		Age	Total (2)	Normal (3)	Anormal	
			No.	%				No.	%
years					*years*				
10	4	4	0	0	33	9,403	9,283	120	1.28
11	179	179	0	0	34	9,388	9,242	146	1.56
12	786	781	5	0.64	35	9,480	9,354	126	1.33
13	1,597	1,589	8	0.50	36	9,271	9,159	112	1.21
14	2,132	2,120	12	0.56	37	9,390	9,273	117	1.25
15	2,160	2,127	33	1.53	38	9,472	9,393	79	0.83
16	1,969	1,954	15	0.76	39	9,204	9,128	76	0.83
17	2,423	2,405	18	0.74	40	9,343	9,228	115	1.23
18	4,867	4,850	17	0.35	41	9,080	8,961	119	1.31
19	8,762	8,739	23	0.26	42	8,294	8,148	146	1.76
20	10,585	10,492	93	0.88	43	7,172	7,033	139	1.94
21	11,491	11,429	62	0.54	44	5,649	5,566	83	1.47
22	11,741	11,680	61	0.52	45	4,129	4,087	42	1.01
23	11,497	11,429	68	0.59	46	3,013	2,980	33	1.10
24	10,967	10,855	112	1.02	47	2,051	2,026	25	1.22
25	10,576	10,502	74	0.70	48	1,287	1,264	23	1.79
26	10,055	9,979	76	0.76	49	815	799	16	1.96
27	9,734	9,636	98	1.01	50	498	483	15	3.01
28	9,611	9,533	78	0.81	51	312	291	21	6.73
29	9,448	9,377	71	0.75	52	201	200	1	0.50
30	9,267	9,205	62	0.67	53	102	99	3	2.94
31	9,136	9,058	78	0.85	54	46	43	3	6.52
32	9,323	9,272	51	0.55	55	28	28	0	0
					56	9	9	0	0
Totals						275,947	273,272	2,675	0.97

intervals at each age will be noted to be very small, varying between 0 and 2 per cent until age 50 is reached. In the last seven years of recorded experience there are only 43 designated potentially anormal intervals out of the total of 1196 intervals. For these years collectively the percentage designated as anormal rises to 3.6 per cent.

When all 2675 so-called anormal intervals are withdrawn, the total distribution of normal intervals is generated. This distribution forms column 3 of Table II. The contour pattern for distribution of these intervals within each year of age over the restricted age range given for all intervals in Figure 3, takes the form given in Figure 4. Careful study of the differences in these two diagrams impresses upon one the very slight effect of withdrawal of the possibly anormal intervals.

Anticipation that certain types of medical interventions will affect the time of onset of the next menstrual period may or may not be justified by experience. In following certain empirical rules for designation of a menstrual interval as potentially anormal, we have clearly risked two dangers. Not only does the qualifying adjective "potentially" tend to be dropped for brevity, but also we

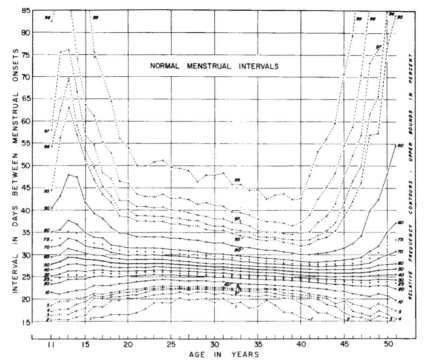

Figure 4. Contours for the frequency distribution of "normal" menstrual intervals changing with age.

inevitably generate a mixture in this small group, for it will include intervals not in fact affected by the type of intervention recorded or accepted as influential. Withdrawal of the possibly anormal intervals, with the attendant hazards of this procedure, has so small an effect that we have accepted the total assembly of all intervals as preferable to the one which by subtle inference becomes cloaked in a drape of normality which is not too well defined. For further analyses of these data we have therefore chosen to use all intervals as recorded.

Both the onset and cessation of menstrual life are known to be variable from one person to another, not only with respect to the age at which each occurs, but also in the extent of time through which the associated instability of menstrual experience extends. Thus the chronologic age scale does not serve well to bring biologic homogeneity to the early or the late years in the preceding charts. Just as the terminal five years of data following age 51 are omitted from the graphs because therein the contours lose all value in a melee of heterogeneity, so also the earliest years must be affected, although in less obvious degree. Below age 13 it is clear that the contours show a change of direction which may well incite speculation concerning causes. Does the variability of menstrual interval really increase after menarche?

The Menstrual Year Scale. Our data for the earliest years of menstrual life

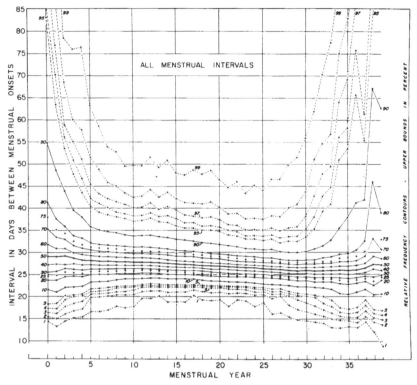

Figure 5. Contours for the frequency distribution of all menstrual intervals changing with year of menstrual experience.

have been assembled almost entirely from the records of daughters of the original collaborators. Thus we deal here with a different group of persons from those establishing patterns in the middle life sector. When these persons are divided into age groups for recorded menstrual experience, there are only 35 persons contributing data at age 11, and only 179 intervals available for the contours. The number of young persons experiencing menstruation rises rapidly with age, so that we have 1597 intervals available for the age 13 distribution. This climb continues steadily to reach its peak of nearly 12,000 intervals at age 22. Thus the influence of individual persons is strong at age 11; lessening as increase in age introduces more persons into this study.

The contour picture by year of menstrual experience can readily be generated for those collaborators whose age at menarche is a matter of record. Figure 5 presents the contours in terms of the "menstrual year" scale for all recorded menstrual intervals through the first four decades of this experience. The aberrant "peaking" of percentile contours about 13 years of age in Figures 3 and 4 is not present in Figure 5. The menstrual year scale thus removes a factor which had distorted the variability picture for menstrual intervals in the earliest years.

It is not entirely reasonable to infer from the effect of using the menstrual year scale that the peaking in Figures 3 and 4 is an artifact of sampling; it is still possible that those who experience menarche at the earliest ages may vary less in menstrual interval at the beginning than those who enter late. As more adequate numbers of cases from menarche onwards become available to us we may inquire more securely into the presence of any relation between chronologic age at menarche and the subsequent pattern of interval variability.

Through the middle years of menstrual experience there is no obvious gain in using the scale of age since menarche. When Figure 5 is superimposed on Figure 3 so that the seventh menstrual year of Figure 5 coincides with chronologic age 20 in Figure 3, the contours also become remarkably alike, indeed almost coincident, for the next 20 years of menstrual experience.

Offsetting its value in the early years, the menstrual age scale introduces devastating effects in its upper reaches. Figure 5 is terminated in its contours with four decades of menstrual experience because the effect of early menopause cases on the interval contours is already clearly apparent in the third decade. After the 25th year of menstrual experience this cumulative diagram for all histories begins to respond to the increasing variability of those who are destined to reach menopause after a relatively short experience in menstruation. Within the fourth decade of menstrual life, this impact is very pronounced and the contours spread rapidly. Yet at menstrual age 35, up to 10 or more years of menstrual experience still await those who will retire from the activity among the last, in terms of age. To cover the full span of menstrual life as at present defined in our records, Figure 5 would be extended beyond the 45th menstrual year and show at least 15 years of very unstable contours.

The Scale of Premenopausal Year. In order to achieve for the years of menopausal experience the homogeneity that the menstrual year scale introduces at the beginning of menstrual life, it is necessary to establish a scale of premenopausal years. This can only be done retrospectively from records of completed menstrual history. We required at least a full calendar year without menstrual flow for menopause to be "confirmed." We have since found this to be somewhat inadequate, for slight cyclic flows have now been recorded in 2 cases after longer intervals of pause. However, one full calendar year of "no flow" seems rigid enough in view of the practicalities of retaining contact with collaborators after apparent menopause.

We have given detailed attention to every confirmed menopause case in our file, extending the coverage at this writing to include the 19 menopause cases in 1962 confirmed at the close of 1963. For the premenopausal scale we set the origin as the calendar year in which the menopause occurs; the penultimate year thus becomes −1, and on this scale we thus move back through time. Assembled for this study are 120 cases of confirmed menopause. For 100 of these the records are complete for the 10 years preceding the menopausal year; only 20 are broken for one or more years. Both sets were analyzed separately. No advantage accrued through using only the 100 unbroken records, so we have used all 1167 person-years of experience available for this analysis.

The latest menopause at present included in our data occurs at 56 years on the conventional scale of age; 5 persons close their histories at this age.

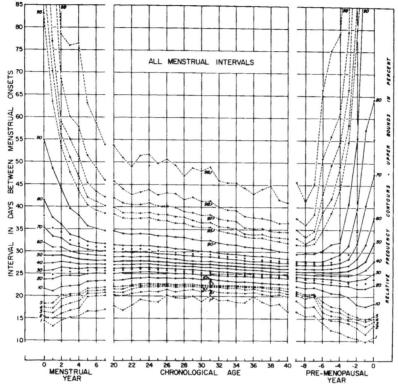

Figure 6. Contours for the frequency distribution of all menstrual intervals in three zones of experience.

Three Zones in Menstrual Life. The contours for the premenopausal time scale are given for the last 10 years on the *right* of Figure 6. This chart likewise presents the early postmenarche years in the panel on the *left*, this part having been transferred directly from Figure 5. Both end zones (the postmenarche and premenopause years) are collated with a "middle life" zone defined in terms of age as it is customarily given. Return to the chronologic age scale for the two central decades of menstrual life has the advantage that personal placement on the chart will be in familiar terms which require no unaccustomed calculation. The points of matching to give continuity of the two terminal zones to the central one with its contrasting stability were chosen simply as the ones where the transition from the menstrual year contours and the premenopausal year contours to the usual age contours as given in Figure 3 seemed in general to be smoothest.

The composite of three age zones as arrayed in Figure 6 may be regarded as an approximation to community experience in menstruation. The span so defined adds up to 38 years, the extreme years scaled as 0, each averaging only six months of experience. The total range reduces to 37 years for those who would consider menstrual year 7 to be repetitious of chronologic age

20. This length of menstrual life, approximating graphically the cumulative menstrual experience of all individuals in a large community, is a little longer than the actual average difference of 36 years between recorded age at menopause and recalled age at menarche for the 120 confirmed menopause cases reported in this study. This is consistent with the view that our menarchial and menopausal zones are weighted statistically in favor of somewhat longer periods for those zones.

The increased variation in menstrual interval immediately following menarche and preceding menopause is well known. It will be new information to many interested scientists and women that the transitions from the comparative regularity of "middle life" occur smoothly over a period of many years for both menarchial and menopausal experience. In the senior years the transition to absolute menopause is very much like a mirror image of the menarchial pattern of change. The menopausal transition, however, is accomplished perhaps a little slower, in eight years instead of seven, one may say. Also, the transition to menopause passes from the most regular period of life (for all women collectively) to the most variable.

In both the menarchial and the menopausal zones there is an increase in short intervals in step with the increase in long intervals. So much compensation in *number* is made for the long intervals by the short ones that the median interval (fiftieth percentile) follows an almost straight line path from menarche to within three years of menopause. It is of considerable interest to note the striking increase in shorter intervals as premenopausal experience is traversed. This increase in very short intervals in premenopause is more marked than the corresponding decrease in the postmenarchial years.

Through the "middle life" of menstrual experience, the median interval between onsets falls with remarkable steadiness for all intervals collectively from approximately 28 to 26 days. The frequency contour lines for deviation by deciles of proportion likewise fall with straight line steadiness, converging noticeably on the central tendency. Our frequencies in this region are so large that even the extreme percentile contours, both low and high, show remarkable stability in their adherence to this general pattern. And it is worthy of repeated emphasis that the period of life of greatest regularity in menstrual periodicity occurs just before the menopausal divergence commences.

The numerical values for a selection of the contours of Figure 6 are given in Table III. It may be noted that at age 40 where the ranges between symmetrically chosen percentiles in general are least, the range of menstrual intervals for the middle 90 per cent is from 21.8 to 32.0 days, or 10.2 days. For the middle 50 per cent, this range spans the 3.5-day interval from 24.4 to 27.9 days.

In its definition of menstrual experience for a community, Figure 6 is *not* a representation of any one personal experience. While the sequence of median values at each age, as indicated in this graph, is definitive of what is central for the cooperating community of persons, the variability of interval shown at each age reflects differences between persons, in addition to variability in

TABLE III

Selected Percentiles for the Distribution of Menstrual Interval by Age in Three Zones of Experience for All Subjects Collectively

Age Scale	Year	No. of Intervals	Percentiles						
			5	10	25 (Q₁)	50 (median)	75 (Q₃)	90	95
Postmenarche.........	0	522	18.3	21.6	24.6	29.1	38.0	54.9	83.1
	1	2,080	18.4	21.1	24.8	29.1	35.2	48.6	63.5
	2	2,435	20.2	22.0	25.6	29.2	34.3	44.0	53.5
	3	2,546	20.4	22.2	25.4	28.7	32.5	39.6	47.7
	4	3,157	20.6	22.4	25.3	28.3	31.8	38.1	43.6
	5	4,909	21.7	23.3	25.7	28.2	31.3	35.8	40.4
	6	7,097	21.8	23.4	25.8	28.0	31.0	35.1	39.2
	7	9,488	22.0	23.5	25.7	28.1	31.0	34.7	38.6
Chronologic..........	20	4,928	22.1	23.5	25.7	27.8	30.6	34.6	38.4
	21	8,692	22.2	23.7	25.8	27.9	30.6	34.0	37.5
	22	10,968	22.5	24.0	25.9	27.9	30.6	33.9	37.4
	23	11,259	22.7	24.1	26.1	27.9	30.6	34.0	37.5
	24	10,904	22.8	24.2	26.0	27.9	30.5	33.9	37.6
	25	10,548	22.7	24.1	25.9	27.8	30.2	33.6	37.1
	26	10,055	22.7	24.1	25.7	27.7	30.1	33.6	36.9
	27	9,734	22.6	24.0	25.7	27.5	29.9	33.3	36.4
	28	9,585	22.7	24.1	25.6	27.4	29.8	33.2	36.4
	29	9,426	22.7	24.0	25.5	27.3	29.6	32.8	35.7
	30	9,255	22.5	23.8	25.3	27.2	29.5	32.5	35.4
	31	9,100	22.6	23.9	25.3	27.2	29.5	32.6	35.5
	32	9,286	22.4	23.6	25.1	27.0	29.2	32.0	34.8
	33	9,340	22.4	23.4	25.0	26.9	29.0	31.7	34.3
	34	9,259	22.4	23.3	24.9	26.8	28.9	31.6	34.0
	35	9,278	22.3	23.3	24.9	26.7	28.7	31.2	33.4
	36	8,957	22.3	23.2	24.8	26.6	28.4	31.0	33.2
	37	8,970	22.2	23.0	24.7	26.5	28.3	30.9	33.2
	38	8,863	22.1	22.9	24.6	26.4	28.2	30.6	32.7
	39	8,412	22.0	22.8	24.5	26.2	28.0	30.2	32.4
	40	8,393	21.8	22.7	24.4	26.2	27.9	30.1	32.0
Premenopause........	−9	1,451	21.1	22.3	24.1	25.6	27.5	29.6	31.7
	−8	1,462	20.5	21.9	23.8	25.5	27.5	29.7	31.5
	−7	1,462	20.6	22.0	23.7	25.5	27.4	29.7	31.9
	−6	1,502	18.9	21.4	23.5	25.5	27.5	30.4	35.1
	−5	1,551	17.8	20.8	23.3	25.5	27.8	31.8	38.8
	−4	1,505	17.5	20.6	23.1	25.6	28.4	32.2	44.2
	−3	1,439	16.2	19.9	23.0	25.8	29.6	40.8	54.7
	−2	1,274	15.4	18.2	22.8	26.6	34.7	55.5	80.0
	−1	915	14.9	17.8	23.0	27.9	48.2		
	0	360	15.6	18.4	23.9	32.2	55.4		

menstrual interval within personal experience. Figure 6 provides a basis for discussion of menstrual interval lengths only in the absence of reliable definition of the individual's average interval and personal characteristics of irregularity. Also, the number of years of each person's menstrual experience is known to be highly individual, and this variability must be distributed among the postmenarchial, middle life, and premenopausal zones, probably in a disproportionate manner.

Hospital record room files continue to testify that not less than 60 per cent of women choose to be recorded in their histories as menstruating "regularly, every 28 days." This erroneous concept may in time be removed through experience in factual recording, or reduced by professional teasing of recollection. The use of Figure 6 as a basis for control of pregnancy through rhythm would be admissible only if a woman knew nothing of her personal rhythm pattern. Rather obviously from Figure 6, the control would then become one of complete continence. Fortunately, the rhythm method of birth control requires each individual to establish a sequence of accurately recorded menstrual onsets if relative safety is to be achieved. The length of this sequence will be shown to be a more critical factor than is generally supposed if conception is to be avoided with a high degree of security.

II. The Average Record

The preceding presentation of frequency distributions in continuous array of intervals between menstrual onsets leaves no doubt that periodicity in human menstruation is characterized by variability rather than by regularity, and that the variability pattern changes throughout menstrual life. In pooling all available intervals from many persons, with their contributions varying from many years of experience to much shorter spans, we have defined the characteristics of interval variation with age solely for a changing community. We have indeed submerged each person in a sea of intervals as we have sought initially to define the characteristics of the principal variable. Only if women differ insignificantly from each other in their individual characteristics of interval variation as they proceed through menstrual life will Figure 6 become a first approximation to biologic law.

Well over 100 years ago, Roberton[17] challenged the commonplace notion of a simple uniformity in menstruation and argued for deviation from a 28-day average as being entirely normal for the individual; in his opinion, such deviation was not any indication in itself of pathology. Since that time, the advance to greater maturity in professional as well as public thinking on this matter has been slow, primarily, no doubt, because of lack of adequate data with which to test Roberton's hypothesis.

Change in Mean Menstrual Interval with Age. The average menstrual interval for each person-year of experience has been calculated for every history of record in this study. The time scales of conventional age and menstrual year were both used for seriation of the results. For coverage of the premenopausal years, manual procedures were followed in these calculations; all others were secured through computer operations. Assembly of the neces-

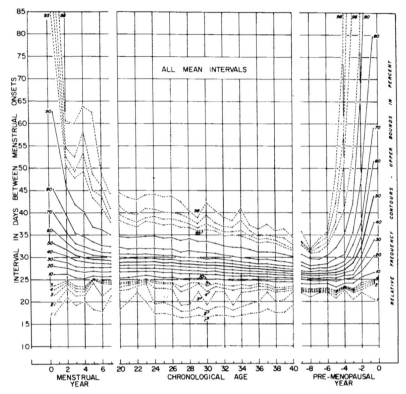

Figure 7. Contours for the distribution of mean intervals for each person-year of experience.

sary segments of these results for our three chosen zones of menstrual life then permitted calculation of the selected pattern of percentiles which are portrayed in Figure 7. Selected numerical values at each age are given in Table IV.

Although each record keeper is represented by a single average in any age class, the sampling stability of that person-year average remains sensitive to the number of menstrual intervals provided by her record that year. This number of intervals per person-year varies from none (only one menstrual onset, perhaps following a birth) to well in excess of the 13 normally expected for 28-day intervals; our highest frequency of 18 intervals in any one year occurs twice.

The contours of Figure 7 are strikingly similar in general pattern to those of the single intervals in Figure 6. Thus the interval experiences of women through menstrual life have much in common. But there are differences in detail which call for careful consideration. It is of incidental interest that the smaller numbers of persons than there were of intervals has led to the more extreme percentile contours being somewhat more irregular in Figure 7 than they are in Figure 6. In the regions outside the 10 and 90 percentile lines particularly, there is a less satisfying continuity of the contours in passing from each menstrual life zone to its successor. Also, the short intervals apparent in Figure 6 are outweighed so effectively by long ones in securing averages that major changes in the low percentile contours occur in each zone as one passes from Figure 6 to Figure 7.

Accepting the median of the personal averages at each age as the typical value for discussion, it may be noted that this midvalue falls from 33 days in the 18 months following menarche to 30 days in the fourth menstrual year. From this age on, through "middle life" and into the eighth premenopausal year, the median continues to decrease very steadily. Between the ages of 20 and 40 years this rate of fall is approximately one tenth of a day per year. The lowest median value of 26.3 days occurs eight years before menopause. Thereafter there is a curvilinear increase in the median until the peak of 44 days is reached in the final 18 months of menstrual experience.

If instead of the median we had used the mean person-year average as the typical value, this pattern of fall would have been through a somewhat higher set of values. This consequence of the positive skewness of every age-specific distribution is numerically defined in Table IV, where the more rapid changes in the postmenarchial and premenopausal years may be noted. Through "'middle life" the decrease in the mean person-year average is from 30.1 to 27.3 days. This decrease occurs chiefly after age 26; there is little change in the mean between ages 20 and 26. The average falls somewhat faster than the median as the skewness of these distributions diminishes.

Which typical value is used is of small consequence to the over-all conclusion. There is continuous change throughout menstrual life, typically a decrease in length of interval from menarche to some years before menopause; the decrease is rapid at first but becomes reasonably steady through the middle years. A minimum is reached on the average of about eight years before menopause, after which the typical menstrual interval lengthens with increasing rapidity. The maximum interval of menstrual life is usually reached just prior to menopause.

Turning to variation in yearly average intervals for individual persons, one notes from the contours in Figure 7 that the skewness of these distributions of person-averages for each year is not as marked as that for the single intervals in Figure 6. Through the two decades of middle life the central 90 per cent of the person-year averages fall within a range which is only 1.5 days less (approximately) than the range at each age for the single intervals. This is a crucial observation, for at least three times this reduction should be expected if women did not differ by more than random sampling expectation in average length of menstrual interval per year. This attests to the individuality of women with respect to their periodicity in menstruation; they differ much more among themselves than can reasonably be ascribed to chance. Thus the range of menstrual intervals in Figure 6 at any age in middle life is in part ascribable to systematic differences between women.

The consistency in contours of the two terminal zones with those of the middle life zone in Figure 7 will be noted. An inference that the indicated

TABLE IV

Selected Typical Values and Percentiles for Person-Year Means of Menstrual Interval by Age in Three Zones of Experience

| Age Scale | Year | N | Mean | Median | Percentiles | | | | | |
					5	10	25	75	90	95
Post-menarche...	0,1	361	36.90	33.08	23.6	26.2	28.6	42.3	62.6	90.0
	2	245	34.09	31.67	24.8	26.3	28.1	37.0	45.9	50.6
	3	253	32.40	30.48	23.6	25.4	27.5	34.1	41.9	47.9
	4	334	31.94	29.94	23.4	25.3	27.2	33.4	40.3	49.2
	5	543	31.22	29.60	25.2	25.9	27.4	32.5	36.8	43.5
	6	736	30.65	29.47	24.8	25.6	27.2	31.9	36.2	41.2
	7	898	30.27	29.26	24.7	25.8	27.3	31.6	35.0	37.9
Chronologic...	20	452	30.09	28.87	24.3	25.4	27.2	31.5	34.7	38.3
	21	775	29.92	28.97	24.5	25.6	27.2	31.3	34.4	37.5
	22	969	29.77	28.96	24.7	25.7	27.2	31.2	34.5	36.8
	23	1013	30.01	28.95	25.2	26.0	27.2	31.3	34.7	38.1
	24	1002	30.18	29.04	24.6	25.7	27.3	31.2	34.8	37.8
	25	1005	29.84	28.75	24.3	25.4	27.1	31.0	34.3	37.2
	26	977	29.99	28.79	24.3	25.5	27.0	31.0	34.4	37.5
	27	963	29.44	28.53	23.3	25.1	26.7	30.6	33.8	36.8
	28	950	29.56	28.49	24.2	25.3	26.7	30.8	34.2	36.7
	29	940	29.26	28.34	24.3	25.2	26.6	30.5	33.6	36.0
	30	916	29.30	28.25	23.5	25.0	26.5	30.3	33.6	36.2
	31	906	29.12	28.23	24.1	25.1	26.6	30.3	33.2	35.9
	32	897	28.70	28.05	23.7	24.9	26.3	29.9	32.5	34.8
	33	877	28.60	27.90	23.5	24.8	26.2	29.7	32.3	35.0
	34	868	28.43	27.64	23.8	24.8	26.1	29.4	32.2	34.9
	35	850	28.22	27.48	23.6	24.9	26.2	29.3	31.8	34.2
	36	812	27.98	27.39	24.0	24.8	26.0	28.9	31.2	33.2
	37	810	27.92	27.26	23.8	24.7	26.0	29.0	31.2	33.5
	38	787	27.76	27.15	23.1	24.4	25.7	28.8	31.1	33.1
	39	748	27.53	26.98	23.3	24.5	25.7	28.6	30.7	32.3
	40	730	27.26	26.80	23.4	24.4	25.6	28.3	30.3	31.6
Pre-menopause..	−9	113	27.04	26.48	23.0	24.1	25.3	28.6	30.7	32.8
	−8	112	26.52	26.29	22.8	24.0	25.1	27.7	29.8	30.9
	−7	116	26.73	26.43	23.0	24.0	25.0	27.9	29.6	31.2
	−6	113	26.88	26.46	23.0	24.1	25.2	28.0	30.4	32.7
	−5	117	28.38	26.60	22.4	23.3	25.0	28.7	32.2	36.5
	−4	118	30.02	27.18	23.5	24.2	25.5	29.9	35.2	40.6
	−3	119	33.20	28.82	22.9	24.2	25.7	34.2	42.1	52.6
	−2	117	43.51	32.41	24.3	25.6	28.0	42.4	65.5	77.9
	−1,0	212	57.14	43.68	24.7	26.6	31.8	70.9	112.7	148.0

individuality prevails throughout menstrual life therefore seems justified; each woman has her own central tendency in menstrual interval throughout reproductive life.

Change in Variability of Menstrual Interval with Age. Study of the change in variability of the intervals between onsets with increasing menstrual maturity may also be made quantitatively. For this purpose we calculated the

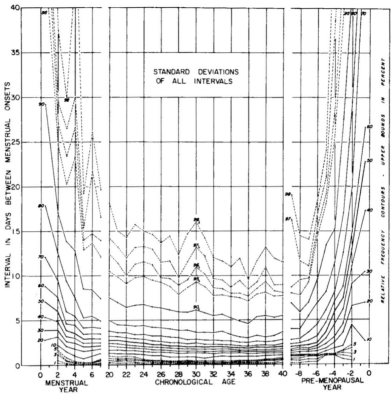

Figure 8. Contours for the distribution of standard deviations of intervals for all person-years of experience.

standard deviations of menstrual interval for each person-year of experience.* The change in form of distribution of this descriptive statistic by age within the three zones of menstrual life is portrayed by the contour method in Figure 8. Numerical values for a selection of these contours are given in Table V.

The median standard deviation for all women at any age will serve to typify variation in interval at the given stage of menstrual experience. The decrease of this median value through middle life, from 2.75 days at age 20 to a minimum value of 1.83 days at age 36, is worthy of remark on at least two counts: (1) the decrease through these ages occurs in very close approximation to a straight line; and (2) the decrease in variability is one of considerable proportion, for the minimum value attained at age 36 is one-third less than the value at age 20.

The range of variabilities at age 36, although at its minimum for all ages,

---

* The number N of menstrual intervals per person-year of experience varies from 2 to 18. To achieve greater comparability of standard deviations as a measure of variability of interval, they were computed as "root-variances," i.e., using $(N-1)$ in the denominator.

TABLE V

Selected Typical Values and Percentiles for Person-Year Standard Deviations of Menstrual Interval by Age in Three Zones of Experience

Age Scale	Year	N	Mean	Median	Percentiles					
					5	10	25	75	90	95
Post- menarche...	0,1	361	11.28	7.16			3.4	14.3		
	2	245	8.65	6.08	1.6	2.3	3.5	11.0	17.1	24.6
	3	253	6.38	3.84	0.8	1.5	2.3	7.0	13.8	20.3
	4	334	6.16	3.58	0.4	1.1	2.1	6.4	12.8	23.3
	5	543	4.37	2.93	0.3	0.7	1.8	4.5	8.5	12.9
	6	736	4.47	2.96	0.3	1.0	1.8	4.9	8.4	13.7
	7	898	4.19	2.92	0.7	1.3	2.0	4.5	7.4	12.1
Chronologic...	20	452	3.94	2.75	1.0	1.3	1.8	4.2	7.6	10.6
	21	775	3.73	2.79	0.9	1.2	1.8	4.0	7.0	9.8
	22	969	3.62	2.64	0.9	1.2	1.8	4.0	6.4	9.1
	23	1013	3.64	2.53	0.8	1.2	1.7	3.8	6.7	9.8
	24	1002	3.61	2.40	0.6	1.1	1.6	3.8	6.7	9.9
	25	1005	3.45	2.28	0.5	1.0	1.5	3.7	6.5	9.5
	26	977	3.47	2.24	0.5	1.0	1.5	3.6	6.4	9.0
	27	963	3:21	2.13	0.4	0.8	1.5	3.6	6.2	8.8
	28	950	3.07	2.11	0.4	0.9	1.4	3.4	6.0	7.9
	29	940	3.17	2.04	0.5	0.9	1.4	3.3	5.9	8.7
	30	916	3.16	2.06	0.4	0.8	1.4	3.2	6.1	9.3
	31	906	2.93	2.00	0.4	0.8	1.4	3.2	5.8	8.8
	32	897	2.86	2.02	0.4	0.9	1.4	3.1	5.5	7.8
	33	877	2.81	2.01	0.4	1.0	1.4	3.1	5.7	7.8
	34	868	2.91	1.95	0.4	0.9	1.4	3.0	5.2	7.7
	35	850	2.67	1.87	0.5	1.0	1.4	2.8	4.9	7.5
	36	812	2.51	1.83	0.5	1.0	1.4	2.7	4.6	7.1
	37	810	2.74	1.92	0.5	1.0	1.4	2.9	5.4	7.9
	38	787	2.85	1.89	0.6	1.0	1.4	2.8	5.5	8.1
	39	748	2.76	1.93	0.6	1.0	1.4	2.8	5.3	7.7
	40	730	2.83	2.00	0.8	1.1	1.4	3.2	5.5	7.7
Pre- menopause..	−9	113	3.15	1.96	1.0	1.1	1.4	3.1	6.9	8.1
	−8	112	3.06	2.11	1.0	1.1	1.6	3.4	5.9	7.8
	−7	116	3.49	2.22	1.0	1.1	1.5	4.3	7.0	9.3
	−6	113	4.35	2.37	1.0	1.1	1.7	6.1	9.6	14.4
	−5	117	6.39	3.60	1.2	1.5	2.1	7.1	13.4	18.1
	−4	118	8.23	5.87	1.2	1.8	2.8	9.5	15.3	25.8
	−3	119	14.24	7.51	1.6	2.1	4.2	14.4	27.6	40.0
	−2	117	19.54	13.03	2.2	4.4	8.2	23.6	44.6	60.5
	−1,0	212	35.49	22.87			9.4	49.3		

is from very nearly regular to standard deviations in excess of 10 days. The central 50 per cent of standard deviations at this age range from 1.4 to 4.6 days. A standard deviation of less than one day holds for the most regular 10 per cent of the women, but at the other extreme this measure of variability exceeds 7.1 days for another 10 per cent. Those who wish an approximation for the full range of variation may choose to use six times the standard deviation as a rough guide.

Special interest centers on the degree to which "regularity" may be called a normal characteristic of menstrual rhythm. Strict interpretation of "regular, every 28 days" calls for a zero S.D., presumably over a span of time long enough to satisfy purposeful requirements. Figure 8 does not provide any information on the frequency of zero S.D's. The basic calculations show that out of the 22,754 S.D.'s computed, 205 (less than 1 per cent of the total) indicated no variation in interval that year. All but one of these zero values belong to histories in which events such as menarche, pregnancy, or menopause reduced the number of menstrual intervals to so few a number (from two to five) that this coincidence was consistent by chance alone with presence of real variation.* The unique case (no. 646) is an exception; her almost complete regularity for two calendar years, with only one 27-day interval breaking the sequence of 28-day intervals, has been mentioned. The chart of her history is included in a later section of this report.

It seems logical to infer that when in giving her medical history a woman says she menstruates "regularly," she uses that term in a broadly relative sense, or she feels she is normal and this is her way of saying so, or she really doesn't know any better answer to give. Indeed, all three may be true concurrently. It is therefore reasonable to accept the word "regular" as used by most women in this connection to mean "relatively regular, as far as I know."

All person-year histories with standard deviations of less than the median value may be considered relatively regular. In Figure 8 (or Table V) it is evident that from the second menstrual year to the second before menopause, this 50 per cent of women fall within a reasonably compact range of smooth contours. The median contour forming the upper bound of this group begins a reasonably straight line decrease in the fifth menstrual year at a value of 2.9 days. After age 36 there is an increase in typical variability; it is slow for about seven years before it begins its upward sweep to menopause.

A more stringent requirement for "regularity" would stipulate a lower percentile as the upper bound of standard deviations. In this connection, satisfaction of many personal preferences is possible through reference to Table V; suffice it here to note that the values for the lowest 10 per cent contour are approximately one half of those given above for the median contour.

Synthesis of an Average History. It is of value for conceptual purposes to attempt to picture the change in interval between onsets through menstrual life for the "average person." The *upper set of dots* in Figure 9 depicts the means of the person-year averages as given in Table IV. The *lower set of dots* likewise defines the mean standard deviations of interval through menstrual life as given in Table V. In this diagram each person who submitted her menstrual record for the appropriate calendar year is represented in the

---

* In calendar years of interrupted histories in which all intervals were identical, two identical values occurred 82 times; 3, 4, and 5 identical intervals occurred with frequencies of 15, 6, and 1, respectively.

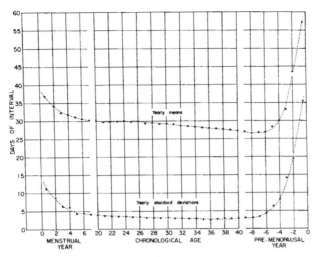

Figure 9. Average person-year means and standard deviations in three zones of experience.

averaging process by a single mean and a single standard deviation, regardless of the number of menstrual periods experienced that year.

An attempt has been made in Figure 9 to provide a reasonable freehand graduation of each set of these annual mean values. It is intended only that these smoothings will permit a simpler focus on the general trends depicted, and thus provide stepping stones to another deriviation.

Tables of the normal curve are frequently used to estimate the ranges of values to be expected for an individual case when both mean and standard deviation are known. This involves an assumption of symmetry in distribution of the variable under consideration. It is more consistent with experience in our study of individual histories that the distribution of menstrual intervals is generally skew. Use of normal curve theory with this variable contributes to error in depicting ranges of variation. We proceed to use normal curve theory in the present connection as a first approximation, well aware of its limitations.

Employing the empirically graduated values from the two lines of Figure 9 as the necessary parameters for normal curve calculations, in Figure 10 we sought, as a first approximation, to generalize the scope of variation in menstrual interval for the "average person" at each age. Contours bounding the central 50 per cent of cases and each extreme 5 per cent, are obtained for a normal curve distribution by multiplying the standard deviation by the factors ± 0.6745 and ± 1.6449, respectively, and adding these results to the mean value. Thus the central 90 per cent of intervals at age 20 would fall between 23.5 and 36.5 days for the average person if they were normally distributed. The range of 13 days embraced by these limits is more useful than the limits themselves when allowance is made for skewness of the distribution.

It is interesting to note in Figure 10 the change in this range with age

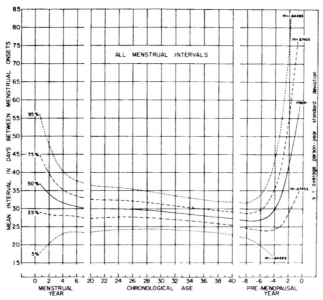

Figure 10. Normal curve contours for the distribution of interval in three zones of experience.

through the more stable years. The range of 13 days for the central 90 per cent at age 20 falls fairly steadily as age increases until a minimum of 9 days is reached on the average at age 36 years. The range remains fairly stable at this minimum for about four years, then it begins to increase rapidly as premenopausal irregularity becomes characteristic.

In the postmenarche and premenopause zones of experience we commend that attention be restricted in Figure 10 to the patterns of change made apparent there. We note that for the "average individual" the change in premenopausal variation is more rapid and attains more extreme values than is the case (inversely) with postmenarchial variation. As more data accumulate in our study, the details of range in these beginning and ending zones of experience may change detectably, but the more general inference of contrast between the two zones is not likely to be affected disturbingly.

Derivation of a more satisfactory basis for calculating frequency contours appropriate to the average case is needed. In our study this basis must be derived from computer-generated results which we await with a patience born of necessity. For the present we must be content with the foregoing gross estimation.

III. The Individual Record

Typical values are great levelers well described by Galton[18] in his reflection on those who

... commonly limit their inquiries to Averages, and do not revel in more comprehensive views. Their souls seem as dull to the charm of variety as that of the native of one of our flat English counties, whose retrospect of Switzerland was that, if its mountains could be thrown into its lakes, two nuisances would be got rid of at once.

We have learned that without extensive attention to individual records when studying menstruation, one will miss features of challenging biologic interest, matters of crucial importance to individual planning.

A comprehensive search of our total file of histories might conceivably produce a record which would agree approximately with the trends given in Figure 9 (Tables IV and V). The tedium attending such a search, and the small likelihood of its being a successful one, commended consideration of alternative approaches. Our data enable the plotting of individual histories over many years for a sizable proportion of our collaborators, who include 687 cases with at least 20 years of recorded history and 213 others with 10 years or more. In graphing over 70 of these histories, chosen for the most part in a statistically random order, we have not found ourselves dulled by monotony. Selections have been made from among these graphs to illustrate herein many fairly common characteristics. However, no one of these graphs throughout its span of menstrual history serves to represent the "average person" of Figure 10.

We lack adequate criteria for assigning breaks between middle life experience and the menarchial and menopausal transition zones for individual histories. To facilitate comparison of histories with each other we can adopt instead the time scale of menstrual year.

Most of our subjects joined this study several years after the menarchial year, in most cases providing their age at menarche by recall. The current calendar year of record for these cases was converted to menstrual year by subtracting age at menarche from age attained in that calendar year. The menstrual year scale in our diagrams may therefore be restored to conventional age attained that year by adding age at menarche to the scaled menstrual year. When date of menarche is known, the calendar year in which it occurs corresponds to the first menstrual year, as above, only if the birthday in that calendar year follows menarche. The menstrual year scale starts with zero when the birthday precedes menarche in the calendar year of reference. Thus the preservation of consistency with the only simple rule applicable when the menarche date is not known generates an inconsistency.

A Complete History of Menstrual Life. Figure 11 presents annual means and standard deviations for case 4754 in terms of the menstrual year scale. This graph may be related to that for the "all persons" average values given in Figure 9 by zones of menstrual experience. Pertinent events affecting menstruation in the history are indicated in Figure 11 (and in all following graphs) by symbols inscribed in relation to the trend lines. As far as possible these symbols have been chosen to be self suggestive: *M*, marriage; *B*, birth; *A*, abortion; *H*, hysterectomy; *U*, urogenital surgery other than *H*; *SA*, surgery, abdominal; *S*, surgery, other; and *X*, deep x-ray treatment.

Three births intervened in the menstrual history represented statistically in Figure 11. Both the means and standard deviations for the years in which these births occurred show marked increases as post partum sequelae. Prior

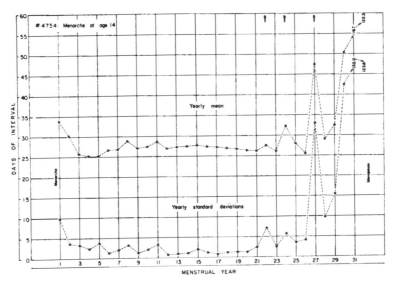

Figure 11. A lifetime trend in average and variability.

to her first pregnancy, case **4754** showed a shorter menstrual interval (by two or more days) than the "average person," and considerably less variability in those intervals. This relative position is reversed after the final birth when a transition to menopause occurs rather quickly. Her total menstrual experience spans **32** years instead of the **38** suggested by the composite graph in Figure 9.

The complete pattern of successive menstrual intervals for case **4754** (a physician) is portrayed in Figure 12. This history, unbroken from menarche to menopause, is unique in our files, and perhaps in the literature. Each solid dot in Figure 12 corresponds to an interval between menstrual onsets of length in days as defined on the vertical scale. The position of each dot relative to the horizontal scale indicates the terminal point of the interval within the calendar year. *Open circles with a dependent arrow* define for the horizontal scale only an initial menstrual onset after a break; a menstrual interval is not generated until another onset occurs. The *open circle* in the year of menarche defines the date of that event. Each interval is linked by a line to its succeeding interval to assist assimilation of the sequential continuity.

Individuality in Typical Interval. The separate panels of Figure 13 present the intervals between onsets for three persons through the same 12 years of age (31 to 42) and of menstrual life (18 to 29). All three persons experienced two pregnancies during this period. These segments of middle life menstrual experience have been selected primarily to illustrate differences between persons in average interval. All are more regular than is usual.

The *lower panel* of Figure 13 shows that case 1772 menstruated very consistently throughout this period at intervals averaging a little over three

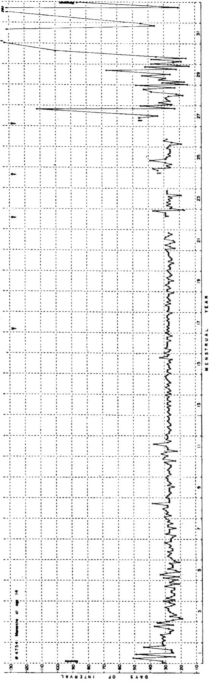

Figure 12. A complete history of menstrual intervals from menarche to menopause.

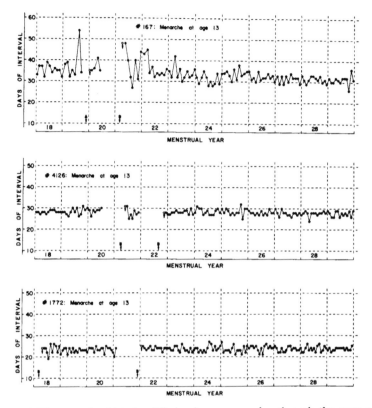

Figure 13. Three regular histories differing in average value through the same years.

weeks. Although almost one third of the intervals were 23 days in length, the remainder varied from 19 to 27 days, giving a total range of nine days. A feature of interest is the lack of any drift toward lower or higher values throughout these 12 years; the average value of 23.5 days is representative throughout the period. The annual standard deviations average 1.19 days.

The *middle panel* of Figure 13 shows a variation pattern very like that in the *lower panel,* but it is centered at 28 days, or five days longer than case 1772. The range of variation is again nine days, from 24 to 32 days. The average annual standard deviation is only slightly higher at 1.26 days. Again, there is no sign of drift toward a lower or higher mean value throughout the 12-year period.

The *top panel* differs in three major respects from those below it. In her 18th menstrual year, case 167 had a cycle length of slightly over five weeks, a full week longer than that in the middle panel and nearly two weeks longer than that in the bottom panel. Through the next 11 years her menstrual interval decreased steadily to approximately 31 days, contrasting sharply therein with the two *lower panels* through the same 12 years. The variability pattern in the *upper panel* is distinctly wider; except for two short increases associated with pregnancy experiences, the tendency is for variability to decrease with the passage of time.

A Contrast in Regularity. Figure 14 presents two histories of very different variability. The *upper panel* depicts the rather short recorded experience through 11 years for case 646. This history is unique in our records in that it alone contains a complete calendar year of experience throughout which menstruation occurred "regularly every 28 days." A single lapse the following year to 27 days spoiled what would have been a two-year constancy. This remarkable regularity is followed by four years of modest variability before the last three years of available records again became impressive for their approach to constancy. It was a disappointment to lose case 646 through an illness that eventually involved hysterectomy. The nearest approach in regularity in any other history available to us contains eight consecutive intervals of the same length.

A contrasting pattern of variability is shown in the *lower panel* of Figure 14. Through the same years of menstrual experience these two cases differ as widely in variability as we can reasonably portray in this format. Over the span of its first 18 menstrual years, the history of case 4884 is not the most variable one in our files. This history is unique, however, in the progressive decrease in variability that occurred through its last dozen years. Through the initial 14 years of record, a median interval of 55 days prevails, the range of variation being from 27 days to 30 weeks. After the third birth (at approximately 33 years of age) the median and variability of interval decreased through the next 12 years until impressive regularity was reached at about a median of essentially 30 days, with a range of seven days. Twice in the 25th menstrual year, two successive intervals of less than 20 days may incite speculation that mid-menstrual bleedings may be proving deceptive of menstruation. However, the durations of flow of 8 and 7 days were within the range of usual menstrual experience.

We turn now from purposeful selections for special expository purposes to consideration of points of interest occurring in more commonplace experience.

The Years Following Menarche. Study of the age-specific menstrual interval distribution statistics (Figures 7 to 9) left no doubt concerning typical trends for the postmenarche transition to middle life stability—shortening intervals and decreasing variability of interval. Following menarche, however, individuality with respect to (1) central trend, (2) amount of variation, and (3) duration of the transition period is very pronounced. A small selection of histories to portray combinations of these three characteristics, all variable over substantial ranges, must inevitably prove incomplete. The following illustrative cases must therefore serve to suggest rather than to define.

Two case histories with clearly demarked menarchial zones are presented in Figure 15. In each experience a period of six or seven years of irregularity preceded an abrupt change to comparative stability. The initial periods of irregularity differ chiefly in that case 7207 (*upper panel*) has twice as many intervals greater than 60 days than has case 7217 (*lower panel*).

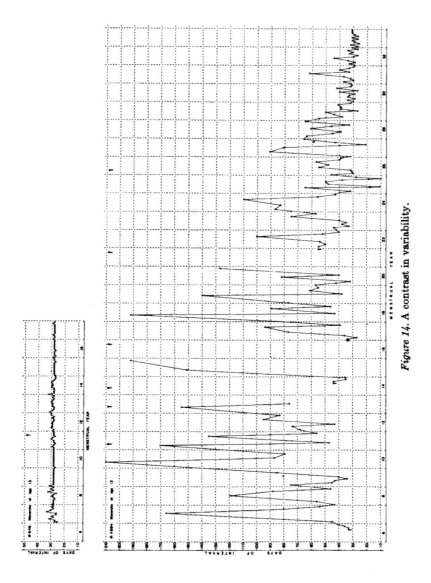

Figure 14. A contrast in variability.

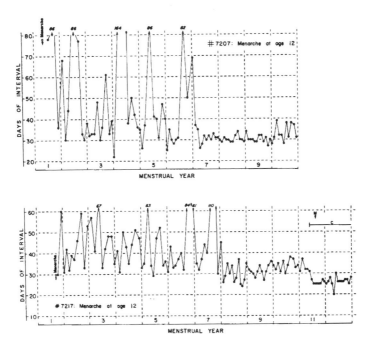

Figure 15. Postmenarche transitions.

After these very irregular years, the variability difference is reversed; case 7207 is more regular than 7217 for three years. Following this period, case 7217 begins to use control drugs and imposes an artificial regularity at an interval value of about 26 days while 7207 becomes more variable.

Figure 16 includes two histories which differ chiefly in duration of their postmenarche transitions. The conversion to relative regularity takes approximately five years for case 7212 (*upper panel*). We suggest it is substantially less, a little more than one year, for case 7200 (*lower panel*). The two-year increase in variability of the latter history after an interlude of relative regularity may well incite speculation that perhaps the short transition was itself predisposing to a limited return of instability. The variability picture in early middle life for these two cases is not widely different; both level off in central tendency at about 28 days with only small differences in variability. Both adopt birth control medication at the time of marriage, but neither woman establishes complete regularity of interval under this regimen.

Both menarchial experiences portrayed in Figure 17 show somewhat atypical experience. The *upper panel* (for case 7238) shows a not particularly uncommon early history in which enough stability is established *ab initio* that transition from menarche to middle life experience is not apparent. After the first year the central trend for this case remains stable for seven years at approximately 25 days; thereafter a somewhat longer typical interval may be in the making.

The pattern in the *lower panel* (for case 7210) also lacks the usual

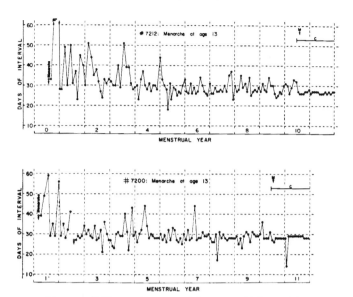

Figure 16. Differing durations of the menarchial transitions.

menarchial transition, but in two major respects this history is sharply different from the one above it. The variability of interval for case 7210 was not only substantially greater than for case 7238 from menarche onwards, but also that variability shows a marked increase from the sixth year on because extreme deviations become so much greater. Thus the history of case 7210 becomes an inversion of what would normally be anticipated in the years covered.

Middle Life and Menopausal Experience. Those of our collaborators for whom menopause or hysterectomy has already terminated menstrual activity have been keeping records for us since reasonably early in middle life. Consequently these histories permit coverage of individual experience through both the central and terminal zones of menstrual life. Selections from a random sample of these terminated histories follow. By way of introduction we first present two histories terminated by hysterectomy, and then a rather long history showing abrupt change within middle life.

The 28 years of menstrual history portrayed for a single woman in Figure 18 (case 1984) is representative of rather high regularity in menstrual interval. Also, the typical interval value falls very steadily over a 26-year period, from about 32 days in her fifth menstrual year to approximately 27 days just before an abrupt change. A full year of alternating long, normal, and short intervals, all with long durations of flow, was judged menopausal by her physician and treated with Enovid. Then a dilatation and curettage (D. & C.) was followed within two weeks by hysterectomy, without any notation in our records of pathology.

Contrast appears in many respects in the history of case 616, shown in Figure 19. After a seemingly normal pattern of variation, about a 28-day

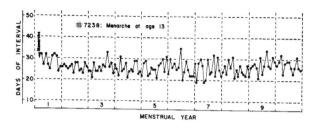

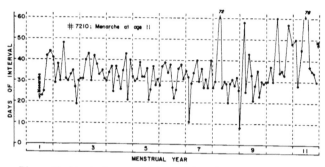

Figure 17. Atypical menarchial transitions into later experience.

median for nearly one year, increasing variability accompanies a progressive increase of about 10 days in interval through the next five or six years. This is followed for eight years by a slower reversal of the previous pattern of change. Then marriage and pregnancies leading to five live births and two recorded abortions are interspersed with five short episodes of essentially regular menstruation before the final pregnancy is followed by three more years of highly regular experience. A menopausal transition seems to be under way in her 33rd menstrual year, evidenced chiefly by the increase of short intervals. Following marriage, the fragmentary trend in this history clearly shows a steady decrease in length of menstrual interval from the mid-30-day level to a premenopausal value about 10 days shorter. Erratic premenopausal intervals appearing in the 34th menstrual year led to Oreton being prescribed as a control medication. A D. & C. then indicated endometrial hyperplasia, which was followed in a few months by hysterectomy.

It seems reasonable to conjecture that the two immediately preceding histories would have ended with menopause a little later had not surgery intervened.

Through the first available 11 years (from 20 to 30 years of age) of the history for case 1855, plotted in Figure 20, high variability in menstrual interval was characteristic. Her marriage at age 24 occurred at about the middle of this period. A sudden change to surprising regularity occurs for one year, regardless of intervening surgery, before pregnancy results in a live birth. This is followed by higher variability in menstrual interval for almost 18 months before another pregnancy. Following the second birth her

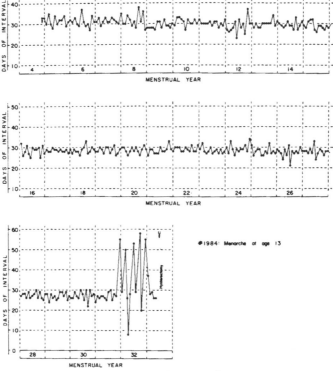

Figure 18. A uniform experience.

menstrual experience became unstable for three years, chiefly in central trend. Her experience for the next 11 years then holds very well indeed to a rather highly regular pattern following the general average trend in its central tendency. The single long interval in her 33rd menstrual year may be an advance signal of menopause. Like many another extremely long isolated interval, it may alternatively indicate an unrecognized pregnancy terminated by a failure in implantation.

We now turn to several confirmed menopause cases which also include a substantial part of experience through middle life.

The final 24 years of menstrual experience for case 5598 are graphed in Figure 21. This history is notable as a highly regular one of practically unchanging central tendency throughout the middle life record. The two long intervals in the 32nd menstrual year occasioned her wonder about onset of menopause; the signs were misleading, for regularity was resumed for nearly four years before recurrences of extreme deviations became close in the characteristic fashion for transition to menopause. Her total menstrual life of 41 years is a rather long one, ranging from 11 to 52 years of age.

Case 64 (Figure 22) shows the more usual type of middle life experience in both decreasing variability and slowly falling central trend. The numerous short intervals extending into the ninth menstrual year may belong to an

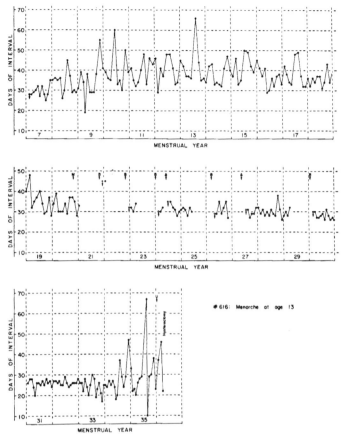

Figure 19. A varied experience.

unusually long menarchial transition period. There is some tendency for similar short intervals to reappear in more scattered fashion well in advance of the usual signs of approach to menopause. A break in the continuity of this record for a year (a record card lost in the mails) adds to the difficulty of conjecture concerning start of the menopausal transition.

Figure 23 (case 627) is again a typical history in that (1) its central trend falls somewhat steadily through the recorded period of middle life, and (2) the variability pattern is about average. Menopause for this case comes after a transition period of about three and one-half years, which is closed with her longest interval. If the increase in number of short intervals is a dependable signal of the approach of menopause, in this case that signal occurred at least one year in advance of the unusually long intervals. Commencing early with menarche at age 11, this menstrual life covered as long a span as is on record within this study.

The history of case 1113, given in Figure 24, illustrates changing variation

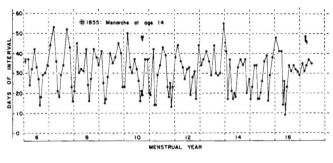

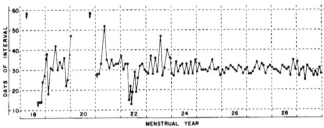

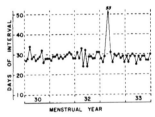

Figure 20. A pattern of changes in variability.

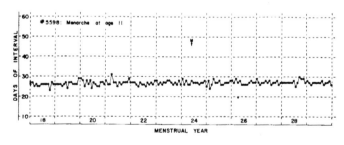

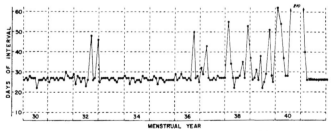

Figure 21. A long experience with very low variability.

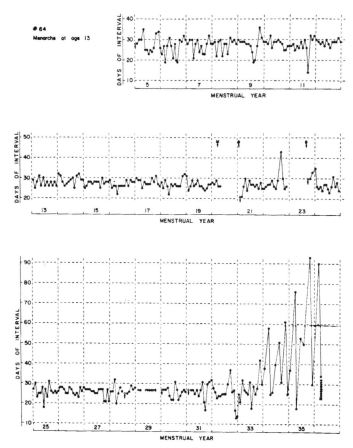

Figure 22. Typical changes through middle life to menopause.

in menstrual intervals through the middle years. The band of high variation, repeatedly reaching a range of 20 days within a few successive months, lies between an earlier period of nearly four years of greater regularity and a following span of nine years in which it settles down again rather abruptly. The transition to menopause was fairly short and somewhat episodic in its clumping of long and short intervals. The age at menopause (54 years) reflects a long menstrual life after a somewhat tardy start.

In Figure 25 we draw together for comparison the final 12 years of menstrual experience of two persons. In the *upper panel* (case 6007) a middle life of rather regular intervals is followed by the shortest transition to menopause so far available in our records. This final period of experience did not exceed 18 months, during which only two long and four short intervals departed from a consistent pattern through 13 preceding years.

The record of case 2595, given in the *lower panel* of Figure 25, presents a very different picture. A relatively short menstrual experience of only 25 years is brought to a close by a long exposure to menopausal instability

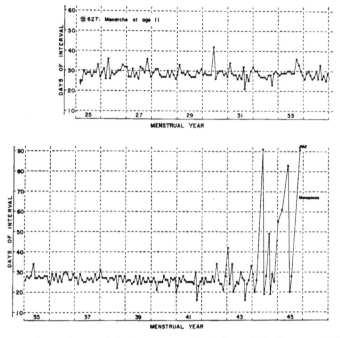

Figure 23. Some characteristic changes through the latter half of menstrual life.

extending over at least eight years. The 10 preceding years of middle life experience as recorded by this person are well represented by the 30 months with which this chart opens. In those 10 years, nine extra short or long intervals occurred sporadically among over 100 others which were confined to a range from 26 to 33 days. The basis on which the judgment of a long menopausal experience is reached is thus well defined. This history does not fall in the continually erratic class well described by the collaborator who wrote: "If it weren't for four children I'd think I had been in menopause my entire life."

DISCUSSION

An analysis of the periodicity our original collaborators *thought* to characterize their menstrual intervals, and its relation to the facts as recorded immediately thereafter, will be presented in a later report. It will suffice here to state that the reasonableness of bypassing recollection as a source of dependable information on menstruation will be amply supported by that analysis. Further comment on the literature summarizing the statements of patients (like those of respondents to questionnaires) may appropriately be confined here to repeating the views expressed by Hartman[19] in his presentation of newer concepts as prepared some 30 years ago:

... these records are scarcely worth the paper they are written on. The data are basically false. Consider how they are secured. An assistant who receives the patient asks

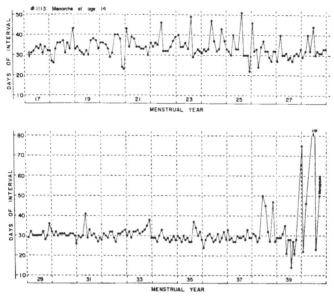

Figure 24. Contrasts precede conformity.

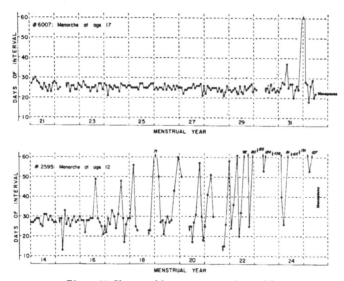

Figure 25. Short and long menopausal transitions.

her: 'Are you regular?' and she answers that she is, because, forsooth, she wants to be and usually thinks she is; ...*

---

* Hartman retained this attitude in his "compendium of human reproduction" entitled "Science and the Safe Period." [20] An early analysis of this disparity between statement and subsequent records in these matters is given by Treloar. [16]

It is of a very different order of importance to discuss here the concordance, or lack of it, between our findings and those of others who have approached the establishment of fact in this basic biologic rhythm as we have. Rather substantial differences in the frequency distributions of menstrual interval may be demonstrated in the studies of recorded menstruations made prior to 1934. These differences in distribution were augmented by the investigations of Fluhmann,[21] Engle and Shelesnyak,[22] Scipiades,[23] Latz and Reiner,[24, 25] and Gunn et al.,[26] in the four following years. All were comprehensively assembled and discussed in 1939 by Arey.[27] Belonging with these now are the more recent contributions of Haman[28] and Goldzieher et al.[29]

The importance of age in the study of menstrual rhythm was first adequately demonstrated by Vollmann, who has given emphasis several times[15], [30-32] to this point with his continuously expanding series of data. More recently, Matsumoto et al.[33] have also presented extensive data for Japanese women, confirming in the Asiatic setting the importance of age as a variable in studies of menstruation. Our specification in detail of the importance of age is fully confirmatory. Resolution of the problems peculiar to the postmenarche and premenopause years in the foregoing pages gives a new emphasis to the importance of "gynecological maturity." (vide Vollmann[32]). The differences which are apparent in the many sets of data which do not take age into account are now clearly ascribable in considerable part to differences in age distribution of the groups of women studied.

An attempt is made in Figure 26 to portray an array of these distributions of menstrual intervals in a single diagram. Cumulative curves are used for simplicity of presentation in Figure 26. There is no difficulty in drawing a smooth curve freehand through all cumulative frequency points for the numerically large series. For the others, curves are drawn as close to the points they link as they can be inscribed smoothly.

The two patterns of lines (broken and continuous) used in Figure 26 are intended to distinguish data of different types. The broken lines themselves differentiate three subgroups: (1) the data of Ogino[6] and Matsumoto[33] for Japanese women; (2) the essentially youthful groups of Fluhmann[21] and Scipiades,[23] and (3) the puberty series of Engle and Shelesnyak.[22] The four fine continuous lines have been selected as boundaries of a shaded area containing an intermingling set of cumulative curves for the data in ten other studies.[2-4, 7, 8, 24, 25, 28-30] The curve for Pratt[4] serves fairly well to define the series which is least variable and also has the highest proportions of cases (shortest intervals in general) at almost all percentage points. It takes segments of the curves from Latz and Reiner,[25] Allen,[7] and Vollmann,[31] however, to provide a reasonable boundary for the distributions characterized by longer intervals and/or more variability of interval. Between these boundaries the remaining curves form a complex of lines which, although they tend to be parallel to some degree, also involve much entangling intersection, making adequate differentiation of them beyond our capability in a small graph. The heavy continous line defining the cumulative curve for the mixture of all person-years of data in this study is in the main within the shaded area.

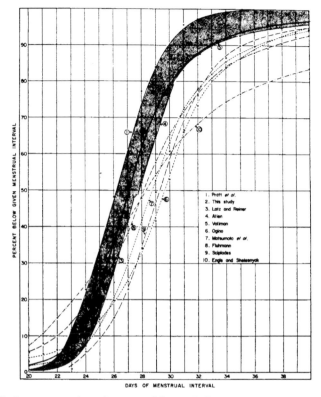

Figure 26. A representation of menstrual interval distributions from the literature.

The mixture of ages, or preferably, of "gynecological maturities," which any large series of menstrual intervals embraces must inevitably determine the form of its cumulative distribution curve. A progressive shift from a curve of the form of no. 10 in Figure 26, through no. 9 and 8 into that of no. 1 at the more regular period of experience, would be completely compatible with what our data indicate if followed progressively from menarche to just before the start of the menopausal transition. Through the years of the latter approach to menopause, the change in form of the maturity-specific curves would occur in the reverse direction and of course with considerably increased speed. We suggest therefore that the differences between all the series of data of reference above for the races of European stock substantially reflect differences in maturity mixture of the subjects involved.

The data for the Japanese women, who for the most part were in the middle years of experience, in our present judgment seem to indicate a substantial shift from the others in characteristic length of menstrual interval toward a longer cycle. The variability pattern of menstrual interval for the Asiatic group through the *central section of the curve* is much akin to that of the European, but the curve does indicate greater frequency in the relatively more deviate intervals, especially the shorter ones. We tentatively infer from this that while the person and her stage of menstrual maturity are major sources of heterogeneity in intervals between menstrual onsets as assembled for groups of subjects, perhaps race (collectively with its correlates) may receive priority over competitors for next place.

It will be observed in Figure 26 that despite the general dispersion of these curves, the median values fall within the relatively small range of 26.3 to 29.7 days. Vastly increased ranges of variation are apparent when pairs of percentile values are chosen toward the extremes of 0 and 100. Thus these distributions are much more alike in their central values than in their dispersions.

It is certainly possible that the factors which lead persons to become record keepers for study purposes are also influential as contributors to the values recorded. We do not claim that our community of collaborators establishes a norm for any population of people other than that of which it is in fact a representative sample. There are tests we can apply to see if we have such a sample from the University of Minnesota student body. We intend to apply such tests in analyses of this question. But this will not resolve any of the problems of how representative such persons are of women generally within the nationality grouping to which they ascribe allegiance, or within the geographic areas where they have resided, or under any other conditions known or speculated to influence menstrual periodicity.

The uncertainties concerning the representativeness of our subjects in their menstruation have a counterbalance in a fact now clearly established. We have been assembling data from very different sources concerning the interval from onset of last menstrual period to birth of the child. In well over 2000 fruitful pregnancies our married collaborators show remarkable agreement in this interval with all other gestational interval data from Caucasian stocks within this nation which we have analyzed. The phenomena of gestation and menstruation have biologic affinities which are suggestive of representativeness in one being kin to the other. Thus, although we are not sure in definition of the breadth of the population of which our community is representative, we do feel that its norms have adequate generality to serve as a basis for comparative studies with other populations or communities of very different ethnic backgrounds, or current geographic environments in their living, or both.

In giving considerable emphasis to the individual history in this study, we depart in some degree from adherence to statistical tradition. The appearance of statistical homogeneity, as portrayed in our sample by the smoothness of the frequency distribution transition throughout menstrual life, must not obscure underlying differences between persons. Homogeneity is relative. Any variation system, no matter how orderly it may be, reflects the operation of a multiplicity of causes, and therein reflects heterogeneity. Only invariant data are absolutely homogeneous. Acknowledgment here of an over-riding importance to be given to each person's variation through time is unquestionably pertinent.

Our description of menstrual cyclicity as a facet of human biology will be turned inward by each individual interested in its implications for conception or contraception. "How does this apply to me?" will be asked much more frequently than the more general alternative: "How does this affect the possibilities for control of the population explosion?" Both questions are basically the same, however. Conception remains very much an individual matter in the human sector of the life kingdom; human sperm are not broadcast as is plant seed to secure the means for human living. The probabilities one faces in these human issues of "to be, or not to be" are not those of populations of persons but of time relationships within an individual's menstrual and coition experiences; *both* of these are crucially personal.

Given the necessary data on gynecologic maturity, any person's record can be aligned within the three definitive scales for age as used in this discussion. But the individuality of each woman with respect to menstrual intervals throughout her years of gynecologic activity is not itself a constant. She *can* be just like the "average woman" as our construct defines it. She *may* alternatively have a life experience which neatly parallels the average change through the years, differing only in a longer or shorter central tendency. But it is certainly *more* likely that her individuality will not be expressed so simply as to be identical with, or parallel to, the general average. There are unlimited possibilities involving both continuous and episodic changes with age, many of which have appeared in our illustrative histories. These characteristics of the individual history bear heavily on the dependability of pregnancy control through use of rhythm only. Successful use of this technique can be the lot of many, but unquestionably these many must still be a minority of all who would seek it. A carefully compiled menstrual history for the individual must ordinarily be essential, and the longer it is the better. But complete success in control can never be guaranteed by reliance on rhythm alone.

CONCLUSIONS

1. There is no substantial justification for the widely held belief that women normally vary in menstrual interval about a value of 28 days common to all. Each woman has her own central trend and variation, both of which change with age. Assemblies of menstrual interval for many persons and covering a wide span of chronologic ages should, however, be expected to average within a few days of the oft-quoted 28.

2. Complete regularity in menstruation through extended time is a myth. Fraenkel's dictum* is much more appropriate than the protests of Knaus. Variation is the rule, exceptions to it in individual cases being of small dura-

---

* Translating from Knaus,[34] we have the view of Fraenkel and an indication of rejoinder by Knaus: "Without having collected a large sample of data on the length of the menstrual cycle, based on menstrual records kept for a long period of time, at any possible occasion Fraenkel repeats his slogan: 'The only regularity in the menstrual cycle is its irregularity.'" One of us dealt with this conflict of fact and fancy two years later (Treloar[16]).

tion. Women apparently use the reply "regular" as they do "28 days" to indicate belief that they are normal in their menstrual characteristics.

3. The first few years of menstrual life, like the last few, are marked usually by a variation pattern of mixed short and long intervals with a characteristic transition into and out of the relatively more regular pattern of middle life. These transitions vary widely in length, but seem to occupy more usually about five to seven years after menarche and about six to eight years before menopause. There is no obvious criterion for ending of the menarchial or beginning of the menopausal transition. On the contour diagrams of changing frequency distributions with age, these two transition zones are very much like mirror images of one another, with both central trend and variation changing in curvilinear forms.

4. The "middle life" zone, which may be said in a general way to occupy about two decades beginning in the vicinity of age 20, is characterized on the average by linear change in both central tendency and variation. The general fall in interval through this age span is of the order of two to three days, depending on whether the median or mean is used for the typical value.

5. The amount of intraperson variation in menstrual interval has been measured for all 22,754 calendar years of experience available for this study. The general trend of variation through menstrual life, as measured by averages of person-year standard deviations, is strikingly curvilinear through the menarchial and menopausal zones, but essentially rectilinear through the middle years. Variation reaches its minimum at approximately 36 years of age on the average, where the mean and median S.D.'s are 2.5 and 1.83 days, respectively. The pronounced upward swing of the typical standard deviation commences about six years later.

6. The pattern of variation in menstrual interval from which probabilities of anticipated intervals could be derived for individual use is clearly a frequency curve of considerable skewness. Thus an estimate of the standard deviation of interval for any person at a given age needs to be supplemented by an estimate of the degree of skewness. Problems involved in such estimation have not been resolved as yet for this study; work on this rather crucial matter is currently in progress.

7. All menstrual histories show individualities that make the norms provided by statistical procedures useful only for comparisons of groups of persons. The characteristics of an individual menstrual history may alter with time and show fluctuating divergences from an average pattern. A woman's personal arrangements that may be influenced by her menstrual cyclicity may be made with greater probability of success the longer the guiding record of her past menstruations. The practice of birth control through use of rhythm methods alone must introduce elements of such uncertainty as to pose serious problems for all persons affected.

We are indebted to every collaborator whose contribution, whatever length it may be, from one year to those still continuing after 30 years, has been an investment in this project. We trust each such investment has been turned to good account.

The analyses reported herein have been greatly aided by the Kimberly-Clark Corporation through a contract with the University of Minnesota, supporting the computer operations and clerical work basic to them. The authors express their gratitude to the officers of both these institutions and to other associates within the University who have contributed so much over the decades. The stimulating efforts of Professor Jacob E. Bearman and Dr. Donald W. Cowan in bringing this study to its present fruition have been particularly helpful.

REFERENCES

1. Foster, F. P. The periodicity and duration of the menstrual flow. *New York M. J.* 49: 610, 1889.
2. Issmer, F. Über die Zeitdauer der menschlichen Schwangerschaft. *Arch. Gynäk.* 35: 310, 1889.
3. King, J. L. Menstrual records and vaginal smears in a selected group of normal women. *Contribut. Embryol.* 18: 79, 1926.
4. Pratt, J. P., Allen, E., Newell, Q. U., and Bland, L. J. Human ova from the uterine tubes. *J. A. M. A.* 93: 834, 1929.
5. Geist, S. H. The variability of menstrual rhythm and character. *Am. J. Obst. & Gynec.* 20: 320, 1930.
6. Ogino, K. Über den Konzeptionstermin des Weibes und seine Anwendung in der Praxis. *Zentralbl. Gynäk.* 56: 721, 1932.
7. Allen, E. The irregularity of the menstrual function. *Am. J. Obst. & Gynec.* 25: 705, 1933.
8. King, J. L. Menstrual intervals. *Am. J. Obst. & Gynec.* 25: 583, 1933.
9. Krieger, E. *Die Menstruation, eine gynakologische Studie.* A. Hirschwald, Berlin, 1869.
10. Kelly, H. A. *Medical Gynecology.* Appleton-Century-Crofts, Inc., New York, 1908.
11. Sanes, K. I. Menstrual statistics. A study based on 4500 menstrual histories. *Am. J. Obst. & Dis. Women & Child.* 73: 93, 1916.
12. Committee of the London Association of the Medical Women's Federation. Menstruation in school girls. A survey based on replies to a questionnaire. *Lancet* 219: 57, 1930.
13. Kosakae, J., Karwanabe, K., Kursishi, Y., and Yamamura, A. Beiträge zur Statistik über die Menstruation de Japanischen Studentin. *Jap. J. Obst. & Gynec.* 16: 141, 1933.
14. Kennedy, W. The menarche and menstrual type; notes on 10,000 case records. *J. Obst. & Gynaec. Brit. Emp.* 40: 792, 1933.
15. Vollmann, R. Variationstatistiche Analyse der Phasen des Genitalzyklus der Frau durch Auswertung des Intermenstrualschmierzes als Indikator für den Ovulationstermin. *Monatsschr. Geburtsh. u. Gynäk.* 110: 115, 1940.
16. Treloar, A. E. Menstruation and birth control. *Gamma Alpha Rec.* 29: 65, 1939.
17. Roberton, J. An inquiry into the natural history of the menstrual function. *Edinburgh M. & Surg. J.* 38: 227, 1832.
18. Galton, F. *Natural Inheritance,* p. 62. The Macmillan Company, London, 1889.
19. Hartman, C. G. *Time of Ovulation in Women,* p. 61. The Williams & Wilkins Co., Baltimore, 1936.
20. Hartman, C. G. *Science and the Safe Period.* The Williams & Wilkins Co., Baltimore, 1962.
21. Fluhmann, C. F. The length of the human menstrual cycle. *Am. J. Obst. & Gynec.* 27: 73, 1934.
22. Engle, E. T., and Shelesnyak, M. C. First menstruation and subsequent menstrual cycles of pubertal girls. *Human Biol.* 6: 431, 1934.
23. Scipiades, E. Beobachtung über den Typus des humanen Menstruationzyklus. *Arch. Gynäk.* 159: 360, 1935.
24. Latz, L. J., and Reiner, E. Natural conception control. *J. A. M. A.* 105: 1241, 1935.
25. Latz, L. J., and Reiner, E. Further studies on the sterile and fertile periods in women. *Illinois M. J.* 71: 210, 1937.

26. Gunn, D. L., Jenkin, P. M., and Gunn, A. L. Menstrual periodicity and statistical observations on a large sample of normal cases. *J. Obst. & Gynaec. Brit. Emp.* 44: 839, 1937.

27. Arey, L. B. The degree of normal menstrual irregularity. *Am. J. Obst. & Gynec.* 37: 12, 1939.

28. Haman, J. O. The length of the menstrual cycle. *Am. J. Obst. & Gynec.* 43: 870, 1942.

29. Goldzieher, J. W., Henkin, A. E., and Hamblen, E. C. Characteristics of the normal menstrual cycle. *Am. J. Obst. & Gynec.* 54: 668, 1947.

30. Vollmann, R. *Fruchtbarkeit und Temperaturkurve der Frau.* Kyklos, Zürich, 1947.

31. Vollmann, R. Die Länge des Pramenstruum in Regression zum alter der Frau. *Gynaecologia* 135: 78, 1953.

32. Vollmann, R. F. Degree of variability of the length of the menstrual cycle in correlation with age of woman. *Gynaecologia* 142: 310, 1956.

33. Matsumoto, S., Nogami, Y., and Ohkuri, S. Statistical studies of menstruation: A criticism of the definition of normal menstruation. *Gunma J. M. Sc.* 11: 294, 1962.

34. Knaus, H. *Die periodische Fruchtbarkeit und Unfructbarkeit des Weibes*, p. 76. Wilhelm Maudrich Buchhandlung und Verlag Wien, 1935.

*This paper has been reproduced by kind permission of
Medical Science Publishing International, Inc.,
Port Washington, New York.*

Commentary on Classic Paper No.8

In this Classic Paper, Treloar, a reproductive anthropomorphist, and his colleagues[1] describe the natural variations that occur in the human menstrual cycle, based not on opinion, but on the statistical analysis of sound data. This paper is particularly important, since, despite vast scientific knowledge of the human female reproductive cycle, as Treloar points out, *The inadequacy of fact concerning this phenomenon, established by scientific enquiry involving complete coverage of human menstrual life, is remarkable.'*

According to Treloar, the majority of women when giving medical histories affirm that they menstruate 'regularly' and 'every 28 days', only a minority suggesting otherwise. The truth, however, is not so clear and again in Treloar's words, *The inference that this pattern attests to one fact alone, wide variability between persons in the menstrual interval, seems to have had appeal only to those few who were not uncomfortable in being unconventional.'*

Earlier animal work, notably by Hitschmann and Adler in 1908[2] and Stockard and Papanicolaou in 1917[3], had laid the foundation for Treloar's important study.

To ascertain the facts behind popular opinion, in 1933, Treloar and his colleagues began a prospective study in school girls and student nurses, and later their own children. They collected information on intra-person variation in menstrual interval over a total of 22 754 calendar years of experience, pre-oral contraception. By statistical evaluation of centiles of intervals, they reached a number of conclusions.

- There is no substantial evidence for the widely held belief that women normally vary in menstrual interval, about a value of 28 days common to all. Each woman has her own central trend and variation, both of which change with age.

- Complete regularity in menstruation through extended time is a myth.

- With regard to menstrual interval, there are three zones in menstrual life: the first few years (post-menarche), a middle life zone from 20 to 40 years, and the last few years (premenopausal).

- All menstrual histories show individualities.

This Classic Paper finally established the truth behind the regularity of the menstrual cycle, or the lack of it, adding an important piece of information in the jigsaw that makes up our understanding of the human reproductive cycle. Robert Battey's paper[4] on oophorectomy in normal women originally established the first link between ovarian hormones and menstruation.

1. Treloar, A.E., Boynton, R.E., Behn, B.G. and Brown, B.W. (1967). Variation of the human menstrual cycle through reproductive life. *Int. J. Fertil.*, **12**, 77

2. Hitschmann, F. and Adler, L. (1908). Der Bau der Uterusschleimhaut des geschlechtsreifen Weibes besonderer Berücksichtigung der Menstruation. *Mschr. Geburt. Gynäk.*, **27**, 1

3. Stockard, C.R. and Papanicolaou, G. N. (1917). The existence of a typical oestrus cycle in the guinea-pig; with the study of its histological and physiological changes. *Am. J. Anat.*, **22**, 225

4. Battey, R. (1872). Normal ovariotomy. *Atlanta Med. Surg. J.*, **10**, 321

The ovary

5. Vesalius, A. (1543). *De Humani Corporis Fabrica*

6. De Graaf, R. (1672). *De mulierum organis generationi inservientibus.* Lugduni Batavorum, *ex. off.* Hackiana

7. Berthold, A.A. (1849). Transplantation der Hoden. *Arch. Anat. Physiol. wiss Med.*, 42–6

8. Knauer, E. (1896). Einige Versuche über Ovarientransplantation beim Kaninchen. *Zentralblatt. Gynäkol.*, **20**, 524

9. Bayliss, W.M. and Starling, E.H. (1904). The chemical regulation of the secretory process. *Proc. R. Soc. Ser. B.*, **73**, 310

Some understanding of the human reproductive system goes back as far as the 17th century, when the Italian scientist, Marcello Malpighi, recognized that the ovary was involved in reproduction. Even earlier than Malpighi, the yellow structure had been recognized by Vesalius[5].

Andreas Vesalius gave an extensive description of the ovary during the autopsy of an 18-year-old girl, performed in 1533 in Brussels. He stated that, during compression of the ovary, a miraculous white but sometimes also yellow or orange-like fluid could escape like a fountain.

In the middle of the 17th century, Regnier De Graaf described extensively the morphology and function of the female reproductive organs[6]. He studied the changes in the ovary in animals after mating and, from these descriptions, it is clear that he observed ovarian special units (later to be known as Graafian follicles), although these were first described by Vesalius. In 1672, De Graaf was the first to describe the corpus luteum[6]. However, it took a further three centuries before detailed descriptions of the human ovary were presented.

In 1849, Berthold[7] found that the typical features of castrated cockerels could be prevented by testicle implantation and a related observation was described by Knauer in 1896[8], namely that transplantation of ovaries prevented uterine atrophy. The term 'hormones' was introduced by Bayliss and Starling[9] in 1904, who described them as '*The active substance secreted into the blood stream or tissue fluids by the ductless or endocrine glands.*'

Shifts of basal body temperature

10. Velde Th. H. van de (1904). *Ueber den Zusamnenhang zwischen Ovarialfunktion, Wellenbewegung und Menstrualblutung und ueber die Entstehung des sogenannten* Mittelschmerzes. (Haarlem, The Netherlands: De Erven F. Bohn)

One of the oldest documented effects of ovarian function on the human body is that of a shift in basal body temperature, originally documented by van de Velde[10] in 1904.

Dr H.A.I.M. Van Leusden, Arnhem, The Netherlands, wrote to us upon our request:

'*In 1904 van de Velde described the biphasic basal body temperature of menstruating women. He meticulously recorded a large amount of data and the reader is impressed by its thoroughness. He was also the first to point to the cyclic ovarian changes causing the rhythm.*

Van de Velde, a pupil of Hector Treub, started his practice as an obstetrician and gynecologist in Haarlem, The Netherlands, in 1904. In 1923 he moved to Switzerland and only then (1926) did he dare to publish Het Volkomen Huwelijk ('The perfect marriage'), a book of unusual frankness for that time.

As early as 1904, he stated that the ovarian stimulus for the temperature rhythm is of a chemical nature. Without any knowledge of progesterone (isolated in 1934), he was on the right trail[10].

In this classic illustration[10], he described how a woman of 37 years expected her menstrual period on January 3rd. The rise in basal body temperature occurred later than expected, however, and she started to menstruate on January 9th (see figure below).'

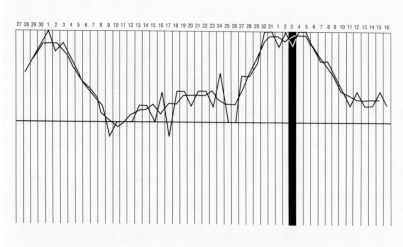

Normal menstruation in a 37-year-old woman. The last temperature wave lasted longer than usual. Also the menstrual bleeding occurred later than expected. The expected day of bleeding on January 3 is blackened[10].
Courtesy of Dr H.A.I.M. Van Leusden, Arnhem, NL

We can 'simply' explain the delayed menstrual period by postponed ovulation. Nowadays, however, we know that menstruation does not predict ovulation, but that menstruation is the result of foregoing ovulation. This paradoxical fact only becomes clear in the 1930s due to the observations of Ogino[11] and Knaus[12].

The era of hormones: endocrinology

Ovarian function

In a classic paper published in 1926, Bernhard Zondek and Selmar Aschheim[13] described their ideas on the function of the human ovary and confirmed the involvement of hormones in the normal functioning of the ovary.

They implanted human ovarian tissue into the mouse and used the induction of estrus and vaginal cornification as a 'bio-assay'. They also examined parts of these specimens histologically and were able to obtain a reasonable idea of the hormonally active sites of the ovary. They concluded

11. Ogino, K. (1930). Ovulationstermin und Konzeptionstermin. *Zentralbl. Gynäkol.*, **54**, 469

12. Knaus, H. (1929). Eine neue Methode zur Bestimmung des Ovulationstermines. *Zentralbl. Gynäkol.*, **53**, 2193

13. Zondek, B. and Aschheim, S. (1926). Zur funktion des Ovariums. *Klin. Wochenschr.*, **10**, 400

14. Marshall, F.H.A. and Jolly, W.A. (1905). Contributions to the physiology of mammalian reproduction. II. The ovary as an organ of internal secretion. *Philos. Trans. R. Soc. Lond. Ser. B.*, **198**, 123

15. Fraenkel, L. (1903). Die Funktion des Corpus Luteum. *Arch. Gynäk.*, **68**, 438

16. Corner, G. and Allen, W.M. (1929). Physiology of the corpus luteum. *Am. J. Physiol.*, **88**, 326

17. Butenandt, A. and Schmidt, J. (1934). Überführung des Pregnandiols in Corpus-Luteum-Hormon. *Berichte d. D. Chem. Gesellschaft*, **67**,1901

18. Marrian, G. F. (1930). The chemistry of oestrin. III. An approved method of preparation and the isolation of active crystalline material. *Biochem. J.*, **24**, 435

19. Butenandt, A. F. J. (1934). Neuere Ergebnisse auf dem Gebiet der Sexualhormone. *Wien Klin. Wschr.*, **47**, 897

20. Adler, L. (1912). Zur Physiologie und Pathologie der Ovarial-funktion. *Arch. Gynäk.*, **95**, 349

21. Stockard, C.R. and Papanicolaou, G.N. (1917). The existence of a typical estrous cycle in the guinea pig – with a study of its histological and physiological changes. *Am. J. Anat.*, **22**, 225

that, 'Theca and granulosa cells produce simultaneously an ovarian hormone.' Zondek and Aschheim received the Nobel Prize in physiology and medicine for their pioneering work in the area of ovarian function.

Progesterone

The importance of progesterone

In the early 1900s, Marshall and Jolly[14], and Fraenkel[15] observed that the removal of corpora lutea from rats and rabbits during the first days of pregnancy resulted in abortion. Corner and Allen[16] confirmed this observation; when using lipid extracts of corpora lutea, they prepared a substance that initiated progestational changes in rabbit endometrium and maintained pregnancy in ovariectomized rabbits. From studies of these crude extracts, identification and later synthesis of active crystalline progesterone evolved[16,17]. In 1930, Guy Marrian[18] prepared crystalline estriol and in 1934, Adolf Butenandt[19] succeeded in producing crystalline progesterone.

Estrogen and progesterone: the urinary sex steroids

Hormonal activity of the ovary was demonstrated by Halban in 1904, when, by subcutaneously transplanting an ovary into castrated guinea pigs, he brought about normal puberty. Injections of ovarian extract in spayed animals evoked sexual activity[20]. Changes of the vaginal epithelium in association with ovulation were reported by Stockard and Papanicolaou[21]. Finally, in 1923, Allen and Doisy[22] first isolated estrogen.

Until 1953, the only estrogens known to be present in human urine were the three classical ones: estradiol, estrone and estriol which had been isolated from various sources such as sow's ovaries, pregnancy urine, placental tissue and horse testis.

Chemical procedures, such as the Kober reaction, fluorometric methods and gas chromatography, were also being developed for the determination of these compounds. Using these techniques, the pattern of estrogen excretion in women with normal menstrual cycles was established[23].

In the first phase of the cycle, pregnanediol values were found to be at or below 1 mg per 24 hours, with values following ovulation between 2 and 4 mg per 24 hours.

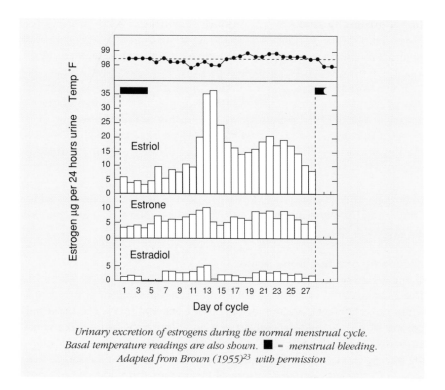

22. Allen, E. and Doisy, E.A. (1923). An ovarian hormone. Preliminary report on its localization, extraction and partial purification. *J. Am. Med. Assoc.*, **81**, 819

23. Brown, J.B. (1955). Urinary excretion of oestrogen during the menstrual cycle. *Lancet*, I, 320

Urinary excretion of estrogens during the normal menstrual cycle. Basal temperature readings are also shown. ■ = *menstrual bleeding. Adapted from Brown (1955)[23] with permission*

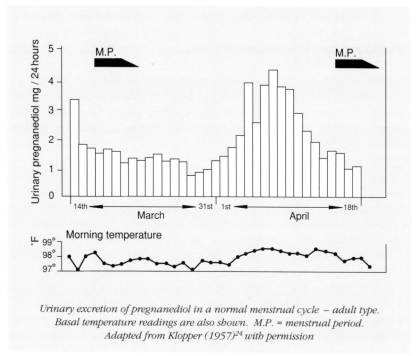

24. Klopper, A. (1957). The excretion of pregnanediol during the normal menstrual cycle. *J. Obstet. Gynaecol. Br. Emp.*, **64**, 504

Urinary excretion of pregnanediol in a normal menstrual cycle – adult type. Basal temperature readings are also shown. M.P. = menstrual period. Adapted from Klopper (1957)[24] with permission

The first longitudinal studies on the menstrual cycle were made by determining the excretion of estrogens and pregnanediol in the urine[23,24].

Gonadotropic hormones

25. Aschheim, S. and Zondek, B. (1927) Hypophysenvorderlappen-hormon und ovarial hormon im Harn von Schwangeren. *Klin. Wochenschr.*, **28**, 1322

In 1927, Aschheim and Zondek[25] reported that ovarian stimulation in the infantile mouse could be provoked by urine from pregnant women, but their conclusion that pregnancy urine contained hypophyseal hormones was proven to be incorrect. It is now clear that hCG (human chorionic gonadotropin) and hypophyseal LH (luteinizing hormone) behave in an identical fashion in biological assays. The discovery of LH and follicle stimulating hormone (FSH) was in part due to the work of Li and colleagues[26,27] who published their work in the 1940s.

26. Li, C. H., Simpson, M. E., Evans, H. M. *et al.* (1940). Interstitial cell stimulating hormone. II. Method of preparation and some physico-chemical studies. *Endocrinology*, **27**, 803

Later, a number of tests were developed, all based on the same principle, namely stimulation of the gonads (toads, frogs, rabbits, rats) and this has led to specific pregnancy tests.

The luteinizing hormone peak

27. Li, C. H., Simpson, M. E. and Evans, H. M. (1949). Isolation of pituitary follicle-stimulating hormone (FSH). *Science*, **109**, 445

The great majority of assays used for the determination of gonadotropic hormones were based on the mouse uterine test and this led to the development of specific methods for the separate determination of FSH and LH, including the use of reference preparations.

Numerous workers reported a peak of LH excretion at midcycle as a relatively constant occurrence. Results from an investigation of 64 normal menstrual cycles from 57 subjects, by Stevens[28], confirmed this observation.

From bio-assay to radio-immunoassay

28. Stevens, V.C. (1967). In Bell, E.T. and Loraine, J.A. (eds.) *Recent Research on Gonadotropic Hormones*, p. 223. (Edinburgh: Churchill Livingstone)

After the reports of Aschheim and Zondek, various qualitative and quantitative biological tests were developed to measure sex hormones, especially in urine. This was followed by an advance that greatly facilitated further research, namely the development of radio-immunological methods in which competitive reactions of labelled and unlabelled hormone take place with hormone antibodies[29].

29. Yalow, R. S. and Berson, S.A. (1960). Immunoassay of endogenous plasma insulin in man. *J. Clin. Invest.*, **39**, 1157

Soon, radio-immunological assays (RIAs) became available for FSH, replacing the ovarian or uterine augmentation tests in mice. Similarly for LH, an RIA was developed superseding the ovarian ascorbic acid, the cholesterol depletion test and the ventral prostatic weight test in rats.

Using radio-immunoassays, longitudinal studies in women confirmed the temporal relationship between estrogen, progesterone and LH. Approximately 10–12 hours before ovulation, an LH peak occurs; 34–36 hours prior to follicle rupture, the LH peak starts to rise. This LH surge initiates the resumption of meiosis in the oocyte, a process that started in fetal life, and luteinization of granulosa cells occurs.

The receptor model

The classic receptor model, which assigned a primary role to receptors in the cytoplasm of the cell, was developed by Jensen and Gorski in 1960 (see Jensen and De Sombre)[30]. This concept was later modified, when the role of a nuclear protein that can change from low to high affinity was identified[31].

Once in the nucleus the hormone–receptor complex binds with DNA resulting in RNA polymerase initiating transcription. Transcription leads to translation and RNA-mediated protein synthesis. Specific stimuli for steroidogenesis in the ovary are the large glycopeptides, FSH and LH, which bind to specific receptors on the cell membrane.

A considerable amount of research has been done to elucidate cell communication, and, in 1971, Earl W. Sutherland[32] received the Nobel Prize for proposing the second messenger, adenosine 3'5'-monophosphate (cyclic AMP), which initiates the synthesis and secretion of estradiol.

From pituitary to hypothalamus releasing hormones

'Believing that the nervous system is something more than a mere system of conducting paths, I formed the hypothesis that nerve cells are true secreting cells ...' (Scott, 1905) [33].

In 1947, it was postulated that hypothalamic hormones regulated the pituitary gland[34]. Later, both Roger Guillemin[35] and Andrew Schally[36] were able to demonstrate that materials with the properties of peptides, purified from ovine and pig hypothalami, stimulated LH and FSH release *in vivo* and *in vitro*. Finally, in 1971, the decapeptide sequence was determined and synthesized. This hypothalamic hormone is now known as the gonadotropin releasing hormone (GnRH) and, in later years, analogues known as GnRH analogues were made which were capable of suppressing ovarian function.

Much has been learned from neuroendocrinology. In the past the pituitary was seen as the master gland, but later on the hypothalamus was recognized as the conductor, exerting its influence through neurotransmitters by a portal vessel network.

From elegant studies in the monkey[37] and the human[38], much insight is now available into the neuroendocrine control of the menstrual cycle.

Gonadotropin production

It has been documented that gonadotropin is produced throughout fetal life, childhood and into adult life[39]. GnRH is detectable in the hypothalamus as early as 10 weeks of gestation and, by 10–13 weeks, FSH and LH are being produced in the pituitary. Peak fetal concentrations of FSH and

30. Jensen, E.V. and De Sombre, E.R. (1973). Estrogen-receptor interaction. *Science*, **182**, 126

31. Walters, M.R. (1985). Steroid hormone receptors and the nucleus. *Endocrinol. Rev.*, **6**, 5121

32. Robson, G. A., Butcher, R.W. and Sutherland, E. W. (1968). Cyclic AMP. *Ann. Rev. Biochem.*, **37**, 149

33. Scott, F.H. (1905). On the metabolism and action of nerve cells. *Brain*, **28**, 506

34. Green, H.P. and Harris, G.W. (1947). The neurovascular link between the neurohypophysis and adenohypophysis. *J. Endocrinol.*, **5**, 136

35. Burgus, R., Butcher, M., Ling, N., Monahan, M., Rivier, J., Fellows, R., Amoss, M., Blackwell, R., Vale, W. and Guillemin, R. (1971). Structure moléculaire du facteur hypothalamique (LRF) d'origine ovine, contrôlant la secretion de l'hormone Gonadotrope Hypophysaire de Luteinisation (LH). *Comptes Rendus de l'Académie des Sciences (Paris)*, **273**, 1611

36. Matsuo, H., Baba, Y., Nair, R.M.G. and Schally, A.V. (1971). Structure of the porcine LH- and FSH - releasing hormone. *Biochem. Biophys. Res. Commun.*, **43**, 1334

37. Knobil, E. (1980). The neuroendocrine control of the menstrual cycle. *Rec. Progr. Horm. Res.*, **36**, 53

38. Yen, S.S.C. and Lein, A. (1976). The apparent paradox of the negative and positive feedback control system on gonadotropin secretion. *Am. J. Obstet. Gynecol.*, **126**, 942

39. Kaplan, S.L., Grunbach, M.M. and Aubert, M.L. (1976). The ontogenesis of pituitary hormones and hypothalamic factors in the human fetus: maturation of central nervous system regulation of anterior pituitary function. *Rec. Prog. Horm. Res.*, **32**, 161

40. Baker, T.G. (1963). A quantitative and cytological study of germ cells in human ovaries. *Proc. R. Soc. Lond. (Biol.)*, **158**, 417

41. Boyar, R., Finkelstein, J., Roffwarg, H., Kapen, S., Weitzmann, E. and Hellman, L. (1972). Synchronization of augmented luteinizing hormone secretion with sleep during puberty. *N. Engl. J. Med.*, **287**, 582

LH occur at about 20 weeks and, remarkably, these levels are high and similar to those which occur postmenopause. It is challenging to combine these hormonal findings with the enormous quantity of germ cells which reach their nadir at the 5th month[40] (see figure below).

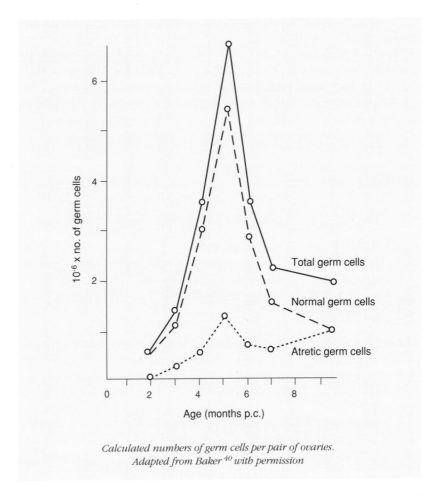

Calculated numbers of germ cells per pair of ovaries. Adapted from Baker [40] with permission

Puberty is linked with the development of episodic LH secretion associated with sleep. The rise of gonadotropins at puberty seems to be independent of the gonadal steroids because the augmented gonadotropin secretion during sleep[41] is also seen in adolescent girls with Turner's syndrome. Thus, maturation at puberty must involve changes in the hypothalamus independent of ovarian steroids.

The concept of the feto-placental unit

The existence of a feto-placental unit for steroid biosynthesis was outlined by Diczfalusy[42,43]. The fetus is able to synthesize cholesterol *de novo* from acetate[44,45]. From cholesterol, the placenta covers the various steps to progesterone. The fetus can transform progesterone into 17-hydroxyprogesterone, hydrocortisone or deoxycorticosterone, corticosterone and aldosterone. The fetus can also initiate the pathways for conversion of cholesterol to dehydroepiandrosterone sulfate (DHEAS). From DHEAS, the placenta converts this androgen precursor into estrogens, of which estriol is the main metabolite excreted in the urine of the mother. The measurement of steroids produced only by the fetus or placenta was expected to give an accurate description of fetal state. But, apart from the lack of estrogen production, the technology of electronic fetal monitoring, ultrasound and amniotic fluid analysis overruled this expectation. Nevertheless, endocrine studies on the feto-placental unit went in parallel with those on the steroidogenesis of the human ovary, which was completely described by the group of Kenneth J. Ryan[46].

Menstrual bleeding

Apart from all our knowledge of hormones, we still do not know much on the precise mechanisms of menstrual bleeding. Markee (1940)[47] studied the menstrual process by transplanting endometrium into the anterior eye chamber of monkeys. He noted that regression of the endometrium was more important for tissue shrinkage than shedding. He described this process as vasoconstriction.

We can now assume that prostaglandins, especially the 2-alpha type, might be the vasoconstrictor acting locally on uterine arteries. Hemostasis is also attained through the formation of hemostatic thrombi[48].

Epilogue

Detailed information is now available on the processes that regulate the menstrual cycle. The ovary, the pituitary and the hypothalamus are recognized as one unit that acts through endocrine, paracrine and autocrine mechanisms. The key events of the regulatory mechanisms are now known. FSH initiates the cycle in response to the estrogen–progesterone ratios of the preceding cycle. From there on, estrogens produced in the follicles maintain follicular sensitivity to FSH by increasing the number of receptors.

Granulosa cells and theca cells work together in steroidogenesis. With high estrogen concentrations, the follicle becomes receptive to LH and finally ovulation is triggered by the LH peak (preceded by a rapid increase of estrogens and progesterone). The corpus luteum also produces estrogens and progesterone and has a life span of its own. Regression of the corpus luteum, in the case where no pregnancy follows, is induced by its own estrogen production and a local luteolytic effect. The tropic hormones are triggered by hormones released from the hypothalamus.

Tropic hormones (FSH, LH, thyroid stimulating hormone and hCG) share a common alpha-chain, a structure of 92 amino acids. The beta-chains differ

42. Diczfalusy, E. (1962). Endocrinology of the foetus. *Acta Obstet. Gynecol. Scand.*, **41** (suppl. 1), 45

43. Diczfalusy, E. (1964). Endocrinological functions of the human foeto-placental unit. *Fed. Proc.*, **23**, 791

44. Mathur, R.S., Archer, D.F., Wiqvist, N. and Diczfalusy, E. (1970). Quantitative assessment of the de novo sterol and steroid synthesis in the human foeto-placental unit. I. Synthesis and secretion of cholesterol and cholesterol sulphate. *Acta Endocrinol.*, **65**, 663

45. Leusden, H.A. van, Siemerink, M., Telegdy, G. and Diczfalusy, E. (1971). Squalene and lanosterol synthesis in the foeto-placental unit at midgestation. *Acta Endocrinol.*, **66**, 711

46. McNatty, K.P., Makris, A., De Grazia, C., Osathanondh, R. and Ryan, K.J. (1979). The production of progesterone, androgens and estrogens by granulosa cells, thecal tissue and stromal tissue from human ovaries in vitro. *J. Clin. Endocrinol. Metab.*, **49**, 687

47. Markee, J.E. (1940). Menstruation in intraocular endometrial transplants in the rhesus monkey. *Contr. Embryol. Carneg. Inst.*, **28**, 219

48. Christiaens, G.C.M.L., Sixma, J.J. and Haspels, A.A. (1980). Morphology of haemostasis in menstrual endometrium.
Br. J. Obstet. Gynaecol.,
87, 425

in amino acid and carbohydrate content and are specific for the ability of the hormone to fit on the receptor. Beta hCG has a large beta-subunit containing a large carbohydrate moiety and 145–150 amino-acids with a unique terminal tail of 28–30 amino acids. This part of the molecule was particularly important in that it allowed the production of highly specific antibodies and radio-immunological assays.

We now know that the tropic hormones are heterogeneous, that they can regulate receptors up and down and that they can regulate adenylate cyclase, the enzyme involved in ATP and cyclic AMP.

All this research, performed by many devoted scientists, has led to numerous applications in reproductive medicine, ranging from the treatment of infertility to oral contraception.

Summary of references

1. Treloar, A.E., Boynton, R.E., Behn, B.G. and Brown, B.W. (1967). Variation of the human menstrual cycle through reproductive life. *Int. J. Fertil.,* **12**, 77

2. Hitschmann, F. and Adler, L. (1908). Der Bau der Uterusschleimhaut des geschlechtsreifen Weibes besonderer Berücksichtigung der Menstruation. *Mschr. Geburt. Gynäk.,* **27,** 1

3. Stockard, C.R. and Papanicoloaou, G.N. (1917). The existence of a typical oestrus cycle in the guinea-pig; with the study of its histological and physiological changes. *Am. J. Anat.,* **22**, 225

4. Battey, R. (1872). Normal ovariotomy. *Atlanta Med. Surg. J.,* **10**, 321

5. Vesalius, A. (1543). De Humani Corporis Fabrica

6. De Graaf, R. (1672). *De mulierum organis generationi inservientibus.* Lugduni Batavorum, *ex. off.* Hackiana

7. Berthold, A.A. (1849). Transplantation der Hoden. *Arch. Anat. Physiol. wiss Med.,* 42–6

8. Knauer, E. (1896). Einige Versuche über Ovarientransplantation beim Kaninchen. *Zentralblatt. Gynäkol.,* **20**, 524

9. Bayliss, W.M. and Starling, E.H. (1904). The chemical regulation of the secretory process. *Proc. R. Soc. Ser. B.,* **73**, 310

10. Velde Th. H. van de (1904). Ueber den Zusamnenhang zwischen Ovarialfunktion, Wellenbewegung und Menstrualblutung und ueber die Entstehung des sogenannten Mittelschmerzes. (Haarlem, The Netherlands: De Erven F. Bohn)

11. Ogino, K. (1930). Ovulationstermin und Konzeptionstermin. *Zentralbl. Gynäkol.,* **54**, 469

12. Knaus, H. (1929). Eine neue Methode zur Bestimmung des Ovulationstermines. *Zentralbl. Gynäkol.,* **53**, 2193

13. Zondek, B. and Aschheim, S. (1926). Zur funktion des Ovariums. *Klin. Wochenschr.,* **10**, 400

14. Marshall, F.H.A. and Jolly, W.A. (1905). Contributions to the physiology of mammalian reproduction. II. The ovary as an organ of internal secretion. *Philos. Trans. R. Soc. Lond. Ser. B.,* **198**, 123

15. Fraenkel, L. (1903). Die Funktion des Corpus Luteum. *Arch. Gynäk.*, **68**, 438

16. Corner, G. and Allen, W.M. (1929). Physiology of the corpus luteum. *Am. J. Physiol.*, **88**, 326

17. Butenandt, A. and Schmidt, J. (1934). Überführung des Pregnandiols in Corpus-Luteum-Hormon. *Berichte d. D. Chem. Gesellschaft,* **67**, 1901

18. Marrian, G.F. (1930). The chemistry of oestrin. III. An approved method of preparation and the isolation of active crystalline material. *Biochem. J.,* **24**, 435

19. Butenandt, A.F.J. (1934). Neuere Ergebnisse auf dem Gebiet der Sexualhormone. *Wien. Klin. Wschr.,* **47**, 897

20. Adler, L. (1912). Zur Physiologie und Pathologie der Ovarial-funktion. *Arch. Gynäk.*, **95**, 349

21. Stockard, C.R. and Papanicolaou, G.N. (1917). The existence of a typical estrous cycle in the guinea pig – with a study of its histological and physiological changes. *Am. J. Anat.*, **22**, 225

22. Allen, E. and Doisy, E.A. (1923). An ovarian hormone. Preliminary report on its localization, extraction and partial purification. *J. Am. Med. Assoc.*, **81**, 819

23. Brown, J.B. (1955). Urinary excretion of oestrogen during the menstrual cycle. *Lancet,* **I**, 320

24. Klopper, A. (1957). The excretion of pregnanediol during the normal menstrual cycle. *J. Obstet. Gynaecol. Br. Emp.*, **64**, 504

25. Aschheim, S. and Zondek, B. (1927). Hypophysenvorderlappen-hor mon und ovarial hormon im Harn von Schwangeren. *Klin.Wochenschr.*, **28**, 1322

26. Li, C.H., Simpson, M.E., Evans, H.M. *et al.* (1940). Interstitial cell stimulating hormone. II. Method of preparation and some physico-chemical studies. *Endocrinology*, **27**, 803

27. Li, C.H., Simpson, M.E. and Evans, H.M. (1949). Isolation of pituitary follicle-stimulating hormone (FSH). *Science*, **109**, 445

28. Stevens, V.C. (1967). In Bell, E.T. and Loraine, J.A.(eds.) *Recent Research on Gonadotropic Hormones*, p.223. (Edinburgh: Churchill Livingstone)

29. Yalow, R.S. and Berson, S.A. (1960). Immunoassay of endogenous plasma insulin in man. *J. Clin. Invest,* **39**, 1157

30. Jensen, E.V. and De Sombre, E.R. (1973). Estrogen–receptor interaction. *Science,* **182**, 126

31. Walters, M.R. (1985). Steroid hormone receptors and the nucleus. *Endocrinol. Rev.,* **6**, 5121

32. Robson, G.A., Butcher, R.W. and Sutherland, E.W. (1968). Cyclic AMP. *Ann. Rev. Biochem.,* **37**, 149

33. Scott, F.H. (1905). On the metabolism and action of nerve cells. *Brain,* **28**, 506

34. Green, H.P. and Harris, G.W. (1947). The neurovascular link between the neurohypophysis and adenohypophysis. *J. Endocrinol.,* **5**, 136

35. Burgus, R., Butcher, M., Ling, N., Monahan, M., Rivier, J., Fellows, R., Amoss, M., Blackwell, R., Vale, W. and Guillemin, R. (1971). Structure moléculaire du facteur hypothalamique (LRF) d'origine ovine, contrôlant la secretion de l'hormone Gonadotrope Hypophysaire de Luteinisation (LH). *Comptes Rendus de l'Académie des Sciences* (*Paris*), **273**, 1611

36. Matsuo, H., Baba, Y., Nair, R.M.G. and Schally, A.V. (1971). Structure of the porcine LH- and FSH-releasing hormone. *Biochem. Biophys. Res. Commun.*, **43**, 1334

37. Knobil, E. (1980). The neuroendocrine control of the menstrual cycle. *Rec. Progr. Horm. Res.*, **36**, 53

38. Yen, S.S.C. and Lein, A. (1976). The apparent paradox of the negative and positive feedback control system on gonadotropin secretion. *Am. J. Obstet. Gynecol.*, **126**, 942

39. Kaplan, S.L., Grunbach, M.M. and Aubert, M.L. (1976). The ontogenesis of pituitary hormones and hypothalamic factors in the human fetus: maturation of central nervous system regulation of anterior pituitary function. *Rec. Prog. Horm. Res.*, **32**, 161

40. Baker, T.G. (1963). A quantitative and cytological study of germ cells in human ovaries. *Proc. R. Soc. Lond. (Biol.)*, **158**, 417

41. Boyar, R., Finkelstein, J., Roffwarg, H., Kapen, S., Weitzmann, E. and Hellman, L. (1972). Synchronization of augmented luteinizing hormone secretion with sleep during puberty. *N. Engl. J. Med.*, **287**, 582

42. Diczfalusy, E. (1962). Endocrinology of the foetus. *Acta Obstet. Gynecol. Scand.*, **41** (suppl. 1), 45

43. Diczfalusy, E. (1964). Endocrinological functions of the human foeto-placental unit. *Fed. Proc.*, **23**, 791

44. Mathur, R.S., Archer, D.F., Wiqvist, N. and Diczfalusy, E. (1970). Quantitative assessment of the de novo sterol and steroid synthesis in the human foeto-placental unit. I. Synthesis and secretion of cholesterol and cholesterol sulphate. *Acta Endocrinol.*, **65**, 663

45. Leusden, H.A. van, Siemerink, M., Telegdy, G. and Diczfalusy, E. (1971). Squalene and lanosterol synthesis in the foeto-placental unit at midgestation. *Acta Endocrinol.*, **66**, 711

46. McNatty, K.P., Makris, A., De Grazia, C., Osathanondh, R. and Ryan, K.J. (1979). The production of progesterone, androgens and estrogens by granulosa cells, thecal tissue and stromal tissue from human ovaries in vitro. *J. Clin. Endocrinol. Metab.*, **49**, 687

47. Markee, J.E. (1940). Menstruation in intraocular endometrial transplants in the rhesus monkey. *Contr. Embryol. Carneg. Inst.*, **28**, 219

48. Christiaens, G.C.M.L., Sixma, J.J. and Haspels, A.A. (1980). Morphology of haemostasis in menstrual endometrium. *Br. J. Obstet. Gynaecol.*, **87**, 425

THE TREATMENT OF INFERTILITY

Classic Paper No.9

Amenorrhea associated with bilateral polycystic ovaries

IRVING F. STEIN AND MICHAEL L. LEVENTHAL

Michael Reese Hospital and Northwestern University Medical School

1. Stein, I.F. and Leventhal, M.L.(1935). Amenorrhea associated with bilateral polycystic ovaries. *Am. J. Obstet. Gynecol.,* **29**, 181

Stein and Leventhal read a paper in 1935 at the meeting of the Central Association of Obstetricians and Gynecologists describing seven cases of women suffering from menstrual disorders, hirsutism and infertility. The ovaries were found to be from two to four times the normal size. The ovarian cortex was hypertrophied with a thick tunica. Wedge resection of the ovaries was recommended. The Stein–Leventhal syndrome now is replaced by the terminology of the Polycystic Ovarian (PCO) syndrome. The prevalence of PCO is approximately one in every 35 females of the reproductive age group. Fertility drugs are now widely used for treatment of infertile couples with *in vitro* fertilization as the last step, mainly due to the increasing age group of infertile women. The ethical issues raised by artificial procreation will probably be a challenge for many years to come.

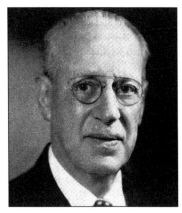

I.F. Stein
Reprinted with permission of Macmillan Publishing Company from Obstetric and Gynecologic Milestones by Harold Speert, MD. Copyright © 1958 Harold Speert, MD.

AMENORRHEA ASSOCIATED WITH BILATERAL
POLYCYSTIC OVARIES*

Irving F. Stein, M.D., and Michael L. Leventhal, M.D.,
Chicago, Ill.

(From Michael Reese Hospital and Northwestern University Medical School)

ACCORDING to leading authoritative works on gynecology, the bilateral polycystic ovary is most commonly found in association with *uterine bleeding* (Fig. 1). This association has been recognized by the medical profession and is not infrequent in occurrence. Endometrial hyperplasia, multiple follicle cysts with granulosa cell lining, and a notable absence of corpora lutea in the ovary are the significant pathologic findings in such cases. The bleeding in these patients is readily explained by the fact that the increase in number of follicles lined by granulosa cells produces an excess of secretion of estrogenic hormone.

According to the same authoritative works, little or no mention is made of bilateral polycystic ovaries accompanied by *amenorrhea,* and inasmuch as we have encountered a series of cases exemplifying the latter conditions, we desire to present the results of our study of them.

Cyst formation in the follicular apparatus of the ovary is very common and is regarded to some extent as a physiologic process. When these structures are visible to the naked eye, they are regarded as cysts; when not, they are called follicles. When this process becomes excessive, persistent or progressive, the ovary becomes enlarged, tense, tender and painful, and produces what has been termed "cystic degen-

*Read at a meeting of the Central Association of Obstetricians and Gynecologists, November 1 to 3, 1934, New Orleans, La.

eration of the ovary,'' and is usually bilateral. The exact cause of this formation is still in doubt; formerly, it was regarded as the result of inflammatory change due to either local infection or that from some distant focus. More recent observations and experiments point to an endocrine causal relationship of the polycystic changes in the ovaries. Furthermore, there are usually no adhesions or other gross or microscopic evidences of inflammation in the ovaries found in these cases. In the series of patients which we observed with bilateral polycystic ovaries and amenorrhea, the ovaries were found to be from two to four times the normal size and while they often maintained their original shape, they were sometimes distinctly globular. In one case, they were flat and soft, the so-called ''oyster ovaries.'' The ovarian cortex was found to be hypertrophied in all of the cases and the tunica thickened, tough, and fibrotic.

The cysts were follicle cysts, near the surface, and almost entirely confined to the cortex, and they contained clear fluid. There were

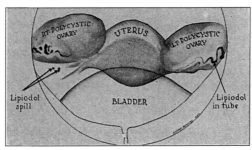

Fig. 1.

from twenty to one hundred cysts in each ovary, varying in size from 1 mm. to about 1.5 cm., but rarely larger. The color of the ovary was oyster gray with bluish areas where the cysts were superficial and appeared on the surface as sago-like bodies. On section, the variation in size of the cysts and the clear fluid contents were revealed. Corpora lutea were sometimes absent and when found, they were very small and deeply placed.

The uteri in these patients were either normal in size or smaller and firmer than normal. The remaining changes observed were those involving the secondary sex characteristics. The breasts presented no characteristic changes except in cases of long-standing amenorrhea when they were small, firm, and pale.

In some patients, there was observed a distinct tendency toward masculinizing changes. A typical rhomboid hairy escutcheon, hair on the face, arms, and legs, and coarse skin was noted. No voice changes have been observed by us. The external genitals in most patients were normal, but in some, the labia minora and clitoris were markedly hypertrophied. Libido is apparently not affected by the changes noted in the ovaries.

CASE REPORTS

CASE 1.—M. G., aged twenty-two, married one and one-half years, gravida o, was first seen Oct. 3, 1928. Her chief complaints were sterility and amenorrhea. Menses began at age of thirteen, irregular, two to seven months, five-day duration, moderate, no pain. She was treated with estrogenic preparations, intramuscularly; she then menstruated irregularly every six or eight weeks; small doses of thyroid extract and calcium were given.

November, 1929: Menstruated about every seven weeks. Examination revealed moderate obesity and slight struma. Bimanual examination: Uterus was 2° retroverted, normal size; right ovary palpable and cystic. January, 1930: Transabdominal pneumoperitoneum (Fig. 2), revealed bilateral cystic ovaries, each ovary appearing as large as the uterine fundus. Operation: May 2, 1930, laparotomy. Uterus was small and both ovaries were polycystic and enlarged, the right more so than the

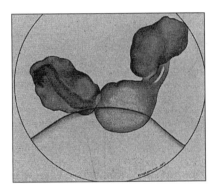 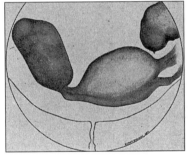

Fig. 2.   Fig. 3.

left. The left also contained a small fibroma. Wedge-resection of both ovaries. Uneventful recovery; discharged from the hospital on the twelfth postoperative day.

Forty-eight hours after operation, slight uterine bleeding occurred, and normal menstrual periods occurred monthly thereafter. Patient became pregnant in October, 1930, and again in February, 1933; both pregnancies were carried to full term and delivered normally. Menstruation since confinement is entirely normal, every twenty-eight days. August, 1934: Follow-up examination showed the uterus and both ovaries to be normal.

Pathologic Report.—Gross: Sections from both ovaries showed numerous cystic cavities varying from 1 mm. to 1 cm. in size. Ovarian tunic was thickened and fibrous. Microscopic: Thick tunic, many cysts varying in size, lined by theca cells; one normally developing graafian follicle; corpus albicans; old corpus luteum; tortuous and dilated blood vessels.

CASE 2.—B. K., aged twenty-nine, married five years, gravida o, was admitted to the hospital Aug. 10, 1931. Her chief complaints were sterility and amenorrhea. Menses began at the age of fifteen, were irregular for several months; no menses *for eight years* prior to first examination. Menstruated twice last year (under our observation) after treatment with estrogenic hormone, intramuscularly. Physical examination: Rigid type; tight coarse skin, hairy face, arms, and legs; masculine escutcheon. Transabdominal pneumoperitoneum; bilateral cystic ovaries almost as large as uterine fundus (Fig. 3). Operation: Wedge-resection of two-thirds to three-fourths of each ovary. Uneventful recovery. Discharged from hospital on thirteenth postoperative day.

Patient has menstruated regularly every twenty-eight days since operation. Follow-up examination in May, 1933: uterus and both ovaries normal; secondary sex characters evidence little improvement; no pregnancy to date.*

Pathologic Report.—Gross: Thick tunic, numerous cystic cavities up to 1 cm. in diameter near surface of ovary (Fig. 4). Microscopic: Tunic thick and fibrous; numerous cysts varying in size, lined by hypertrophied theca layer. Granulosa cells were scarce. Small (old) corpora albicantia. No corpora lutea.

CASE 3.—L. C., aged twenty-one, married two years, gravida o, was first seen April 24, 1929. Her chief complaints were amenorrhea and sterility. Menses began at the age of thirteen, were always irregular, one- to nine-month intervals, usually six months, lasting for five or six days, scant; no pain. Treatment was

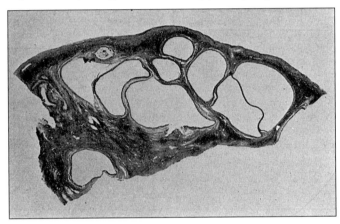

Fig. 4.—Photomicrograph (6 diameters) of section of wedge removed from ovary (Case 2).

given over a period of four years with estrogenic hormone preparations, intramuscularly, and thyroid extract by mouth. In December, 1929, patient had x-ray stimulation of ovaries with no results. In October, 1931, she became pregnant, and was delivered of a normal child at term, August, 1932. Following this, she had four normal periods at regular intervals followed by amenorrhea of one year and nine months. During this time, she was treated with estrogenic hormone preparations without benefit. Examination revealed a short, well-proportioned young woman; breasts normal, masculine escutcheon, long labia minora and hypertrophied clitoris. Bimanual examination showed normal sized uterus, both ovaries enlarged, globular and tender.

July 6, 1933: Transabdominal pneumoperitoneum and intrauterine lipiodol instillation showed both ovaries enlarged and elongated; tubes patent. Uterine contour was normal (Fig. 5). Oct. 14, 1933: Operation: Bilateral wedge-resection of about three-fourths of both ovaries, each of which was 5 by 7 cm. in diameter; the capsule was very thick and leathery. Uneventful postoperative course; discharged from hospital on twelfth day. Patient menstruated forty-eight hours after opera-

---

*This patient is now (Jan. 30, 1935) three months pregnant.

tion and has had regular monthly periods for the past year. Check-up examination in September, 1934, showed the uterus and both ovaries normal to palpation.

Pathologic Report.—Gross: Thick tunic; numerous cysts up to 1 cm. in diameter. Microscopic: Moderately thick tunic; numerous cysts, some lined with granulosa cells, others with theca cells; some corpora albicantia; no corpora lutea; tortuous, large and thickened blood vessels.

CASE 4.—H. W., aged twenty-three, married three years, gravida o, was first examined Jan. 3, 1933. Her chief complaints were sterility and amenorrhea, Menses began at the age of fifteen, were irregular, one to six months, usually three to four months; three- to four-day duration; profuse with clots and cramps. Last menstruation occurred six months previous to admission. No contraception for two years. Treated with estrogenic hormone intramuscularly and orally. Examination: Patient was large, obese with feminine escutcheon and large flabby breasts. Uterus normal; palpable left ovary was enlarged and cystic. Feb. 15, 1933: Transuterine pneumoperitoneum and lipiodol instillation showed the uterus to be normal in size; both ovaries were enlarged and cystic; fallopian tubes were patent (Fig. 6). Mar. 11, 1933: Operation: Bilateral wedge-resection of ovaries which were so large that

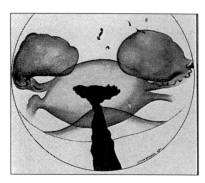 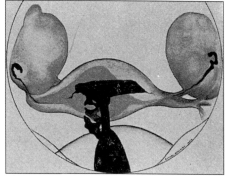

Fig. 5. Fig. 6.

more than three-fourths of each was removed, leaving the hilus approximately the size of a normal ovary.

The patient made an uneventful recovery and was discharged on the tenth post-operative day. She menstruated on the sixth day and regularly every twenty-eight days thereafter for the past year and one-half. Bimanual examination in March, 1934, revealed a normal genital status.

Pathologic Report.—Gross: Each section showed several cysts up to 1.5 cm. in diameter. Microscopic: The ovary appeared normal; tunica moderately thickened and below were multiple small cysts; some lined with granulosa cells, others with theca cells. Normal cystic follicles; small corpora albicantia; cluster of granulosa cells evidently the edge of a normal follicle. No corpora lutea. In one portion was a small papillary cystadenoma. Tortuous and thickened blood vessels.

CASE 5.—O. B., aged twenty-five, married one and one-half years, gravida o, was first seen in the clinic Jan. 9, 1933. Her chief complaints were irregular menses and sterility. Menses began at the age of fifteen, two- to three-month intervals, painful, duration three days. Last menstruation Dec. 29, 1932. Examination: Male escutcheon, hairy thighs, breasts normal. Bimanual: Cystic swelling of right ovary palpable, but not left. Uterus was small. Transuterine pneumoperitoneum and lipiodol instillation: Both ovaries cystic; right larger than left; tubes patent to gas and filled with lipiodol (Fig. 7). Operation: Wedge-resection of one-half to two-thirds of both ovaries which were polycystic; the uterus was found to be small, firm, and slightly bicornuate.

Uneventful postoperative course; patient was discharged on the tenth day. Menstruation occurred on the fourth postoperative day, and regularly each month thereafter. Follow-up examination in September, 1934; uterus and ovaries found normal on palpation.

Pathologic Report.—Gross: Thick tunic; numerous cysts varying in size up to 1.5 cm. Hemorrhagic stroma. Microscopic: Moderately thickened tunic; recent corpus luteum with hemorrhagic corpus luteum cyst; many cysts lined by theca cells. Large corpus albicans; edematous vascular stroma with hemorrhage.

CASE 6.—E. A., aged thirty-three, married fifteen years, gravida ii, was admitted to the hospital Oct. 23, 1933. Her chief complaints were irregular menses for nine years, abnormal hairy growth for three years, and pain in groin for three years. Menses began at the age of twelve, regular until ten years ago, since then, five- to nine-month intervals, becoming longer. Menses were scant, lasting three or four days with no pain. Hairy growth on face, back, arms, and legs for past three years,

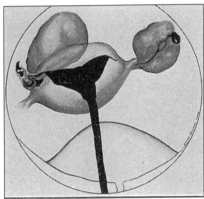

Fig. 7.

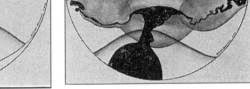

Fig. 8.

becoming more noticeable. Pain in both lower quadrants for three years, with lower abdominal pain accompanying the menstrual moliminia even in the absence of bleeding. Gained 15 pounds in past year; weight, 175. Examination: short, obese, male escutcheon, hair on body and face; pendulous breasts. Uterus normal in size; both ovaries enlarged, cystic, tender. Transuterine pneumoperitoneum and lipiodol instillation: Both ovaries were enlarged, uterus was normal, and fallopian tubes were patent (Fig. 8). Operation: Bilateral wedge-resection of about one-half of each ovary, which contained multiple cortical cysts.

Uneventful recovery, discharged on thirteenth postoperative day. Uterine bleeding occurred on fifth postoperative day and menstruation recurred monthly thereafter (eleven months). Follow-up examination in June, 1934: No evidence of reformation of cysts, genital status normal.

Pathologic Report.—Gross: Thick tunic; numerous cystic cavities varying in size up to 1.5 cm. Microscopic: Tunic thickened in some sections and normal in others. Normal follicle with maturating ovum near surface. Large theca cyst with corpus albicans; recent corpus luteum.

CASE 7.—M. B., aged twenty, single, was admitted to the hospital Aug. 29, 1933. Her chief complaints were amenorrhea and pain in both lower quadrants for one year. Menses began at fourteen years of age, always irregular, six weeks to four months, usually two months, seven-day duration, moderate, occasional clots, no dysmenorrhea. Physical examination revealed a tall, thin girl, with muddy complexion; facial acne; scant breast development. Rectal examination showed the uterus to be erect, and of normal size. The left ovary was cystic and from 7 to 8 cm. in length. The right ovary was cystic and 5 cm. long. Transabdominal pneumoperitoneum on Aug. 30, 1933. Bilateral polycystic ovaries, each as large as the normal uterine fundus (Fig. 9). Operation: Wedge-resection of the cystic portion of each ovary. Patient made an uneventful recovery and was discharged from the hospital on the ninth postoperative day. Menstruation has been regular since operation, and pain has been relieved. Patient was married a few months after operation and has remained in good health. She has moved to a distant city and reported in October, 1934, that she was in good health and that menstruation had recurred monthly.

Pathologic Report.—Gross: Sections of ovaries showed numerous cysts; and hemorrhagic and edematous stroma. Microscopic: Moderately thickened tunic; large corpus luteum cyst; numerous cysts lined by theca cells; follicle cysts with granulosa cell lining. Corpora albicantia; dilated blood vessels and very vascular stroma.

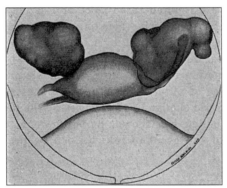

Fig. 9.

DIAGNOSIS AND TREATMENT

The diagnosis of polycystic ovaries is made only after careful and repeated examinations. The history of irregular menses with or without pain gives little clue to the ovarian condition and a bimanual or rectal examination may not always reveal the presence of polycystic ovaries. Due to the fact that the ovaries often show transient enlargements incident to physiologic changes, one must not arrive at hasty judgments. Furthermore, in cases of flat "oyster ovaries," it is sometimes difficult to palpate the pathologic enlargement. Conflicting opinions are not infrequent concerning the presence of these swellings.

The diagnosis is greatly enhanced in cases of ovarian swellings by the use of pneumoroentgenography, as one of us has previously described. We been able to demonstrate the bilateral ovarian enlargements by this method when palpatory findings were doubtful or disputed. The shadow of the normal ovary usually appears on the film to be about one-fourth of the size of that of the uterine corpus. When the ovary is polycystic, it appears from three-fourths to as large as the uterine shadow. This method of diagnosis has been of especial value when there was a difference of opinion concerning the presence of ovarian pathology. The film evidence is convincing as may be seen in the accompanying illustrations. After using pneumoroentgenographic diagnosis for more than ten years, we feel that we are qualified to endorse it as a most valuable aid in gynecology, and especially so in recognizing relatively small ovarian swellings which may escape detection on bimanual examination.

The treatment of amenorrhea and sterility in the group of patients under consideration was at first conservative, using endocrine preparations; eventually the treatment became surgical. In some of the earlier cases, injections of various endocrine preparations were made in an effort to adjust the menstrual cycle. Estrogenic hormone preparations which were reputed to be more or less potent were administered intramuscularly. Uterine bleeding occurred as a result of this treatment in some instances, but it is impossible to say whether this was true menstruation or anovular bleeding. At any rate, no lasting restoration of function followed these treatments and no pregnancies occurred. The use of anterior pituitary-like substances was avoided in order that a cystic change in the ovaries might not be thereby provoked, for, as Zondek has shown, hyperhormonal amenorrhea with overstimulation of the graafian follicles can be produced by the injection of prolan.

In the patients referred to in this series, we have resected from one-half to three-fourths of each ovary by wedge-resection, thereby removing the cortex containing the cysts, and have sutured the hilus with the finest catgut. The immediate results have been entirely satisfactory. All of the patients recovered uneventfully, and were discharged from the hospital from the ninth to the thirteenth postoperative days. Uterine bleeding occurred on the third to the fifth postoperative day and menstruation occurred monthly thereafter in every case. Our first patient, operated upon four years ago, has given birth to two children since operation.

DISCUSSION

The ovarian change in bilateral cystic ovaries is most probably a *result* of some hormonal stimulation and very likely relates to the anterior lobe of the pituitary gland. Geist reported fifty cases in which "antuitrin-S" was injected in large doses a few days prior to operation for fibroids. At operation, the ovaries showed definite changes. While the follicles did not grow in size, they were greatly increased in number. Geist described the additional changes in the ovary which varied in intensity in direct relationship to the amount of hormone injected. He quotes the work of Mandelstamm and Tschackowsky who likewise produced polycystic ovaries in women by the use of anterior pituitary-like substances.

Oddly enough, the surgical treatment directed to the ovary in our series adjusted the endocrine balance to the extent of restoring normal menstruation and the reproductive function. Theoretically, one would expect that if the cystic portion of the ovary were removed without also removing the abnormal stimulus which produced the ovarian change, the same factors would still be operative, resulting in reformation of the polycystic change. Thus far, this has not been our experience although we have observed our patients over a period of from one to four years since operation.

Whenever one attempts to correlate the function or dysfunction with the structure of any of the endocrine glands, one is apt to encounter grave difficulties, due to the recognized instability of the normal anatomy of all glands of internal secretion. The association of amenorrhea with polycystic ovaries in our series is no exception to this statement. The pathologist is unable to conclude from a study of the sections taken from the ovaries in our patients that amenorrhea was a symptom. He can demonstrate no anatomic structure or characteristic change in the ovary which enables him to describe the clinical picture. The only consistent pathologic finding is the presence of follicle cysts lined by theca cells (Table I). The fact remains, however, that when we remove the cystic portion of the ovaries which to all appearances are the same as those observed in patients with uterine bleeding, normal function is restored to the sex apparatus.

It is unlikely that polycystic ovaries are congenital for the condition develops as a rule after the patient has menstruated more or less regularly for a period of years. The amenorrhea is usually secondary. It is also unlikely, for reasons stated above, that the multiple cyst formation is explained on the basis of inflammatory change. That hormones play a rôle in the polycystic change in the ovaries is extremely plausible in the light of our present-day conception of sex physiology. Whether it results from an excessive production of anterior pituitary sex hormone or not is debatable.

It is reasonable to assume that a *mechanical* factor operates actually to produce the most significant symptoms, namely: amenorrhea and sterility. The overproduction of cystic follicles which crowd the ovarian cortex but which do not rupture on the surface of the ovary, together with the presence of a thickened tunic, prevents the immature follicles from ripening and reaching the surface. It is possible that some of these follicles develop, and being impeded in their pathway to the surface of the ovary, may rupture into the cysts. We have ob-

TABLE I. BILATERAL POLYCYSTIC OVARIES WITH AMENORRHEA. HISTOPATHOLOGIC FINDINGS

	TUNICA	STROMA	BLOOD VESSELS	NORMAL FOLLICLES	FOLLICLE CYSTS THECA	FOLLICLE CYSTS GRANULOSA	CORPORA LUTEA	CORPORA ALBICANTIA	TUMOR
1	Thick		Tortuous Distended	Few	Many		Recent	Many, old	
2	Thick		Tortuous Thick		Many			Few, old, small	
3	Thick				Many	Few		Few, small	
4	Normal to moderately thick		Tortuous Distended	One in section	Many			Many, small	Early papillary cystadenoma
5	Moderately thick	Edematous Vascular	Hyperplasia		Many	Few	Recent with c.l. cyst	Large, recent cyst	
6	Normal to moderately thick			Few	Many	Few	One, recent	Many	
7	Moderately thick	Vascular	Dilated		Many		c.l. cyst	Many	

served, in one of our sections, a normal maturing follicle just below and adjacent to a thin-walled theca cyst, so situated that if the follicle ruptured at all, its contained ovum would be discharged into the cyst cavity. This may account for the finding of small corpora lutea and albicantia even in the absence of menstruation. Ordinarily no corpora lutea would be formed unless the graafian follicles reached the surface of the ovary and ruptured. In further substantiation of the mechanical theory, we observed that by removing the cystic cortex which formed the barrier, physiologic function was restored. Apparently the incisional scar in the ovary is of no significance.

SUMMARY AND CONCLUSIONS

1. A series of seven cases is herewith reported in which amenorrhea was associated with the presence of bilateral polycystic ovaries.

2. Bilateral polycystic ovaries are most likely the result of hormonal influences and not the result of inflammatory change.

3. The diagnosis of ovarian pathology is greatly facilitated by the use of pneumoroentgenography.

4. The treatment of the amenorrhea with estrogenic hormone in the patients referred to proved unsatisfactory.

5. Surgical treatment, consisting of wedge-resection of the cystic cortex of the ovaries, was successful in completely restoring physiologic function. Menstruation in every instance became normal and remianed so during the period of observation. Pregnancy followed in two patients.

6. It is our belief that a mechanical crowding of the cortex by cysts interferes with the progress of the normal graafian follicles to the surface of the ovary. This mechanical factor may account for the symptoms of amenorrhea and sterility.

7. Recurrence of the polycystic change in the ovary was not found in the follow-up examinations in any of the patients in this series.

REFERENCES

Zondek, B.: Arch. f. Gynäk. 144: 131, 1930. *Mandelstamm and Tschaikowsky:* Arch. f. Gynäk. 151: 686, 1932. *Kraus, E. J.:* Arch. f. Gynäk. 153: 383, 1933. *Geist, S. H.:* AM. J. OBST. & GYNEC. 26: 588, 1933. *Fluhmann, C. F.:* AM. J. OBST. & GYNEC. 27: 588, 1933. *Gertel:* Outlines of Pathology, Montreal, 1927, Renouf Publ. Co. *Stein, I. F.:* Med. Clin. N. Am. ''Sterility,'' September, 1924. *Stein, I. F.:* Surg. Gynec. Obst. 42: 83, 1926. *Stein, I. F.:* Surg. Gynec. Obst. 55: 207, 1932. *Goodall, J.:* Curtis' Obstetrics and Gynecology 3: 1933, W. B. Saunders Company. *Graves, Wm. P.:* Gynecology, Philadelphia, 1916, W. B. Saunders Company. *Crossen, H. S.:* Diseases of Women, St. Louis, 1930, The C. V. Mosby Co. *Allen, Edgar:* Sex and Internal Secretions, Baltimore, 1932, Williams and Wilkins Co. *Mazer and Goldstein:* Clinical Endocrinology in the Female, Philadelphia, 1931, W. B. Saunders Co.

*We are greatly indebted to Dr. Otto Saphir for valuable assistance in the study and interpretation of the ovarian tissue changes.

Commentary on Classic Paper No.9

In 1935, Stein and Leventhal[1] described seven patients with polycystic ovaries. In this classic paper, they described a syndrome which consisted of 'menstrual irregularity featuring amenorrhea, a history of sterility, masculine type hirsutism and, less consistently, retarded breast development and obesity'.

Stein and Leventhal thought that 'mechanical crowding of the cortex by cysts interferes with the progress of the normal graafian follicles to the surface of the ovary'. This theory was supported by clinical evidence when wedge resection of the ovaries was successfully achieved, restoring physiological function and resulting in pregnancy in two patients.

Interest in this subject was in fact raised when, as early as 1844, Chereau[2] described sclerocystic changes in the human ovary. Fifty years later, in 1895, a report was published by Waldo of a young patient with severe pain in the lower abdomen. Cystic degeneration of the ovaries was found and small cysts were removed. Within a year, however, the patient returned and at laparotomy the same cystic changes of the ovaries were again observed. In 1914, Goldspohn[3] discussed extensively the resection of ovaries.

The role of androgens in ovarian function

During the Second World War Gaarenstroom and de Jongh[4] at the University of Leiden (The Netherlands) studied the influences of gonadotropins and sex steroids on the gonads of rats. These researchers remained active during the 5 years of German occupation. In well-designed experiments they found evidence for a local and crucial role of androgens on follicle maturation and ovulation in the rat.

From their studies, they formed a theory regarding the synthesis of androgens – *It was proved that androgenic substance is indeed formed in the ovary under the influence of chorionic gonadotrophin, even when the hypophysis has been removed.*

'Given together with estrone, testosterone produces follicles with cavities in hypophysectomized rats, without theca development and without luteinization. These cavities differ from normal ones: the ova die, the granulosa-elements lose their coherence. The combination of necrosis of the ovum and disintegration of the granulosa led to the name N.D. follicles' (N indicates necrosis of the ovum and D, disintegration of the granulosa).

1. Stein, I.F. and Leventhal, M.L.(1935). Amenorrhea associated with bilateral polycystic ovaries. *Am. J. Obstet. Gynecol.*, **29**, 181

2. Chereau, A. (1844). *Memoires pour Servir a L'etude des Maladies des Ovaries.* (Paris: Fortin Masson and Cie)

3. Goldspohn, A. (1914). Resection of ovaries. *Am. J. Obstet. Gynecol.*, **70**, 934

4. Gaarenstroom, J.H. and Jongh, S.E. de (1946). A contribution to the knowledge of the influences of gonadotropic and sex hormones on the gonads of rats. (Amsterdam: Elsevier Publishing Company Inc.)

In their research, Gaarenstroom and de Jongh touched upon the role of androgens, so important in the polycystic ovary syndrome.

The polycystic ovary syndrome

5. Yen, S.S.C., Chaney, C. and Judd, H.L. (1976). Functional aberrations of the hypothalamic–pituitary system in polycystic ovary syndrome: a consideration of the pathogenesis. In James, V.H.T., Serie, M. and Giusti, G. (eds.) *The Endocrine Functions of the Human Ovary*, p. 373. (London: London Academic Press)

6. Chang, R.J. (1984). Ovarian steroid excretion in polycystic ovarian disease. *Sem. Reprod. Endocrinol.*, **2**, 244

7. Burger, C.W., Korsten, T., Kessel, H. Van, Dop. P.A. Van, Carom, J.M. and Schoemaker, J. (1985). Pulsatile luteinizing hormone patterns in the follicular phase of the menstrual cycle, polycystic ovarian disease (PCOD) and non-PCOD secondary amenorrhea. *J. Clin. Endocrinol. Metab.*, **61**, 1126

The polycystic ovary syndrome is a common problem in gynecological endocrinology/infertility. The classic definition of the syndrome is obesity with amenorrhea and hirsutism, as described by Stein and Leventhal[1]. In this syndrome, both luteinizing hormone (LH) and testosterone levels are raised. Removal of a wedge of ovarian tissue, as pioneered by Stein and Leventhal, has been shown to restore ovulation.

A proposed mechanism for persistent anovulation in the polycystic ovary syndrome was presented by Yen and co-workers[5] in 1976, as a 'self-perpetuating' cycle. They proposed that the high LH/follicle stimulating hormone (FSH) ratio is due to a constant estrogen feedback on the hypothalamopituitary system. Excessive LH release leads to an increase in 17α-hydroxyprogesterone, the precursor for ovarian and adrenal androgen production. The high androgen production also results in excessive amounts of substrate for conversion of androgen to estrogen by adipose tissues. The high levels of estrogen augment the secretion of gonadotropin releasing hormone (GnRH) by the pituitary, resulting in cyclical follicular maturation with chronic anovulation. Excessive estrogen also suppresses FSH.

It is now recognized that it is clinically more useful to consider various spectra of anovulation with various symptomatologies and probably etiologies. In patients with persistent anovulation, the daily production of estrogen and androgen is increased depending on LH stimulation[6]. The higher level of LH secretion increases the production of androstenedione in the ovary (theca cells) resulting in a higher peripheral conversion to estrone. The excess production of androstenedione and 17-hydroxyprogesterone and testosterone in this syndrome is derived primarily from the ovary. The persistence of abnormal androgen secretion suggests that separation of ovarian from adrenal function has been achieved, being mutually exclusive[6].

Anovulatory women with polycystic ovaries have been observed by Burger and colleagues to have a higher LH pulse amplitude when compared to the mid-follicular phase of ovulatory women[7].

The hormone of the anterior pituitary

The importance to fertility of a hormone produced by the anterior pituitary first came to light in the 1920s with the work of Drs Bernhard Zondek and Selmar Aschheim at the Universitäts-Frauenklinik of the Charité in Berlin.

In 1926, Zondek had implanted pieces of the hypophyseal anterior lobe of cows and humans, into infertile mice. Approximately 100 hours later estrus was observed, with stimulation of the ovaries and uterus. Aschheim and Zondek[8] recognized that the pituitary hormone stimulated ovarian follicles and the corpus luteum. The secondary effect of this ovarian activity was found in reactions of the vaginal wall.

By 1930, Zondek had already discovered that urine from postmenopausal women was a source for gonadotropins that later became known as FSH and LH. In 1958, Gemzell and colleagues[9] reported that FSH from human pituitaries when administered to amenorrheic women produced follicular growth and estrogen secretion. Lunenfeld and co-workers[10] showed that FSH extracted from menopausal urine was clinically active.

8. Zondek, B. and Aschheim, S. (1927). Das Hormon des Hypo-physenvorderlappens. *Klin. Wschr.*, **6**, F248

9. Gemzell, C.A., Diczfalusy, E. and Tillinger, G. (1958). Clinical effect of human pituitary follicle stimulating hormone (FSH). *J. Clin. Endocrinol.*, **18**, 1333

10. Lunenfeld, B., Menzi, A. and Volet, B. (1960). Clinical effects of human postmenopausal gonadotrophin. In 1st International Congress of Endocrinology, p.587. (Copenhagen)

11. Gemzell, C.A., Diczfalusy, E. and Tillinger, G. (1960). Human pituitary follicle stimulating hormone (FSH). I. Clinical effect of a partly purified preparation. *Ciba Found. Colloq. Endocrinol.*, **13**, 191

12. Donini, P., Puzzuoli, D. and Montezemolo, R. (1964). Purification of gonadotrophin from human menopausal urine. *Acta Endocrinol.*, **45**, 321

CLINICAL EFFECTS OF HUMAN POSTMENOPAUSAL GONADOTROPHIN

Bruno Lunenfeld, Annette Menzi and Blaise Volet

Clinique universitaire gynécologie et d'obstétrique, Geneva, Switzerland, and Clinical Research Group, Government Hospital, Tel-Hashomer, Israel

A purified gonadotrophin preparation from pooled human menopausal urine (Pergonal, furnished by the courtesy of Dr. P. Donini of the Istituto Farmacologico Serono, Roma) has been investigated.

Local and general effects as well as ovarian and testicular responses were studied in impotent and sterile men and in amenorrheic women. No local or generalized tonic, irritative or pyrogenic effects were noted. The results depended largely on the condition of the gonads prior to treatment. In primary amenorrhea of pituitary origin, 150 U/d (one unit is defined as the activity equivalent, in the mouse uterus test, to 1.0 mg of the International Reference Preparation for Human Menopausal Gonadotrophin) produce follicular stimulation as noted by the increase in oestrogen output and laparoscopy. Urinary 17-ketosteroids and cortico-steroids were not affected.

The use of this preparation in functional tests of ovarian responsiveness is discussed. It is suggested to treat amenorrheic women with 150 U/d, for four days, and to follow vaginal smears and oestrogen excretion.

A significant increase in the percentage of cornified cells and pycnotic nuclei and in urinary oestrogens will suggest amenorrhea of pituitary origin.

The report from Lunenfeld and colleagues on the clinical activity of FSH extracted from menopausal urine[10]

The first pregnancy following the use of extracted human pituitary gonadotropin preparation was reported by Gemzell and colleagues[11] in 1960. The purification of gonadotropins was achieved by Donini and co-workers[12] and, today, gonadotropins play an important part in the treatment of infertility.

Clomiphene citrate

Clomiphene citrate

Diethylstilbestrol

Adapted from Speroff, L., Glass, R. H. and Kase, N. G. (1989).
Clinical Gynecologic Endocrinology and Fertility, 4th edn.
(Baltimore: Williams and Wilkins) with permission

13. Clark, J.H. and Markaverich, B.M. (1982). The agonistic–antagonistic properties of clomiphene: a review. *Pharmacol. Therap.*, **15**, 467

14. Mikkelson, Th.J., Kroboth, P.D., Cameron, W.J., Dittert, L.W., Chungi, V. and Manberg, P.J. (1986). Single-dose pharmacokinetics of clomiphene citrate in normal volunteers. *Fertil. Steril.*, **46**, 392

15. Cornel, M.C., Kate, L.P. ten and Meerman, G.J. te (1990). Association between ovulation stimulation, in vitro fertilization and neural tube defects. *Teratology*, **42**, 201

Clomiphene, an orally active non-steroidal agent that has a resemblance to diethylstilbestrol (DES), was first synthesized in 1956 and introduced for clinical trials in 1960.

Clomiphene inhibits the action of the intracellular estrogen receptors in the hypothalamus. Clomiphene's antiestrogenic properties mean that it non-competitively binds to the hypothalamic estrogen receptors, thereby preventing a correct interpretation of the endogenous estrogen levels. In an attempt to increase estrogen levels, FSH and LH pulse frequency is increased, stimulating ovarian follicle growth and eventual ovulation[13].

Despite its effectiveness, the clinical use of clomiphene in the treatment of infertility is not without concern because of its long half-life (up to 1 month after 50 mg orally)[14]. Cornel and colleagues have published epidemiological data suggesting that the risk for neural tube defects may be raised[15]. These reports sound a warning against the too liberal use of clomiphene in infertility treatment.

Prolactin

Prolactin was discovered by Stricker and Greuter[16] in 1930 and isolated by Riddle and colleagues[17] in 1933. In the treatment of infertility, menstrual disturbances in combination with galactorrhea had attracted considerable clinical interest which led to work on prolactin in the 1960s and 70s. In the 1960s, much research was aimed at purifying prolactin and lead to the development of a radioimmunoassay by Hwang and co-workers[18] in 1971 for prolactin.

As an off-shoot of this line of research, an ergot alkaloid (ergocryptine) called bromocryptine was discovered by Flückinger and Wagner[19] that could inhibit selectively prolactin secretion. In 1974, Rune Rolland and colleagues[20] successfully treated three patients exhibiting galactorrhea and menstrual disturbances with bromocryptine. Plasma concentrations of prolactin were lowered and normal cyclic ovarian activity was restored. One pregnancy was observed during treatment.

Bromocryptine has become the reference dopamine agonist which directly stimulates dopamine receptors to inhibit pituitary prolactin, permitting secretion of FSH and LH and restoring the menstrual cycle.

Since this discovery, numerous women with hyperprolactinemia have been treated in this way, as have many cases of pituitary adenomas during pregnancy[21]. Because of this treatment, many adenomas of the pituitary gland now do not have to be removed by neurosurgery.

Priming of ovaries and *in vitro* fertilization

The 1970s witnessed a dramatic new approach to the treatment of infertility with the pioneering work on *in vitro* fertilization (IVF) of Steptoe and Edwards[22], for infertility. In the beginning, success was achieved by utilizing non-stimulated cycles. Oocyte maturation was monitored by the measurement of LH at 3-hour intervals and by oocyte retrieval accompanied by laparotomy. To increase the success rate, human menopausal gonadotropins were used to develop multiple ovarian follicles. Unfortunately, success was not achieved instantly and the first attempt resulted in an ectopic embryo that had to be removed at 13 weeks' gestation. Nevertheless, Steptoe and Edwards continued their efforts, which were rewarded in 1978 with the first live-born baby after IVF.

16. Stricker, P. and Greuter, F. (1930). Action du lobe antérieur de l'hypophyse sur la montée laiteuse. *C. R. Soc. Biol. (Paris)*, **99**, 1978

17. Riddle, O., Bates, R.W. and Dykshorn, S.W. (1933). The preparation, identification and assay of prolactin – a hormone of the anterior pituitary. *Am. J. Physiol.*, **105**, 191

18. Hwang, P., Guyda, H. and Friesen, H. (1971). A radio-immuno-assay for human prolactin. *Proc. Natl. Acad. Sci. USA*, **68**, 1902

19. Flückinger, E. and Wagner, H.R. (1969). 2-Br-α-ergocryptine: Beeinflussung von Fertilität und Laktation der Ratte. *Experientia*, **24**, 1130

20. Rolland, R., Schellekens, L.A. and Lequin, R.M. (1974). Successful treatment of galactorrhoea and amenorrhoea and subsequent restoration of ovarian function by a new ergot alkaloid 2-bromo-α-ergocryptine. *Clin. Endocrinol.*, **3**, 155

Letters to the Editor

BIRTH AFTER THE REIMPLANTATION OF A HUMAN EMBRYO

SIR,—We wish to report that one of our patients, a 30-year-old nulliparous married woman, was safely delivered by cæsarean section on July 25, 1978, of a normal healthy infant girl weighing 2700 g. The patient had been referred to one of us (P.C.S.) in 1976 with a history of 9 years' infertility, tubal occlusions, and unsuccessful salpingostomies done in 1970 with excision of the ampullæ of both oviducts followed by persistent tubal blockages. Laparoscopy in February, 1977, revealed grossly distorted tubal remnants with occlusion and peritubal and ovarian adhesions. Laparotomy in August, 1977, was done with excision of the remains of both tubes, adhesolysis, and suspension of the ovaries in good position for oocyte recovery.

Pregnancy was established after laparoscopic recovery of an oocyte on Nov. 10, 1977, in-vitro fertilisation and normal cleavage in culture media, and the reimplantation of the 8-cell embryo into the uterus $2\frac{1}{2}$ days later. Amniocentesis at 16 weeks' pregnancy revealed normal α-fetoprotein levels, with no chromosome abnormalities in a 46 XX fetus. On the day of delivery the mother was 38 weeks and 5 days by dates from her last menstrual period, and she had pre-eclamptic toxæmia. Blood-pressure was fluctuating around 140/95, œdema involved both legs up to knee level together with the abdomen, back, hands, and face; the blood-uric-acid was 390 µmol/l, and albumin 0·5 g/l of urine. Ultrasonic scanning and radiographic appearances showed that the fetus had grown slowly for several weeks from week 30. Blood-œstriols and human placental lactogen levels also dropped below the normal levels during this period. However, the fetus grew considerably during the last 10 days before delivery while placental function improved greatly. On the day of delivery the biparietal diameter had reached 9·6 cm, and 5 ml of amniotic fluid was removed safely under sonic control. The lecithin: sphingomyelin ratio was 3·9:1, indicative of maturity and a low risk of the respiratory-distress syndrome.

We hope to publish further medical and scientific details in your columns at a later date.

Department of
  Obstetrics and Gynæcology,
General Hospital,
Oldham OL1 2JH   P. C. STEPTOE

University Physiology Laboratory,
Cambridge CB2 3EG   R. G. EDWARDS

The report of the first live-born baby after in vitro fertilization.
Reproduced from Lancet (1978)[22] with permission

This work formed the basis for the current work in IVF worldwide. A combination of ovarian suppression by gonadotropin releasing hormone analogs followed by controlled ovarian hyperstimulation with gonadotropins including LH stimulation, has allowed optimum control of superovulation and timing of oocyte retrieval.

A further advance has been in the area of FSH. Because FSH preparations had a low purity, recombinant human FSH (rhFSH) was developed using genetically engineered cells, in which the genes coded for rhFSH units. Two recent case histories[23,24] have described the use of genetically engineered FSH, resulting in successful IVF and embryo transfer. Even after menopause, adequate uterine receptivity can be achieved to allow implantation of transferred embryos[25].

Ethical issues

It is not surprising that successful development of IVF has brought with it medical/ethical problems. As early in its development as 1984, a Report of the Committee of Inquiry into Human Fertilization and Embryology, the so-called 'Warnock Committee', expressed concern and tried to set rules and regulations, especially for embryo research.

Concern about frozen embryos was not only expressed in medical journals, but reached Wall Street as well as the newspapers in Australia! Here the ethical issues became headlines in 1984 with news that the world's first test-tube 'orphans' were in a deep freeze in a Melbourne laboratory – awaiting a life or death decision following the sudden death of their multi-millionaire Californian parents.

Modesty

In 1987, Lilford and Dalton[26] stated that *'many doctors and lay people think that the great technical advances in the past 20 years in treating infertility have led to high success rates in treatment, but this is a myth'*. These authors calculated that, at the maximum, one out of three couples might conceive as a result of medical intervention. The same statement might hold for all the therapeutic and diagnostic techniques that are available for infertility 'work-up'. From these, the rather simple technique of investigating cervical mucus in the fertile period after intercourse[27] should not be forgotten, because of its high prognostic value and its 'simplicity'.

21. Jewelewicz, R. and van de Wiele, R.L. (1980). Clinical course and outcome of pregnancy in twenty-five patients with pituitary micro-adenomas. *Am. J. Obstet. Gynecol.*, **136**, 339

22. Steptoe, P.C. and Edwards, R.G. (1978). Birth after reimplantation of a human embryo. *Lancet*, **1**, 336

23. Devroey, P., Steirteghem, A. van, Mannaerts, B. and Coelingh Bennink, H. (1992). Successful in vitro fertilisation and embryo transfer after treatment with recombinant human FSH. *Lancet*, **339**, 1170

24. Germond, M., Dessole, S., Senn, A., Loumaye, E., Howles, C. and Beltrami, V. (1992). Successful in vitro fertilisation and embryo transfer after treatment with recombinant human FSH. *Lancet*, **339**, 1170

25. Sauer, M.V., Paulson, R.J. and Lobo, R.A. (1993). Pregnancy after age 50: application of oocyte donation to women after natural menopause. *Lancet*, **341**, 321

26. Lilford, R.J. and Dalton, M.E. (1987). Effectiveness of the treatment for infertility. *Br. Med. J.*, **295**, 155

Concern

27. Sims, J.M. (1868). Illustrations of the value of the microscope in the treatment of the sterile condition. *Br. Med. J.,* **2**, 492

28. Derom, C., Vlietinck, R., Derom, R., van den Berghe, H. and Thiery, M. (1987). Increased monozygotic twinning rate after ovulation induction. *Lancet,* **1**, 1236

29. Whittemore, A.S., Harris, R., Itnyre, J. and the Collaborative Ovarian Cancer Group (1992). Characteristics relating to ovarian cancer risk: collaborative analysis of twelve US case–control studies. *Am. J. Epidemiol.,* **136**, 1184 and 1204

30. Willemsen, W., Kruitwagen, R., Bastiaans, B. and Rolland, R. (1993). Ovarian stimulation and granulosa-cell tumour. *Lancet,* **341**, 986

31. Regan, L., Owen, E.J. and Jacobs, H.S. (1990). Hypersecretion of luteinising hormone, infertility and miscarriage. *Lancet,* **336**, 1141

After artificial induction of ovulation, multiple pregnancies are reported to occur in 14–16% of cases. Also, monozygotic twinning rates are increased after ovulation induction[28].

Some concern has been raised by the small fraction of the excess ovarian cancer risk among nulliparous women with infertility and the use of fertility drugs[29]. This was also suggested for ovarian stimulation and granulosa-cell tumors[30]. Such concern should lead to more detailed investigations while drug surveillance remains necessary to prove or disprove these findings.

Another major challenge when treating infertility in women with polycystic ovary syndrome is the high miscarriage rate of 30%, shown by Regan and colleagues[31] to be a particular problem in women with raised LH levels.

Epilogue

Since the original publication of Stein and Leventhal[1] in 1935, research into the treatment of infertility has progressed in diverse ways, with some considerable success. The study of anovulation has revealed a subset of women with polycystic ovary syndrome who have a certain set of homonal characteristics typified by excessive LH release and constant estrogen production. The reason for the higher androgen production in this disease was also found, probably resulting from an ovarian and adrenal origin.

A logical approach to the treatment of this condition followed, namely ovarian suppression with the emphasis on androgen suppression, using dexamethasone and stimulation of ovarian folliculogenesis using clomiphene citrate. The discovery of a dopamine agonist from the ergot family has enabled clinicians to treat menstrual cycle abnormalities due to hyperprolactinemia, restoring fertility. Even prolactinomas of the pituitary gland now can be reduced in size and medication can be continued during pregnancy.

The discovery of hormones from the anterior pituitary gland led to the development of gonadotropin preparations and their use to stimulate the ovaries. This finding led to ovulation induction and now together with LHRH agonists for timing, forms the basis of the program for IVF centers. Finally, purification of FSH using recombinant technology has opened the possibility of having available pure natural FSH without LH activity and this has been shown to be successful in inducing pregnancy.

The ethical issues raised by artificial procreation have now become a major area of interest, and will probably be a challenge for many years to come.

Summary of references

1. Stein, I.F. and Leventhal, M.L. (1935). Amenorrhea associated with bilateral polycystic ovaries. *Am. J. Obstet. Gynecol.*, **29**, 181

2. Chereau, A. (1844). *Memoires pour Servir a L'etude des Maladies des Ovaries.* (Paris: Fortin Masson and Cie)

3. Goldspohn, A. (1914). Resection of ovaries. *Am. J. Obstet. Gynecol.*, **70**, 934

4. Gaarenstroom, J.H. and Jongh, S.E. de (1946). A contribution to the knowledge of the influences of gonadotropic and sex hormones on the gonads of rats. (Amsterdam: Elsevier Publishing Company Inc)

5. Yen, S.S.C., Chaney, C. and Judd, H.L. (1976). Functional aberrations of the hypothalamic–pituitary system in polycystic ovary syndrome: a consideration of the pathogenesis. In James, V.H.T., Serio, M. and Giusti, G.(eds.) *The Endocrine Functions of the Human Ovary*, p.373. (London: London Academic Press)

6. Chang, R.J. (1984). Ovarian steroid excretion in polycystic ovarian disease. *Sem. Reprod. Endocrinol.*, **2**, 244

7. Burger, C.W., Korsten, T., Kessel, H. Van, Dop, P.A. Van, Carom, J.M. and Schoemaker, J. (1985). Pulsatile luteinizing hormone patterns in the follicular phase of the menstrual cycle, polycystic ovarian disease (PCOD) and non-PCOD secondary amenorrhea. *J. Clin. Endocrinol. Metab.*, **61**, 1126

8. Zondek, B. and Aschheim, S. (1927). Das Hormon des Hypophysenvorderlappens. *Klin.Wschr.*, **6**, F248

9. Gemzell, C.A., Diczfalusy, E. and Tillinger, G. (1958). Clinical effect of human pituitary follicle stimulating hormone (FSH). *J. Clin. Endocrinol.*, **18**, 1333

10. Lunenfeld, B., Menzi, A. and Volet, B. (1960). Clinical effects of human postmenopausal gonadotrophin. In *1st International Congress of Endocrinology*, p.587. (Copenhagen)

11. Gemzell, C.A., Diczfalusy, E. and Tillinger, G. (1960). Human pituitary follicle stimulating hormone (FSH). I. Clinical effect of a partly purified preparation. *Ciba Found. Colloq. Endocrinol.*, **13**, 191

12. Donini, P., Puzzuoli, D. and Montezemolo, R. (1964). Purification of gonadotrophin from human menopausal urine. *Acta Endocrinol.*, **45**, 321

13. Clark, J.H. and Markaverich, B.M. (1982). The agonistic–antagonistic properties of clomiphene: a review. *Pharmacol. Therap.*, **15**, 467

14. Mikkelson, Th.J., Kroboth, P.D., Cameron, W.J., Dittert, L.W., Chungi, V. and Manberg, P.J. (1986). Single-dose pharmacokinetics of clomiphene citrate in normal volunteers. *Fertil. Steril.*, **46**, 392–6

15. Cornel, M.C., Kate, L.P. ten and Meerman, G.J. te (1990). Association between ovulation stimulation, in vitro fertilization and neural tube defects. *Teratology*, **42**, 201

16. Stricker, P. and Greuter, F. (1930). Action du lobe antérieur de l'hypophyse sur la montée laiteuse. *C. R. Soc. Biol. (Paris)*, **99**, 1978

17. Riddle, O., Bates, R.W. and Dykshorn, S.W. (1933). The preparation, identification and assay of prolactin – a hormone of the anterior pituitary. *Am. J. Physiol.,* **105**, 191

18. Hwang, P., Guyda, H. and Friesen, H. (1971). A radio-immunoassay for human prolactin. *Proc. Natl. Acad. Sci. USA,* **68**, 1902

19. Flückinger, E. and Wagner, H.R. (1969). 2-Br-α-ergocryptine: Beeinflussung von Fertilität und Laktation der Ratte. *Experientia,* **24**, 1130

20. Rolland, R., Schellekens, L.A. and Lequin, R.M. (1974). Successful treatment of galactorrhoea and amenorrhoea and subsequent restoration of ovarian function by a new ergot alkaloid 2-bromo-α-ergocryptine. *Clin. Endocrinol.,* **3**, 155

21. Jewelewicz, R. and van de Wiele, R.L. (1980). Clinical course and outcome of pregnancy in twenty-five patients with pituitary micro-adenomas. *Am. J. Obstet. Gynecol.,* **136**, 339

22. Steptoe, P.C. and Edwards, R.G. (1978). Birth after reimplantation of a human embryo. *Lancet,* **1**, 336

23. Devroey, P., Steirteghem, A. van, Mannaerts, B. and Coelingh Bennink, H. (1992). Successful in vitro fertilisation and embryo transfer after treatment with recombinant human FSH. *Lancet,* **339**, 1170

24. Germond, M., Dessole, S., Senn A., Loumaye, E., Howles, C. and Beltrami, V. (1992). Successful in vitro fertilisation and embryo transfer after treatment with recombinant human FSH. *Lancet,* **339**, 1170

25. Sauer, M.V., Paulson, R.J. and Lobo, R.A. (1993). Pregnancy after age 50: application of oocyte donation to women after natural menopause. *Lancet,* **341**, 321

26. Lilford, R.J. and Dalton, M.E. (1987). Effectiveness of treatment for infertility. *Br. Med. J.,* **295**, 155

27. Sims, J.M. (1868). Illustrations of the value of the microscope in the treatment of the sterile condition. *Br. Med. J.,* **2**, 492

28. Derom, C., Vlietinck, R., Derom, R., van den Berghe, H. and Thiery, M. (1987). Increased monozygotic twinning rate after ovulation induction. *Lancet,* **1**, 1236

29. Whittemore, A.S., Harris, R., Itnyre, J. and the Collaborative Ovarian Cancer Group (1992). Characteristics relating to ovarian cancer risk: collaborative analysis of twelve US case–control studies. *Am. J. Epidemiol.,* **136**, 1184 and 1204

30. Willemsen, W., Kruitwagen, R., Bastiaans, B. and Rolland, R. (1993). Ovarian stimulation and granulosa-cell tumour. *Lancet,* **341**, 986

31. Regan, L., Owen, E.J. and Jacobs, H.S. (1990). Hypersecretion of luteinising hormone, infertility and miscarriage. *Lancet,* **336**, 1141

ENDOMETRIOSIS

Classic
Paper
No.10

Peritoneal endometriosis due to the menstrual dissemination of endometrial tissue into the peritoneal cavity

JOHN A. SAMPSON

Albany Hospital and Albany Medical College, Albany, New York

1. Sampson, J.A. (1927). Peritoneal endometriosis due to the menstrual dissemination of endometrial tissue into the peritoneal cavity.
Am. J. Obstet. Gynecol.,
14, 422

Sampson published a series of papers between 1921 and 1940 on endometriosis. His careful observations demonstrated that retrograde menstruation and implantation of endometrium into the peritoneal cavity was most likely.

Endometriosis now is increasingly seen in clinics because of gynecological complaints and/or infertility. Despite an enormous research effort, the real pathogenesis is not known. Age and absence of a 'continuous pregnant' state seem to be predominant factors within this multifactorial disease. Fortunately sex steroids and gonadotropin releasing hormone agonists are available to treat symptoms and prevent surgery up to the menopause.

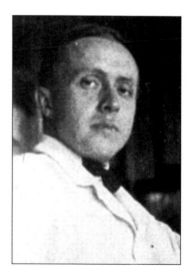

Original Communications[*]

PERITONEAL ENDOMETRIOSIS DUE TO THE MENSTRUAL DISSEMINATION OF ENDOMETRIAL TISSUE INTO THE PERITONEAL CAVITY

By John A. Sampson, M.D., Albany, N. Y.

(From the Gynecologic and Pathologic Departments of the Albany Hospital and the Albany Medical College)

AT THE meeting of the American Gynecological Society in 1921, the writer presented a paper[1] on perforating hemorrhagic cysts of the ovary and their relation to pelvic adenomas of endometrial type. Twenty-three of these cysts were reported at that time. In fourteen of them, a histologic study had been made of the peritoneal lesions, apparently resulting from the escape of the contents of the cysts into the peritoneal cavity. Endometrial tissue was found in thirteen. I concluded that the hemorrhagic ovarian cysts, associated with the peritoneal lesions containing endometrial tissue, were endometrial cysts filled with menstrual blood and that the peritoneal endometriosis arose from the escape of the cyst contents into the pelvis and the resulting peritoneal reaction. In view of the theories which have arisen to explain the origin of the peritoneal endometriosis associated with these cysts, the following quotation from that paper may be of interest.

The question naturally arises: in what way do the contents of the cyst or ovary cause the development of these adenomas? Is it due to some specific irritant present in the cyst contents which stimulates the peritoneal endothelium to a metaplasia with the development of endometrial tissue typical both in structure and function? Some may assert that dormant endometrial epithelium may be present in the tissues soiled by the contents of the cyst and this is stimulated to further growth. It seems to me that the conditions found in many of these specimens are analogous to the implantation of ovarian papilloma or cancer on the peritoneal surfaces of the pelvis from the rupture of an ovarian tumor containing these growths.

At that time I believed that the ovary was the principal, if not the only, source of the peritoneal implantations which arose from endometrial tissue disseminated by the menstrual perforation of an endometrial cyst or by the menstrual reaction of endometrial tissue on the surface of that organ. Up to that time only a few peritoneal lesions had been observed by me without demonstrable endometrial tissue in the ovary. An attempt was made to explain these on the basis that they had arisen from the implantations of endometrial tissue, derived from small

[*]The current issue of the Journal is devoted to the first part of the Transactions of the Fifty-second Annual Meeting of the American Gynecological Society, held at Hot Springs, Va., May 23, 24, 25, 1927. The discussions on the papers presented will be incorporated in part in the next issue of the Journal.

422

endometrial foci in the ovary, and that the latter had either been destroyed by menstrual reactions or else were so small that they had been overlooked.

Later studies convinced me that peritoneal endometriosis frequently occurred without endometrial tissue in the ovaries, and some other way by which this tissue might reach the peritoneal cavity was sought. Blood was observed escaping through the abdominal ostia of the tubes of patients operated upon during menstruation. Bits of endometrial tissue were found in the lumina of some of these tubes. The frequent close anatomic relation between the distribution of the peritoneal lesions and the fimbriated ends of the tubes was observed at operation. It was found that the tubes were usually patent in patients with peritoneal

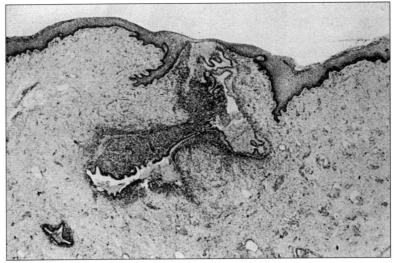

Fig. 1.—Photomicrograph (x 25) of a portion of the posterior vaginal wall with a submucous endometrial cavity about to rupture into the vagina (Case 4 of previous article[2]). The patient had peritoneal endometriosis fusing the anterior surface of the uterus with the bladder, and a similar lesion obliterating the bottom of the posterior culdesac with invasion of the rectosigmoid and the posterior vaginal wall. The cavity contains blood and bits of endometrial tissue; operation on the second day of menstruation. The vaginal mucosa over the cavity is very thin and had the operation been deferred subsequent menstruations of the endometrial tissue lining this cavity undoubtedly would lead to a rupture through the attenuated vaginal mucosa with the discharge of the menstrual contents of the cavity into the vagina. The actual rupture of two similar cavities of the vaginal wall into veins was observed in this case and embolic implantations of endometrial tissue in near-by vessels was found (Figs. 58, 59, 60, 61 and 66 of previous article[2]). It is conceivable that similar endometrial cavities situated in the ovary or in any other pelvic structure, whose endometrial lining reacted to menstruation, might rupture and discharge their contents into the peritoneal cavity and also that implantations of endometrial tissue might occur on the peritoneum just as they occurred in the veins of this patient.

endometriosis. All these data, together with the indication that, at times, endometrial tissue escaped into the peritoneal cavity from other sources than menstruating tissue in the ovary, pointed to the backflow of menstrual blood from the uterine cavity through the tubes as one of these sources and also to epithelium escaping from the tubal mucosa as another. The purpose of this paper is to present the evidence indicating the origin of peritoneal endometriosis from the implantation of endometrial tissue disseminated by menstruation. Its origin from other sources will be considered in a later article.

If it is true that peritoneal endometriosis arises from the implantation of endometrial tissue carried by menstrual blood escaping from endometrial foci in the ovary and also from the uterine cavity through the tubes, the following three suggestions or theories present themselves.

1. Peritoneal endometriosis might be caused by menstrual blood escaping from endometrial tissue on or in other pelvic organs and structures than the ovary.

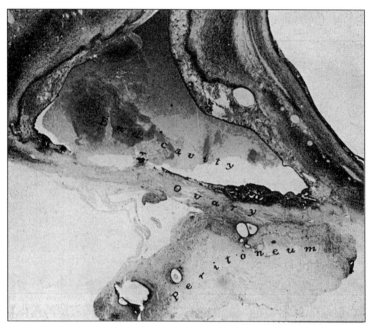

Fig. 2.—Photomicrograph (x 10) of a portion of the ovary adherent to the posterior layer of the broad ligament. Uterus, right tube, and ovary removed for a large leiomyoma on the second day of menstruation (Case 1 of previous article[2]). The ovary was firmly adherent by its *lateral surface* to the posterior layer of the broad ligament. Peritoneal endometriosis was present in the structures about the ovary and in the posterior culdesac. The right tube and ovary, together with the portion of the peritoneum attached to the latter, were carefully removed and placed in formalin before attempting to remove the uterus. A typical endometrial cyst or cavity, filled with blood, is shown and also endometrial lesions in the peritoneum adherent to the surface of the ovary. The endometrial tissue lining the cyst and that in the peritoneum must have had a common origin or one was secondary to the other. Could the peritoneal endometriosis possibly have arisen from the escape of the contents of the endometrial cyst into the pelvis?

2. Endometrial tissue in the ovary might arise from the implantation of bits of that tissue carried by menstrual blood escaping through the tubes and also from endometrial foci on other pelvic organs or structures.

3. The peritoneal endometriosis, so often associated with endometrial tissue in the ovaries and apparently secondary to the latter, at times, might have arisen from some other source.

I greatly appreciate the interest shown by others in those observations and theories and relish most of all their objections and criticisms. The latter are stimulating and will make for a better understanding of the entire subject. I fully realize that the implantation theory does not account for all instances of ectopic endometrium-like tissue in the pelvis and that menstruation is only one means of disseminating that tissue. I value the opinion of those who believe in the differentiation of celomic epithelium as a source of endometrial tissue in the ovary and peritoneum. In spite of the increasing acceptance of the serosal or celomic epithelial origin of peritoneal endometriosis, I believe that bits of endometrial tissue, carried by menstrual blood escaping into the peritoneal cavity, at times, become implanted on the peritoneum and thereby constitute one source of peritoneal endometriosis, just as the implantation of cancer cells on the peritoneum constitutes one cause of peritoneal carcinosis. I

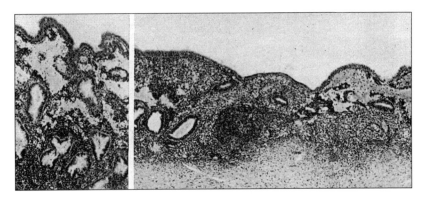

Fig. 3.—Two photomicrographs (x 60), the first of a portion of the menstruating mucosa lining the uterine cavity and the second of the endometrial lining of the cyst shown in Fig. 2. Both show the same reaction to menstruation.

believe that menstrual blood escapes into the peritoneal cavity from the following sources:

1. The menstrual rupture or perforation of the wall of an endometrial cavity (cyst), most frequently seen in the ovary.

2. The menstrual reaction of endometrial tissue, growing on the peritoneal surface of the ovary or any other pelvic organ or structure.

3. A backflow, through the tubes, from the uterine cavity and also from the menstrual reaction of the tubal mucosa.

All phases of this theory, as to the implantation on the peritoneum of endometrial and tubal tissue disseminated by menstruation, must be considered seriously, if each of the following statements can be shown to be true or even possibly true.

1. Whenever endometrial tissue reacts to menstruation this reaction is the same whether in that lining the uterine cavity or situated at a dis-

tance from it, and, at times, bits of this tissue are set free in menstrual blood and may be carried (disseminated) by the latter from these foci.

2. Endometrial tissue, disseminated by menstruation, is sometimes alive and will continue to grow, if transferred to situations suited to its growth.

3. The peritoneum is suited to the growth of endometrial tissue.

4. Menstrual blood, carrying with it bits of endometrial tissue, at times, escapes from ectopic endometrial foci into the peritoneal cavity.

5. Occasionally menstrual blood escapes from the uterine cavity into the tubes. Bits of endometrial tissue have been found in blood in the lumina of the tubes of menstruating uteri. Sometimes the lumen of the

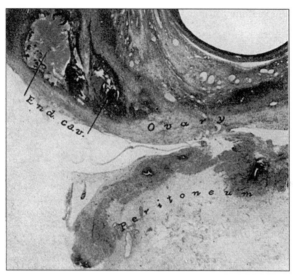

Fig. 4.—Photomicrograph (x 10) of a portion of the ovary and adherent peritoneum shown in Fig. 2 at another level. The endometrial cyst or cavity of the ovary contains blood with bits of endometrial tissue set free by the menstrual reaction of its lining, just as they are set free in menstrual blood arising from the mucosa lining the uterine cavity (see next illustration). Should such a cyst rupture during menstruation, its contents (blood and endometrial tissue) would escape into the peritoneal cavity and might cause adhesions. What would be the possible origin of any endometrial tissue in structures adherent to the ovary, such as the peritoneum shown in this illustration?

interstitial portion of the tube is of sufficient size to permit bits of endometrial tissue to pass through it.

6. The lesions of peritoneal endometriosis often occur in situations and under conditions indicating their origin from the above mentioned sources.

7. The local reaction of the peritoneum to the endometrial tissue in peritoneal endometriosis is similar to the local reaction of the peritoneum to the cancer in peritoneal carcinosis of implantation origin.

THE MENSTRUAL DISSEMINATION OF ENDOMETRIAL TISSUE

The histologic study of uteri, removed during the various stages of the menstrual cycle and in which the veins have been injected, demonstrates the mechanism by which endometrial tissue may be disseminated from that organ (See previous article).[2] The uterine mucosa contains venous capillaries which sometimes are dilated to form sinuses. These sinuses empty into similar sinuses (endothelial lined spaces without definite walls) of the myometrium and the latter empty into the arcuate veins which convey the venous blood from the uterine tissue into the venous circulation outside of that organ. During menstruation the venous capillaries of the mucosa rupture and blood escapes into the sur-

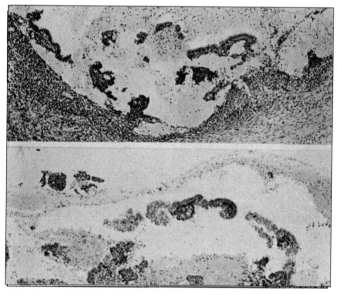

Fig. 5.—Two photomicrographs (x 60), the upper one of the menstrual contents of the endometrial cavity of the ovary shown in Fig. 4 and the other of the uterine cavity. They are much alike. Blood and fragments of endometrial tissue are present in both, histologically in a fair state of preservation and possibly as capable of living, if transferred to a suitable situation, as endometrial emboli disseminated into veins during menstruation.

rounding tissue and bits of the latter are set free in the extravasated blood. This blood breaks through the surface epithelium of the mucosa into the uterine cavity, often carrying with it bits of endometrial tissue suspended in that blood. These studies suggest that extravasated menstrual blood in the uterine mucosa, at times, might escape back into the lumen of the ruptured capillaries and sinuses from which it came and carry with it (disseminate) endometrial tissue into the venous circulation of the uterus. This actually occurs as has been shown.[2]

The histologic study of the endometrial tissue of a direct or primary endometriosis (so-called adenomyoma arising from the direct invasion of the uterine wall by the mucosa lining its cavity) shows that this tissue contains venous capillaries (Fig. 12 of previous article[2]) similar to those of the mucosa lining the uterine cavity and that the reaction to menstruation of this misplaced endometrial tissue is similar to that of the former, except that it is not as constant or as general as that of the uterine mucosa. The endometrial tissue of a direct endometriosis, in its invasion of the myometrium often penetrates the spaces occupied by the

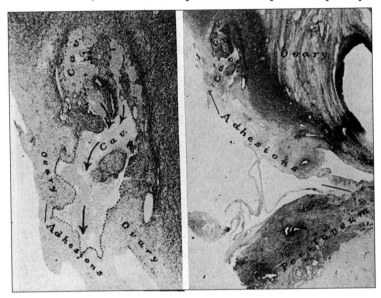

Fig. 6.—Two photomicrographs (x 25 and 10) of a portion of the right ovary and adherent peritoneum shown in the preceding illustrations, at another level. The endometrial cavity of the ovary appears much smaller and nearer the surface of the ovary. It is similar to the endometrial cavity of the vaginal wall shown in Fig. 1. Both patients were operated upon the second day of menstruation and both endometrial cavities contained blood and bits of endometrial tissue. The endometrial cavity of the vaginal wall was about to rupture and discharge its menstrual contents into the vagina. The endometrial cavity of the ovary had possibly ruptured into the peritoneal cavity at a previous menstruation and was closed by newly-formed connective tissue (adhesions) growing over it, as shown by the fibroblastic character of the adhesions covering the ragged rent in the wall of the cavity. The "rent" in the wall of the cavity and the inner surface of the adhesions covering it have been accentuated by dotted lines. These adhesions (see second photomicrograph) are continuous with similar adhesions uniting the lateral surface of the ovary to the posterior layer of the broad ligament. We have evidence that the adhesions uniting the ovary to the peritoneum might have arisen from the escape of the menstrual contents of the endometrial cavity of the ovary and that bits of endometrial tissue are often present in menstrual blood. Endometrial tissue is "embedded" in the peritoneum adherent to the ovary. Could there be any relation between the endometrial tissue escaping from the cavity of the ovary and that "embedded" in the peritoneum adherent to it?

vessels and sinuses of the uterine wall but is separated from the lumina of the latter by their endothelial lining. This has been emphasized by Robert Meyer[3] and Kitai in their descriptions of the relation of misplaced endometrial tissue to the lymphatics of the uterine wall. The study of specimens, in which the veins have been injected, has convinced me that the majority of the vessels of the uterine wall, which previously I had considered to be lymphatics, are venous sinuses. It might be assumed that in the menstrual reaction of this misplaced endometrial tissue, bits of it might escape into its own venous capillaries and even into the lumen of a sinus of the uterine wall along which the endometrial tissue sometimes grows in an extra- or retroendothelial course. I have

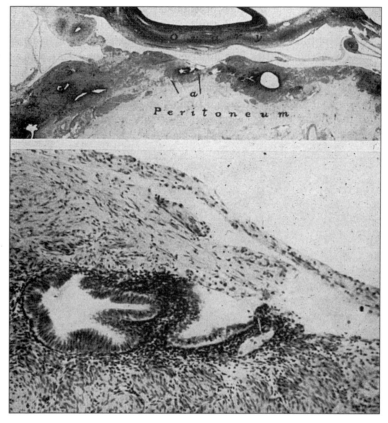

Fig. 7.—Two photomicrographs, the first (x 10) of a portion of the posterior layer of the broad ligament adherent to the lateral surface of the ovary. The adhesions indicate that there had been a reaction to some irritant escaping into the peritoneal cavity. Fig. 6 indicates that blood might have escaped into the peritoneal cavity from the menstrual reaction of endometrial tissue in the ovary. A peritoneal endometriosis is present and if it were caused by the escape of menstrual blood from the ovary, the endometrial tissue of the endometriosis must have arisen, either from a metaplasia of the peritoneal mesothelium due to some specific stimulant in menstrual blood and not found in other well-known peritoneal irritants, or else from the actual implantation of bits of endometrial tissue often present in menstrual blood. There is a hyperplasia of the peritoneum about the endometrial foci. For a higher magnification of the endometrial "deposit" indicated by a, see the next photomicrograph.

The second photomicrograph (x 130) is of the endometrial lesion indicated by a of the preceding illustration. The tissues of the peritoneum are growing over (embedding) the endometrial tissue. The fibroblastic character of the peritoneum covering the endometrial tissue shows that it is of recent origin and histologically it is the same as that of the adhesions covering the rent in the wall of the ovarian endometrial cavity (Fig. 6). This suggests that possibly they are of the same age. The reaction of the peritoneum to the endometrial tissue in this instance is similar to that sometimes found in peritoneal carcinosis of implantation origin. I believe that we are justified in stating that peritoneal endometriosis, at times, arises from the implantation of endometrial tissue carried by menstrual blood escaping from endometrial foci in the ovary, and probably did in this instance. If so, some of the endometrial tissue, set free by menstruation, must have been alive.

not definitely demonstrated this in a careful study of many sections from many blocks of tissues from uteri with a direct endometriosis which were removed during menstruation, but I believe that either it has been seen by others or will be found. The same applies to misplaced endometrial tissue of other origin than a direct invasion of the uterine wall by its mucosa. In one instance of endometriosis of the culdesac, presenting in the posterior vaginal vault (a so-called adenomyoma of the rectovaginal septum) the actual escape of the menstrual contents of two ectopic endometrial cavities into adjacent veins was found. As a result of this observation I believe that a similar condition occasionally may arise in any situation, where endometrial tissue reacts to menstruation.

Since bits of the uterine mucosa, at times, escape into the venous circulation of the uterus during menstruation, certain questions arise. What is its pathologic and clinical significance? Could it possibly give rise

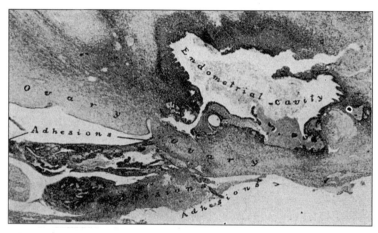

Fig. 8.—Photomicrograph (x 20) of the opposite end of the endometrial cavity shown in Fig 6. Endometrial tissue is enmeshed in adhesions on the surface of the ovary. Many sections were studied from this portion of the "block" and positive evidence of a perforation of the wall of the cavity was not found in this situation. If endometrial tissue had escaped from or had invaded the ovary at this place, the repair has been so complete that the portal of exit or entrance has been effaced.

to metastatic or embolic endometrial lesions not only in the uterine wall but also outside of that organ?

EVIDENCE OF THE VIABILITY OF ENDOMETRIAL TISSUE DISSEMINATED BY MENSTRUATION

If endometrial tissue disseminated by menstruation is "thrown off to die" and is either actually "dead or dying," as has been so emphatically stated by Novak,[4] that phase of the implantation theory is likewise just as dead. If endometrial tissue disseminated by menstruation is sometimes alive and capable of growing, if transferred to suitable situations, we might expect to find embolic lesions of this tissue in the vessels of the uterine wall and even outside of that organ. If these lesions were found, they would furnish very strong evidence that they might have arisen from the implantation of endometrial emboli cast off by menstruation into the venous circulation.

I have recently reported[2] two such cases. Both patients were operated upon during their menstrual period. Bits of endometrial tissue were found in the venous sinuses of both uteri. An embolic or metastatic growth of endometrial tissue was found in a venous sinus of one uterus and many such lesions in the other uterus. Sufficiently complete serial sections showed that these growths either arose from or were implanted on the walls or linings of these vessels and did not arise from the invasion of the latter by endometrial tissue from without. These embolic-like

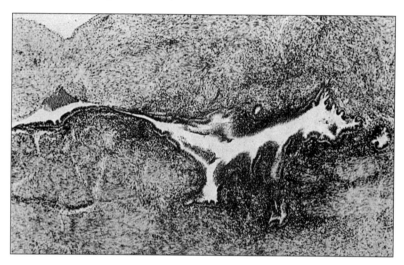

Fig. 9.—Photomicrograph (x 60) of an endometrial cavity of the posterior layer of the broad ligament adherent to the ovary. Blood is present in this cavity, and portions of its endometrial lining show the same reaction to menstruation (but not as marked) as that found in the mucosa lining the uterine cavity and the cyst of the ovary (Fig. 5).

growths of endometrial tissue must have originated either from a localized metaplasia of the endothelial lining of the veins and venous sinuses or else from the actual anchoring and implantation of bits of endometrial tissue similar to those found floating about in some of the vessels of the uterus. While an endometriosis of the direct type was present in a portion of the wall of each uterus, the distribution of the embolic lesions, as well as other histologic findings, indicated that the endometrial emboli, primarily responsible for the metastatic lesions, probably came from the mucosa lining the uterine cavity. Even if these emboli had been derived from the endometrial tissue of a direct endometriosis of the uterine wall, some traumatism would be necessary to rupture the endothelial lining of its veins and disseminate bits of endometrial tissue into their lumina. The reaction to menstruation is the most evident cause of such an injury.

Could bits of endometrial tissue escape into the venous circulation from the mucosa lining the uterine cavity by any other means than as a result of a menstrual reaction? We look to two other possible causes of this phenomenon, curettage and the termination of pregnancy by abortion or labor. Neither of the two patients, mentioned above, had ever been curetted and only one had been pregnant and that fourteen years before her operation.

Many interesting endometrial lesions were present in an endometriosis of the posterior vaginal wall of the second case. An endometrial cavity filled with menstrual blood and containing bits of endometrial tissue had

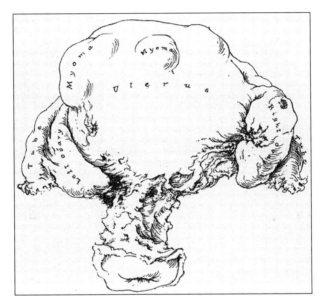

Fig. 10.—Posterior view of the uterus, tubes and ovaries (x ⅔) removed for an extensive peritoneal endometriosis, fusing the posterior surface of the cervix with the sigmoid, thus obliterating the bottom of the culdesac. The uterus contains multiple leiomyomas; both tubes were *patent*. The right ovary is adherent by its *under surface* to the posterior surface of the uterus and the broad ligament of that side. The left ovary is adherent by its *lateral surface* to the posterior layer of the broad ligament. An attempt was made to remove the uterus, tubes, and ovaries without disturbing the attachment of the ovaries to their adjacent structures. This was only partially successful (see Figs. 11 and 13). The patient, fifty-three years old, was married but had never been pregnant.

almost eroded the overlying vaginal mucosa and was about to rupture and discharge its menstrual contents into the vagina (Fig. 1). From the study of this lesion, one could readily understand how a similar endometrial cavity in the ovary or any other pelvic structure might rupture and disseminate its menstrual contents into the peritoneal cavity. We could also understand that a similar endometrial lesion might rupture into an adjoining lymph vessel or capillary during its reaction to menstruation. The operation occurred on the second day of the menstrual period. Bits of endometrial tissue were found lying free in the veins about other endometrial cavities of the vaginal wall and embolic growths of endometrial tissue were also present in these vessels. The actual escape of the menstrual contents of two of these cavities into a vein was seen. I can see only one correct interpretation of the etiology of the embolic endometrial lesions in the veins about these endometrial cavities and that is they arose from the implantation of endometrial tissue, disseminated into the veins from the menstrual rupture of the walls of the endometrial cavities into these vessels. If so, endometrial tissue disseminated by menstruation in this instance must have been alive and capable of growing, when transferred to suitable situations.

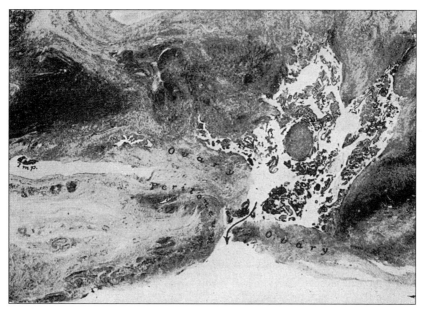

Fig. 11.—Photomicrograph (x 10) of a portion of the left ovary adherent by its lateral surface to the posterior layer of the broad ligament (Fig. 10). An endometrial cyst or cavity of the ovary, filled with fragments of endometrial tissue, is shown. Its wall is torn (see arrow) apparently due to the trauma of the operation and probably at the site of a previous perforation which had been subsequently closed by the fusion of the ovary with the posterior layer of the broad ligament at this point. An implantation-like patch of endometrial tissue (*imp.*) is situated on the lateral surface of the ovary and is similar to the fragments of endometrial tissue in the cavity and that filling the opening in its wall. This endometrial "implant" seems to be of more recent origin than the endometrial cavity, and, from the evidence presented in this section, might have arisen from tissue escaping through the perforation of the latter.

As a result of these studies in the menstrual dissemination of endometrial tissue into the venous circulation, the following three conclusions were drawn:

1. Fragments of endometrial tissue, at times, are disseminated into the venous circulation during menstruation from the mucosa lining the uterine cavity and also from ectopic endometrial foci.

2. Metastatic or embolic endometriosis may arise from the implantation of these emboli in near-by veins.

3. Endometrial tissue set free by menstruation, therefore, is sometimes not only alive but may actually grow, if transferred to situations favorable to its existence.

I might add a fourth conclusion. The veins and venous sinuses of the uterine and vaginal walls, under certain conditions, are favorable to the existence (growth) of endometrial tissue disseminated by menstruation.

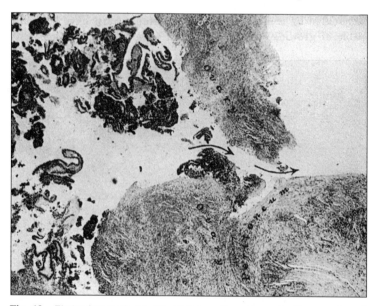

Fig. 12.—Photomicrograph (x 25) of the section, shown in the preceding illustration, at the site of the perforation of the endometrial cavity. The fusion of the fold of the peritoneum with the surface of the ovary indicates a reaction to some irritant escaping into the peritoneal cavity. The opening in the cyst wall indicates that this irritant may have been its contents. The endometrial "plug" filling the opening and attached to (implanted on) its sides suggests that this fragment of endometrial tissue had failed to escape through the perforation and was retained in this situation, or the endometrial lining of the cyst had grown out through the opening. Similar bits of endometrial tissue escaping from the cyst might have become implanted in other places, as the surface of the ovary (see *imp.* of the preceding illustration), the posterior surface of the uterus (Fig. 14), and even causing the peritoneal endometriosis, thus fusing the uterus with the sigmoid. The reaction of the endometrial lining of the cyst to menstruation would be the most likely cause of a perforation of the wall of the cyst.

EVIDENCE OF THE SUITABILITY OF THE PERITONEUM TO THE GROWTH OF ENDOMETRIAL TISSUE

If it can be shown that endometrial and tubal tissue will not grow on the peritoneum and cannot become implanted on it, no part of the implantation theory as an explanation of a cause of peritoneal endometriosis can be considered.

A study of the lesions of peritoneal endometriosis convinces one that endometrial tissue can and does grow on the pelvic peritoneum and also on the peritoneal surface of other structures which may be in the pelvic cavity but primarily did not arise in it, such as the appendix, the cecum, loops of the small intestine, and their mesenteries. We must conclude that the visceral and parietal peritoneum is suited to the growth of endometrial tissue, whatever the origin of the latter may be.

Jacobson[5] has shown by his experimental work in rabbits and monkeys that bits of the uterine mucosa of these animals, when scattered in their peritoneal cavities, give rise to a peritoneal endometriosis similar to that found in human beings. It is natural to assume that the endometrial

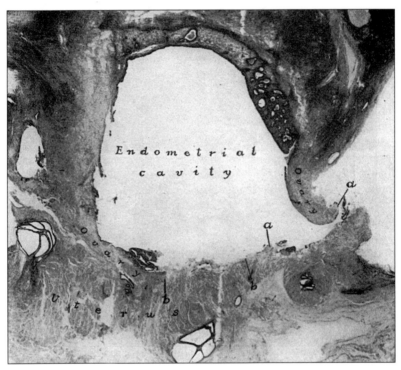

Fig. 13.—Photomicrograph (x 10) of a portion of the right ovary adherent to the posterior surface of the uterus (Fig. 10). An endometrial cyst or cavity of the ovary is shown with its wall *a*, torn from its former attachment to the uterus at *a* by the trauma of the operation. The chocolate-like contents of the hematoma or cyst escaped at that time. There is a gap *b-b* in the portion of the wall of the cyst adherent to the uterus. This gap is filled by the posterior surface of the uterus, thus completing or closing the endometrial cavity. This condition can be explained either by the rupture or by perforation of an endometrial cyst, and the subsequent closure of the opening by the ovary becoming adherent to the uterus or else endometrial tissue developing on the surface of the ovary caused adhesions (possibly due to its menstrual reaction) which fused the ovary to the uterus, and an endometrial cavity developed in this situation. In either instance menstrual blood might have escaped into the peritoneal cavity and a peritoneal endometriosis developed, as indicated by the "deposits" of endometrial tissue on the surface of and embedded in the uterine wall (see also Fig. 15).

tissue in these lesions arose from the implantation of the endometrial tissue "sown" on the surface of the peritoneum.

If bits of endometrial tissue, carried by menstrual blood escaping into the venous circulation of the uterus sometimes become implanted on the

endothelial surface of the veins and venous sinuses of the uterine wall
and a like condition arises in the vaginal veins from the menstrual reaction of the mucosa of ectopic endometrial cavities in that situation, we
might infer that bits of endometrial tissue, carried by menstrual blood
escaping into the peritoneal cavity from any source, might become implanted on the mesothelial surface of the peritoneum and give rise to at
least some of the lesions of peritoneal endometriosis.

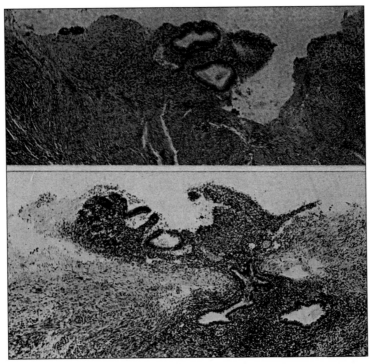

Figs. 14 and 15.—Two photomicrographs (x 60) of implantation-like lesions on
the posterior surface of the uterus. The first was situated beneath the distal pole
of the adherent left ovary shown in Fig. 10, and would seem to be of more recent
origin than the endometrial cavity of the ovary with evidence of perforation shown
in Fig. 11. Similar lesions were also present on the lateral surface of the ovary.
The second was situated near the right ovary (Figs. 10 and 13) also with evidence
of rupture of its endometrial cavity and dissemination of its contents into the
pelvis. If these near-by lesions arose from the escape of the contents of the endometrial cavities of the ovaries, the endometriosis of the culdesac might have had a
similar origin.

The peritoneum of rabbits and monkeys evidently is adapted to the
implantation of endometrial tissue disseminated in the peritoneal cavities
of these animals, but is the peritoneum of women adapted to the implantation of this or any other tissue escaping into their peritoneal cavities?

Cancer escaping into the peritoneal cavity sometimes becomes implanted on the surface of the peritoneum, causing the lesions of peritoneal carcinosis. Could endometrial tissue escaping into the peritoneal
cavity sometimes become implanted on the surface of the peritoneum

and cause the lesions of peritoneal endometriosis? Some will say "cancer is invasive and metastasizes by other channels." Endometrial tissue is sometimes also invasive and mestasizes by vascular channels.

We have shown that the peritoneum is suited to the growth of endometrial tissue, and it will be difficult to deny that endometrial tissue can become implanted on the peritoneum, if it can be demonstrated that this tissue escapes into the peritoneal cavity and the lesions of peritoneal endometriosis occur in situations and under conditions indicating their possible origin from such a source.

THE MENSTRUAL DISSEMINATION OF ENDOMETRIAL TISSUE INTO THE PERITONEAL CAVITY FROM ECTOPIC ENDOMETRIAL FOCI

Evidence has been presented of the viability of endometrial tissue disseminated by menstruation and that it will grow when transferred to suitable situations. We have shown that the peritoneum is suited to the growth of endometrial tissue and furthermore that cancer becomes implanted on it. We might infer that endometrial tissue which, at times, is invasive and metastasizes through vascular channels might also become implanted on the peritoneum. Should it be shown that endometrial tissue carried by menstrual blood escapes into the peritoneal cavity from any source, we would have strong presumptive evidence that under favorable conditions this tissue might become implanted on the peritoneum and cause peritoneal endometriosis. Should these lesions occur in situations and under conditions indicating or even suggesting their origin from such a source, this evidence would be still stronger.

Three possible sources from which menstrual blood might escape into the peritoneal cavity may be considered.

1. The menstrual rupture or perforation of the wall of an endometrial cavity (cyst), most frequently seen in the ovary.

2. The menstrual reaction of endometrial tissue growing on the peritoneal surface of the ovary or any pelvic organ or structure.

3. A back flow through the tubes from the uterus and also possibly from the menstrual reaction of the tubal mucosa.

We know that endometrial cavities in the vaginal wall, at times, rupture into the vaginal canal during menstruation and occasionally must discharge bits of endometrial tissue with the menstrual blood. (Fig. 1). Similar cavities in the abdominal scars of patients with endometriosis in that situation sometimes rupture and discharge blood at the menstrual period. We could infer that like cavities (cysts) in the ovary or in any pelvic organ or structure, at times, must rupture into the peritoneal cavity during menstruation. The study, at operation, of endometrial cysts or hematomas of the ovary shows that the ovary is usually adherent by its *lateral* or *under* surface to the side of the pelvis, posterior layer of the broad ligament, or the posterior surface of the uterus (Figs. 2,

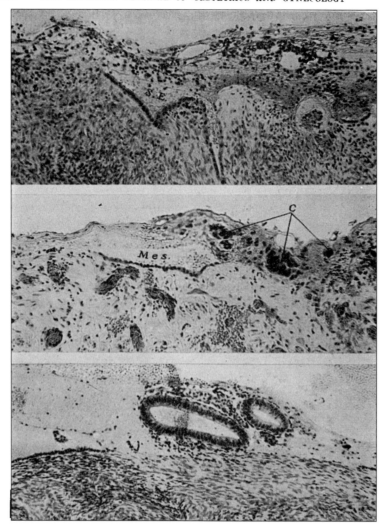

Fig. 16.—Photomicrograph (x 130) showing the reaction of the surface of the ovary to gonorrheal infection escaping through the tubes. An inflammatory exudate is present on the surface of that organ which consists of fibrin, leucocytes and wandering cells derived from the tissues of the ovary. The greater portion of the surface epithelium has disappeared. In the center of the photomicrograph it (*s.e.*) is still present and the exudate has arched over it. If the irritation had continued, the exudate would be replaced by granulation tissue and later by connective tissue with resulting thickening of the ovary or adhesion to adjacent structures. As the result of this reaction to infection, many interesting gland-like structures and cavities lined by the surface epithelium of the ovary arise from the inclusion of this epithelium and its subsequent growth, but they never develop into peritoneal carcinosis or true peritoneal endometriosis.

Fig. 17.—Photomicrograph (x 130) showing the reaction of the surface of the parietal peritoneum to the implantation of cancer, secondary to ovarian cancer. The exudate of Fig. 17, replaced by granulation tissue, is arched over the portion of the mesothelium (*mes.*) which has not disappeared, just as the exudate in Fig. 16 is arched over the surface epithelium of the ovary. Clumps of cancer cells (*c*) caught in the exudate now appear enmeshed in the granulation tissue. As a result of the peritoneal reactions in the implantation of cancer, many interesting lesions result.

Fig. 18.—Photomicrograph (x 130) showing the reaction of the surface of the ovary to the "implantation" of endometrial tissue. Multiple endometrial lesions were

10, 11 and 12). On freeing the ovary, the hematoma or cyst usually ruptures at the apparent seat of a previous perforation and its chocolate-like contents escape into the pelvis (Figs. 19 and 26). Adhesions are always present and often in situations easily soiled by material which might have escaped from a perforation of the ovarian cyst or hematoma. Endometrial tissue is often present in these adhesions and invades the structures involved by them. The question naturally arises: What is the relation between the endometrial tissue lining the cyst of the ovary and that scattered about in the implantation-like lesions of the associated peritoneal endometriosis?

The endometrial tissue in the ovary and that in the peritoneal lesions must have had a common origin or else one is secondary to the other. Should those involving the peritoneum arise from the escape of the con-

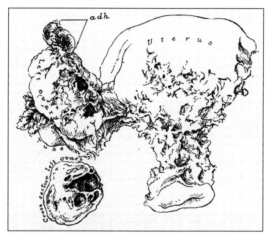

Fig. 19.—Posterior view of the uterus and left tube and ovary (x ⅔). The uterus was retroflexed and firmly adherent due to an extensive peritoneal endometriosis. The uterus, left tube, and ovary were removed and a portion of the right ovary was resected. An endometriosis superficially involved the greater portion of the posterior surface of the uterus. The left ovary was firmly adherent by its *lateral* and *under surfaces* to the posterior layer of the broad ligament and the posterior surface of the uterus. On freeing the ovary the characteristic chocolate-like contents of the ovarian hematoma escaped, possibly through the site of a previous perforation of the hematoma (see cross-section of the ovary). The ovary has been lifted up in order to show the adhesions and endometrial lesions on its *under* and *lateral surfaces*. Both tubes were *patent*. For photomicrographs of sections of the ovaries and uterus, see Figs. 20, 22, 23, and 24. The patient, thirty-six years old, had one child.

tents of the cyst, they must be due either to the stimulation of the peritoneum by some specific element of the cyst contents or else to the implantation of bits of endometrial tissue carried by the contents of the cyst escaping into the peritoneal cavity.

present on the *lateral surface* of the right ovary (see Fig. 29). The endometrial tissue in this illustration may have been derived either from the implantation of similar tissue from other endometrial lesions on the ovary (Fig. 30), from endometrial or tubal tissue escaping through the tubes (both were patent) or from a localized metaplasia of the surface epithelium of the ovary. The surface epithelium is intact at both ends of the illustration, but has disappeared beneath the endometrial tissue. The latter is enmeshed in an exudate somewhat similar to those shown in Figs. 16 and 17. Histologically it resembles an implantation lesion.

Clinical observations have taught us that these cysts sometimes rupture or perforate during menstruation and some of their contents escape into the pelvic cavity. A histologic study of ovarian endometrial cysts, removed during menstruation, demonstrates that the lining of these cysts sometimes reacts to menstruation, as does the mucosa lining the uterine cavity (Figs. 2 and 3), and bits of its endometrial tissue are disseminated into the cavity of the cyst. See Figs. 4 and 5. Therefore, they would be carried into the peritoneal cavity on rupture of the cyst. We have indications that endometrial tissue disseminated by menstruation is sometimes alive and will grow when transferred to suitable situations and also that the peritoneum is suited to the growth of endometrial tissue. Furthermore, the lesions of peritoneal endometriosis often occur in situations and under conditions indicating their origin from the escape of the contents of these cysts into the peritoneal cavity. The peritoneal reac-

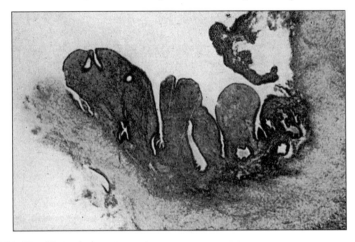

Fig. 20.—Photomicrograph (x 25) showing the lining of an endometrial cavity of the left ovary of Fig. 19 and near the apparent site of a previous perforation. Typical endometrial tissue is present.

tion to this tissue is similar to that of peritoneal carcinosis of implantation origin. We, therefore, have sufficient evidence to believe that peritoneal endometriosis sometimes arises from the implantation of endometrial tissue carried by menstrual blood escaping through a perforation of an endometrial (cavity) cyst of the ovary or any other pelvic structure. (Figs. 6, 10, 19, and 26.)

Endometrial tissue has been found growing on the surfaces of all of the pelvic organs and structures, including the cecum, appendix, loops of the small intestines, sigmoid, and their mesenteries. The patches of endometrial tissue on the ovary nearly always occur on the *lateral* and *under surfaces* of that organ, and these surfaces when they contain endometrial tissue are usually adherent to adjacent structures. The endometrial tissue on the other organs and structures also is often surrounded by adhesions. Some of these patches of endometrial tissue, at times, evidently react to menstruation, just as does the uterine mucosa (Figs. 48, 49, and 50). Menstrual blood occasionally must escape from some of these endometrial foci into the peritoneal cavity. There are, therefore, strong indications that peritoneal endometriosis, at times, spreads in this manner. Because these foci are usually small and are often associated with adhesions and become embedded in the underlying organ

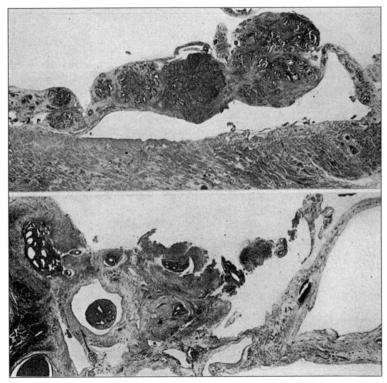

Figs. 21 and 22.—Two photomicrographs (x 10), the first of adhesions on the surface of the uterus, from a patient with peritoneal carcinosis secondary to ovarian cancer. It is but an exaggeration of the condition shown in Fig. 17. Bits of cancer had been caught in the exudate arising from the reaction of the peritoneum to cancer cells escaping into the peritoneal cavity. The subsequent transformation of the exudate into granulation tissue and then connective tissue, together with the growth of the cancer cells, evidently caused the lesion shown here. Compare with Figs. 22, 23, and 24.

The second is of adhesions extending from the left ovary to the uterus, from a patient with peritoneal endometriosis associated with (or secondary to) ovarian endometriosis, with evidence that an endometrial cyst might have ruptured into the peritoneal cavity (Fig. 19). A portion of the ovary is shown at the left with endometrial tissue embedded in it. The origin of the endometrial tissue in these adhesions would seem to be similar to that of cancer in the adhesion of Fig. 21 and the latter was of implantation origin. See also Figs. 23 and 24.

or structure, the opportunity for the menstrual dissemination of endometrial tissue from them probably is not very great except early in their existence.

THE MENSTRUAL DISSEMINATION OF ENDOMETRIAL TISSUE THROUGH THE TUBES FROM THE UTERINE CAVITY

Objections have been made to the theory that bits of endometrial tissue are carried by menstrual blood escaping through the tubes and become implanted on the visceral and parietal peritoneum. The following are the more important of these objections:

1. Menstrual blood rarely, if ever, escapes from the uterine cavity into the tubes.

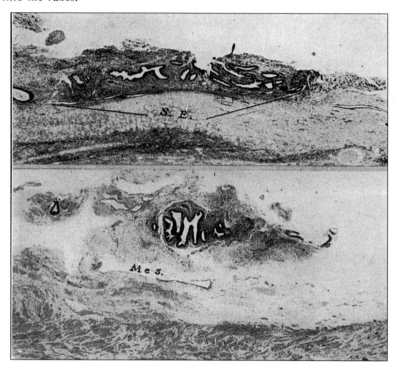

Figs. 23 and 24.—Two photomicrographs (x 25), the first of a patch of endometrial tissue on the *lateral surface* of the ovary (Fig. 19). An inclusion of the surface epithelium of the ovary is shown at *s.e.* The endometrial tissue is situated above it and evidently in ovarian tissue which has arched over the surface epithelium of the ovary as in the peritoneal reactions shown in Figs. 16, 17, and 21.

The second is of adhesions on the posterior surface of the uterus (Fig. 19), containing endometrial tissue. There has been a peritoneal reaction to some irritant causing adhesions and a mesothelial inclusion (*mes.*), the latter due to granulation tissue arching over the mesothelial surface of the peritoneum. Endometrial tissue is embedded in the adhesions above the mesothelial inclusion just as cancer of implantation origin becomes embedded in the adhesions of peritoneal carcinosis (Fig. 21). The peritoneal endometrial lesions possibly are of more recent origin than the endometrial cyst of the ovary and from evidence found at operation, it would seem that they might have arisen from the escape of the contents of the ovarian cyst into the pelvis (Fig. 19):

2. The lumen of the interstitial portion of the tube is too small for bits of endometrial tissue to pass through it.

3. Endometrial tissue, set free by menstruation, is dead or dying and therefore incapable of implantation.

4. Several days must be required for endometrial tissue to be carried from the uterine cavity through the tubes, and, therefore, there is little chance that "such degenerative tissue" after "probably many days of continuing degeneration and autolysis should grow where it falls." Novak.[4]

Novak[6] states that my theory would be greatly strengthened, if I could demonstrate two things.

1. The capacity of the degenerated endometrium given off at menstruation to grow in tissue culture.

2. The capacity of such endometrium to grow in the peritoneum or ovary of the human being or perhaps even of one of the lower animals.

I have examined menstrual blood obtained both from the vagina and also from the cavities of uteri removed at operation. The endometrial tissue obtained from these sources did not always show degenerative

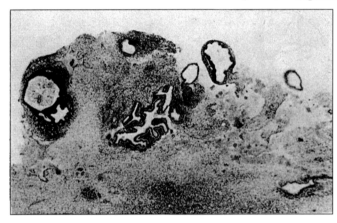

Fig. 25.—Photomicrograph (x 25) of a portion of the right ovary (case of Fig. 19). An apparent endometrial lesion was situated on its *lateral surface*. It is evidently of more recent origin than the endometrial cyst of the opposite ovary (see Fig. 19). Should the endometrial tissue in this case have arisen from the differentiation of celomic epithelium due to its stimulation by an ovarian hormone, we should expect that these lesions would all be of the same age.

changes, but frequently presented a normal appearance (Fig. 47). This, however, does not prove that it is alive and capable of growing, even if transferred to suitable situations. Evidence has already been given to show that endometrial tissue disseminated by menstruation into the venous circulation, at times, becomes implanted in the sinuses of the uterine wall and in one instance in veins about endometrial cavities in the posterior vaginal wall. Evidence has also been presented to show that endometrial cavities (cysts) of the ovary, at times, discharge their contents, containing endometrial tissue cast off by menstruation, into the pelvis and that peritoneal implantations of this tissue arise from this source. It has also been demonstrated by this and other observations that the visceral and parietal peritoneum is suited to the growth of endometrial tissue.

If bits of endometrial tissue could be carried through the interstitial portion of the tubes by menstrual blood escaping from the uterine cavity into these ducts and not spend too long a time in their transit, one would expect that peritoneal implantations of this tissue might occur from this source.

Over twelve years ago I began a series of experiments to determine the shape of the uterine cavity in normal and in pathologic conditions. The technic was as follows: the uterus removed at operation or autopsy was placed in a basin of warm water and then filled with melted gelatin (about 15 per cent) containing in suspension bismuth subcarbonate or barium sulphate. This was introduced through the cervical canal by means of a syringe. After filling the uterine cavity the syringe was withdrawn, the cervix clamped in order to prevent the escape of the injection mass and the specimen placed in cold water until the gelatin

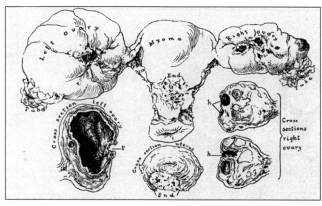

Fig. 26.—Uterus, tubes, and ovaries (x ½). The uterus was retroflexed and adherent due to peritoneal endometriosis. An intramural leiomyoma is present in the posterior wall of the body of the uterus. An endometriosis involved the uterus at the junction of the body and the cervix, invading its wall (see Fig. 28). The left ovary was adherent by its *lateral surface* to the side of the pelvis. On freeing it, the chocolate-like contents of the ovarian hematoma escaped, possibly through the site of a previous perforation of the hematoma (see also cross-section of the ovary). The right ovary was adherent by its *lateral surface* to the posterior layer of the broad ligament. Multiple endometrial lesions involved the posterior surface of the right ovary (see cross-sections of the ovary and Fig. 27). Both tubes were patent. The patient, thirty-one years old, was married but had never been pregnant.

had solidified. The uterus then was fixed in formalin. On filling the uterine cavity, the mass would usually easily escape through the tubes, if the latter were patent. Roentgenograms (especially stereoscopic ones) of the hardened uterus enabled one to obtain a clear picture of the form of the uterine cavity under various conditions and also of the course and relative diameters of the interstitial portions of the tubes. Many uteri were studied in this manner. In some the interstitial portion of the tubes appeared as a mere thread in the roentgenograms and in others as a relatively large canal. The results of some of these studies[7] were presented before this society nine years ago. Two of the illustrations of that paper are again reproduced, one showing a uterus with very

narrow interstitial portions of the tubes and the other with dilated ones
(Figs. 40 and 41). I suggested at that time that menstrual blood under
favorable conditions might escape through the tubes into the peritoneal
cavity. Since then I have been greatly interested in the menstrual
regurgitation of blood into the tubes and have operated upon many
patients during their menstrual period and have occasionally observed
this phenomenon (eight cases). I have also found endometrial tissue

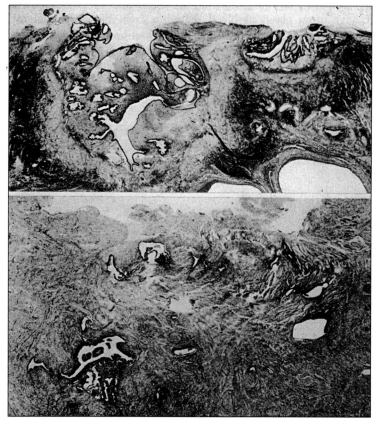

Figs. 27 and 28.—Two photomicrographs (x 10), the first shows some of the
endometrial lesions of the right ovary of the preceding illustration. They are evidently of more recent origin than the endometrial hematoma of the opposite ovary.
The second is of the endometriosis of the posterior uterine wall. There is apparently an invasion of the uterine wall from tissue implanted or developing on its
peritoneal surface. If the former, it might have been derived from endometrial
tissue escaping either from the ovary or from the tubes; both of the latter were
patent.

in the lumina of tubes removed during menstruation. It seemed to
me that the blood in the tubes in these eight cases came from the
uterine cavity. It was present in both tubes in each instance. However,
the source of endometrial tissue in the lumina of the tubes is a debatable
one and if it can be shown that the interstitial portion of the tubes is

always so small that bits of endometrial tissue cannot pass through it, the peritoneal implantation of endometrial tissue from this source can be eliminated.

The roentgenograms of the injected uteri suggested that the interstitial portion of some tubes is sufficiently great to permit bits of endometrial tissue to pass through it (Figs. 40, 41, and 42). Can it be proved that blood escaping from the uterine cavity into the tubes will actually carry with it bits of endometrial tissue?

I have often observed blood dripping from the abdominal ostia of the tubes in abdominal operations which had been preceded by a curettage of the uterus. I do not understand just why this should occur. Bits of endometrial tissue, apparently set free by the curette, were

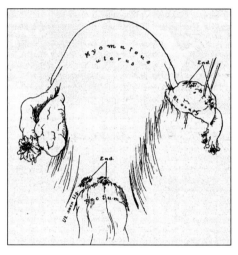

Fig. 29.—Uterus (containing a submucous leiomyoma), tubes, and ovaries drawn upwards (x ⅓), showing a peritoneal endometriosis obliterating the bottom of the culdesac and involving the left uterosacral ligament (Fig. 31). Multiple endometrial lesions are present on the *lateral surface* of the right ovary (Figs. 18 and 30). Both tubes were *patent*. The peritoneal endometriosis in the culdesac is in a situation easily soiled by material escaping from the tubes or ovaries, and that of the right ovary is on a surface of that organ, which would readily be contaminated by material escaping from the tube. The lateral surface of the ovary normally lies against the posterior layer of the broad ligament or side of the pelvis and thus a crevice is formed which would retain any material lodging in it. The lesions are situated on the dependent portion of the ovary, namely, the bottom of the crevice. The patient, forty-five years old, was single.

found in the lumina of tubes which had been removed and some of those pieces were larger than similar pieces of endometrial tissue set free by menstruation (Figs. 44 and 46). If endometrial tissue set free by curettage is carried by blood escaping from the uterine cavity into the tubes, similar tissue set free by menstruation might be carried with menstrual blood escaping from the uterine cavity into the tubes. Also, the time required for menstrual blood to go from the uterine cavity into the tubes might be very short, not several days but a few moments and possibly no longer than that taken by uterine bleeding from a curettage.

These observations demonstrate that blood escaping from the uterine cavity into the tubes, at times, can carry with it bits of endometrial tissue and that the time required for this may be very short.

Fragments of endometrial tissue have been found in the lumina of tubes removed at operation. What is the possible origin of this tissue? I believe that endometrial tissue in the lumen of the tube may arise from the following sources; (1) artefacts; (2) carried by blood escaping from the uterine cavity during or after curettage; (3) from the menstrual reaction of endometrial tissue forming a part of the tubal mucosa; (4) from ectopic endometrial tissue in the pelvis (Novak); (5) carried by blood escaping into the tubes from the uterine cavity during menstruation.

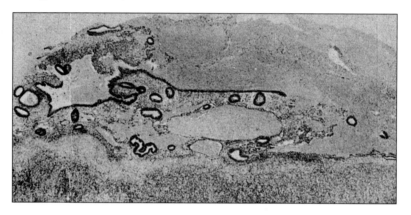

Fig. 30.—Photomicrograph (x 25) of a portion of the right ovary (Fig. 19). Typical endometrial tissue is present. In the menstrual reaction of this tissue bits of it might be set free, escape in the culdesac, or lodge in any of its natural pockets. They might also lodge on other portions of the ovary. Multiple endometrial lesions in different stages of development were present on the lateral surface of this ovary (see Fig. 19). They are often found on the peritoneal surface of structures adjacent to such an ovary. It is conceivable that such lesions on the surface of the ovary primarily might have arisen from endometrial tissue escaping through the tubes.

For some time I have been interested in the study of the menstrual dissemination of endometrial tissue into the venous circulation. Bits of the uterine mucosa were found in the veins and sinuses of menstruating uteri. A careful study of these sections and the technic of embedding the blocks, from which they were cut, convinced me that some of these findings were due to artefacts. The menstruating uterine mucosa is very friable; fragments break off during the embedding of the blocks of the uterus and some of these may lodge in the gaping veins and sinuses of the uterine wall. They appear as endometrial emboli in the stained sections (see Figs. 19, 20, and 21 of previous article[2]). If, however, fragments of the uterine mucosa are found surrounded by blood in a vessel or attached to its wall by fibrin, it is evident that it reached this situation before the tissues were fixed. It occurred to me that bits of endometrial tissue floating about in the embedding solutions could lodge in the lumen of the ampulla of the tube as readily as in the gaping vessels of the uterine wall. A "block" of the ampulla of the tube would furnish a very convenient "basket" for any scraps of tissue floating about in the embedding solutions which were small enough to enter its lumen. Bits of uterine mucosa and barium sulphate were purposely placed in the solutions, in which blocks of tubes were being embedded. Both barium sulphate and pieces of uterine mucosa were found in sections from some of these tubes (Fig. 39). Just as faulty technic sometimes plays an important rôle in placing (disseminating) bits of endometrial tissue in the lumina of the gaping vessels of the uterine wall, it may also place such tissue in

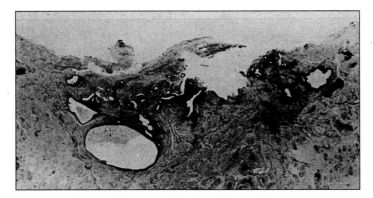

Fig. 31.—Photomicrograph (x 10) of the endometriosis of the left uterosacral ligament (Fig. 29). The endometrial tissue evidently has invaded this structure from its peritoneal surface. It was in a situation easily soiled by material escaping from the ovaries or the tubes. It must have arisen either by metaplasia of the peritoneum or from an implantation of endometrial tissue.

the lumen of the fallopian tube. It is difficult to estimate to what extent artefacts and curettage of the uterus have contributed to the etiology of the endometrial tissue in the tubes which have been described in the literature of this subject. This is a problem for each laboratory worker to decide for himself.

The histologic picture of tubes with bits of endometrial tissue set free by curettage differs from that of tubes containing endometrial tissue due to artefacts. In the latter the endometrial tissue lies free in the lumen of the tube (Fig. 39), while in the former it is embedded in blood (Fig. 46) which has obviously come from the uterine cavity, unless the blood has escaped from the tube after its removal. In recent years I have ligated the distal ends of tubes containing blood before removing them. An interesting problem arises and that is the fate of endometrial tissue carried by blood escaping into the tubes during curettage.   Could it sometimes be retained in the lumen of the tube and even live and actually increase in size or may it escape into the peritoneal cavity and sometimes become implanted on the pelvic peritoneum? Davis[8] has reported an interesting case suggesting the latter.

Theoretically it is possible for bits of endometrial tissue to be set free in the lumen of the tube from the reaction of the tubal mucosa to menstruation (Fig. 58).

Novak has published photomicrographs of sections of tubes showing endometrial tissue in their lumina and offers the theory that this tissue might have come from ectopic endometrial tissue in the pelvis and entered the tube through its abdominal ostium, just as the ovum and

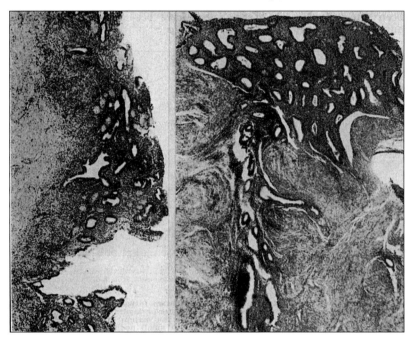

Fig. 32.—Two photomicrographs (x 25), the first of the lateral surface of the left ovary and the other of the adjacent peritoneum.   The left ovary was adherent by its *lateral surface* to the side of the pelvis.   Both *tubes* were *patent*.   The peritoneal endometriosis was situated in the peritoneum adherent to the ovary.   It would seem that the endometriosis of the ovary and of the peritoneum must have had either a common origin or one was secondary to the other.   Both were in a situation readily soiled by material escaping from the patent left tube.   The opposite tube and ovary were normal.   Another peritoneal implantation-like lesion was present in the culdesac near the left uterosacral ligament (accidental findings in resection of the sigmoid for cancer in a patient, forty-nine years old, married, but who never had been pregnant).

particles of cancer in peritoneal carcinosis are known to enter the tubes.   I believe that this occasionally might occur from the rupture of an endometrial cyst (cavity) and also from the menstrual reaction of endometrial tissue growing on the surface of the ovary and other pelvic structures.   Endometrial tissue on the ovary nearly always occurs on the *lateral* and *under surfaces* of that organ and the surface containing this tissue is usually adherent to adjacent structures, such as the side of the pelvis, the posterior layer of the broad ligament or the posterior surface of the uterus. On account of these adhesions it is difficult for bits of endometrial tissue to be set free even by a menstrual reaction so that they could escape into the tubes. However, I believe that it sometimes occurs and that they may escape into the lumen of the tubes.

During the last five years I have studied the material from 293 patients with peritoneal lesions containing endometrium-like tissue. In many of these cases one and sometimes both tubes and ovaries have been removed. In nearly all of the cases, in which one or both tubes have been removed, sections of the tubes have been examined. In some

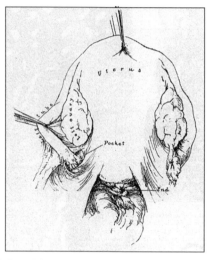

Fig. 33.—View of the pelvic contents, uterus drawn forward (x ½). The fimbriae of the left tube were lightly adherent to the posterior layer of the broad ligament. In a shallow peritoneal pocket directly beneath the ostium of the tube, the endometrial lesion shown in Fig. 34 was obtained. A small nodule (end) is situated in the culdesac. Both ovaries appeared normal and both *tubes* were *patent*. Prior to the operation the uterus was retroflexed. The patient, thirty-four years old, was married and had children.

only one block was cut from the tube and only two or three sections from each block were studied. In other instances two or more blocks from the tube or tubes were made and many sections were studied from each block. The purpose of these studies was threefold: (1) to detect fragments of endometrial tissue in the lumen of the tube; (2) to seek evidence of a menstrual reaction of the tubal mucosa; (3) to compare the histologic structure of the tubal mucosa with that of the associated ectopic endometrial tissue. I have encountered only three instances (Figs. 46, 53, and 55) of fragments of endometrial tissue in the lumen of tubes from these cases and all three patients were menstruating at the time of the operation. Blood was observed in both tubes in each instance at the time of the operation and it was apparently coming from the uterus. At the time I thought (and still believe) that the pieces of endometrial tissue in the tubes were probably carried by the blood coming from the uterine cavity, as blood escaping from the uterine cavity during curettage sometimes carries with it endometrial tissue.

Let us consider the possible sources of blood in the lumina of the tubes of patients operated upon during menstruation: (1) the tubal mucosa; (2) the uterine cavity as the result of curettage; (3) drawn into the tube through its abdominal ostium from blood in the pelvis; (4) as a back flow from blood in the uterine cavity.

Bleeding occasionally occurs during menstruation from ectopic patches of uterine mucosa in the tubal lining (Fig. 58). Should menstruating

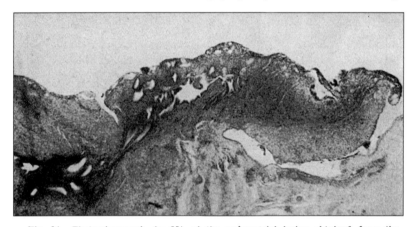

Fig. 34.—Photomicrograph (x 25) of the endometrial lesion obtained from the peritoneal pocket beneath the ostium of the adherent left tube of Fig. 33. Endometrial tissue implanted or developing on the surface of the peritoneum has invaded its deeper structures. It would seem to have arisen from material escaping from the tube. Is it an implantation of endometrial tissue or a metaplasia of the peritoneum arising from stimulation of the latter by some specific material escaping from the tube?

uteri be curetted prior to abdominal operations, one would expect to find blood in the lumina of the tubes in some of these cases, just as it occurs in the tubes of nonmenstruating uteri following curettage.

One would also expect that blood in the pelvic cavity from any source might be drawn into the tube through its abdominal ostium. This last year I operated upon a patient, apparently during her menstrual period. There was a large amount of blood in the pelvis and it could be seen dripping from the right tube which was only slightly larger than the opposite one. The left tube appeared normal and on stripping it blood did not escape from its ostium. The bleeding tube was removed and was found to contain the remains of a very early pregnancy. I have since examined the opposite patent tube in two other cases of tubal pregnancy and was unable to detect any blood in them. I have found it in the opposite tube when the fimbriated end has been occluded. These observations are too few to be of any great value.

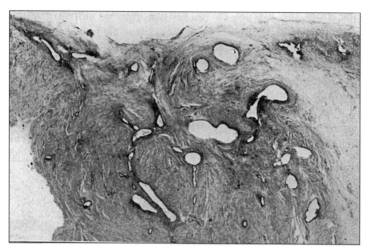

Fig. 35.—Photomicrograph (x 10) of the nodule removed from the culdesac of Fig. 33. It is apparently an older lesion than that shown in Fig. 34. It must have arisen from an earlier implantation of endometrial tissue or an earlier specific stimulation of the peritoneal mesothelium.

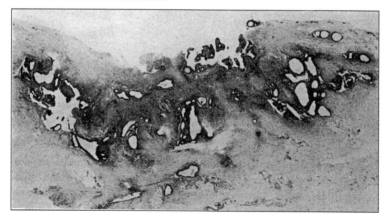

Fig. 36.—Photomicrograph (x 10) of a "patch" of endometriosis in the peritoneum of the side of the pelvis, very close to the ostium of the patent left tube and directly over the ureter, as was the peritoneal endometriosis of Fig. 32. A similar lesion involved the left uterosacral ligament. Both ovaries were normal and both tubes were patent. The patient, forty-two years old, had children. It is an implantation-like lesion in a situation easily soiled by material escaping from the patent left tube.

When blood is found at operation in the tubes of menstruating uteri and apparently is increased by compressing the uterus, this blood probably came from the uterine cavity and, at times, must carry with it bits of endometrial tissue set free by menstruation.

In four instances in which blood was observed by me, escaping from the tubes of patients operated upon during menstruation, there was no indication for the removal of the tubes other than the desire to study their contents. Blood was collected from the tubes by stripping them from the uterus towards their fimbriated end. The blood was spread on slides, dried, fixed, and stained by various methods. Epithelium-like cells were found in these preparations and also clumps of cells resembling the stroma of the uterine mucosa. There are certain valid

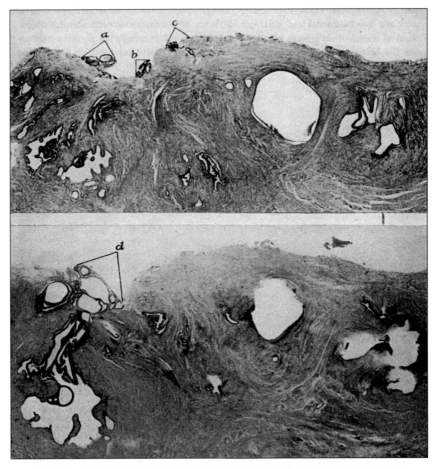

Fig. 37.—Two photomicrographs (x 10) of sections of an endometriosis of the posterior uterine wall at different levels of the same block. Typical endometrial tissue is growing on the peritoneal surface of the uterus at *a* and *b*. Lesion *a* is a part of the endometrial tissue of *d* on the peritoneal surface of the uterus shown in the lower photomicrograph. The latter apparently has invaded the deeper tissues of the uterine wall, causing a so-called adenomyoma. For a higher magnification of the lesion indicated by *c* of the upper photomicrograph, see next illustration. The patient, fifty years old, was single. The uterus was retroflexed and contained multiple leiomyomas. Both *tubes* were *patent* and both ovaries appeared normal. The left ovary was removed and endometrial tissue was not found in it. Implantation-like patches of peritoneal endometriosis were present on the posterior surface of the lower portion of the body of the uterus and in the posterior culdesac in situations easily soiled by material escaping from the patent tubes.

objections to this method. One is that trauma of stripping the tubes may dislodge some of the tubal mucosa and the other is the difficulty we (Dr. L. A. Sutton who was interested in this problem and myself) experienced in identifying the cells in these specimens. In all four cases blood was present in both tubes and in none of them was a peritoneal endometriosis present or any evident endometrial tissue on the surface of the ovaries.

In four other cases one or both tubes were removed with the uterus.

CASE I.—Peritoneal endometriosis with an adherent, retroflexed uterus. Endometrial lesions were present on the lateral surface of the ovary, the posterior surface of the uterus, and on the cecum. Blood was observed escaping from both tubes on exposing the pelvic organs at the operation. The uterus, right tube and ovary

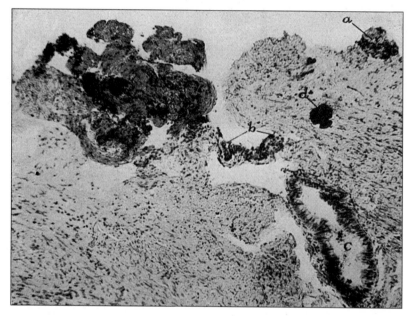

Fig. 38.—Photomicrograph (x 130) of the peritoneal lesion indicated by c of the preceding illustration. The surface of the uterus shows a reaction to some irritant. At a a piece of tissue consisting of fibrin and "dead cells" is adherent to the uterus. A larger mass of similar tissue is present to the left. At b endometrium-like cells have grown over or are attached to a "bridge" of newly-formed tissue. Possibly these cells were derived from similar cells in the necrotic mass above them and to the left, which had not died. Endometrial tissue c is becoming embedded in the uterine wall by the tissue of the latter growing over it. Lesion d probably represents a mass of cells which are dead. This and other sections from the same block suggest a peritoneal reaction to endometrial tissue added to (implanted on) the posterior surface of the uterus. The greater portion of this tissue in this photomicrograph is dead, but some lived (that in contact with the surface of the uterus) with a resulting endometriosis.

were removed. Unfortunately, the distal end of the tube was not ligated and most of the blood in the tube escaped during the manipulation of the operation. Epithelium and tissue resembling endometrial stroma were found in the lumen of the tube, adherent to the surface of the tubal mucosa. From the nature of the peritoneal lesions and those in the ovary I do not believe that endometrial tissue in the tube could have come from these (Figs. 51, 52, and 53).

CASE 2.—Retroflexed uterus containing multiple small leiomyomas. On exposing the pelvic organs at operation blood was observed escaping from both tubes and apparently coming from the uterus. Two small hemorrhagic blebs were present on the under surface of the left ovary. Blood was not observed escaping from these. The fimbriated ends of both tubes were first ligated and also the uterine end of the right tube, then the uterus, left tube and ovary, and right tube were removed. This case was reported in a previous article.[9] Strips of epithelium, a gland, and fragments of endometrial stroma mixed with blood were found in the lumen of one of the tubes. These were identical in their structure and staining reaction with those present in the mucosa of the uterus from which a large amount of tissue had been cast off by menstruation. The ovarian lesion consisted of two

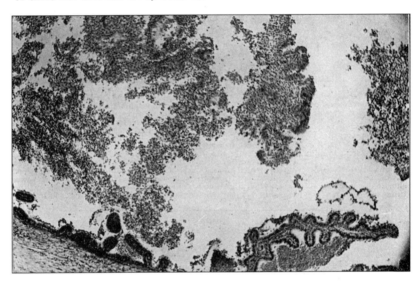

Fig. 39.—Photomicrograph (x 60) showing endometrial tissue free in the lumen of the tube due to an "artefact." Since bits of endometrial tissue floating about in the embedding solutions easily lodge in the empty vessels of blocks of the uterine wall carried through these solutions (see Figs. 19, 20 and 21 of previous article[2]), similar scraps in these solutions might find a "block" of the ampulla of the tube a very convenient "basket" in which to drop. Bits of endometrial tissue and barium sulphate were purposely placed in the embedding solutions through which "blocks" of the tubes were being carried and these were found in sections of the tubes. In a study of endometrial or any other foreign tissue in the lumen of the tube an artefact should be considered, and, if possible, eliminated.

small blebs lined by epithelium of endometrial type with very little stroma and no glands. In places a small amount of the epithelial lining had been cast off by an apparent menstrual reaction or from the trauma of the operation, but not enough to account for that present in the tube nor did it resemble this as closely as did the mucosa lining the uterine cavity. The blood in the tubes was apparently coming from the uterus and carried with it endometrial tissue. It might be claimed that the endometrial tissue was forced into the tubes by the manipulation of the uterus during the operation, but blood was in the tubes prior to the handling of the uterus (Figs. 54, 55, and 56).

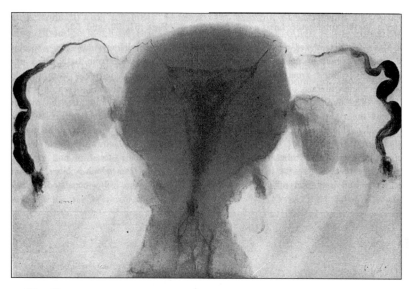

Fig. 40.—Roentgenogram (x ⅔) of the uterus, tubes, and ovaries after filling the uterine cavity with gelatine containing bismuth subcarbonate. The mass readily escaped from the uterine cavity into the tubes. The uterus, tubes, and ovaries were removed for uterine bleeding due to myofibrosis (illustration published[7] in 1918). The interstitial portions of the tubes appear as mere threads, but even so, small bits of endometrial tissue might be carried into the tubes by blood escaping from the uterine cavity during curettage and menstruation (see Fig. 42). The specimen was hardened in formalin, before taking the roentgenogram, which would narrow the lumen of the tube. The uterus was placed, anterior surface downward, on a piece of waxed cardboard, beneath which was the photographic plate in two light-proof envelopes. Therefore, the distance from the tubes to the photographic plate was short. This would cause only a slight enlargement of the apparent lumen of the tube, possibly not compensating for the shrinkage due to hardening the specimen.

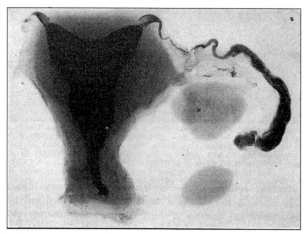

Fig. 41.—Roentgenogram (x ⅔) similar to the preceding. The uterus and one tube and ovary were removed for multiple small uterine leiomyomas. The lumen of the interstitial portion of the tube is much greater than that of the preceding specimen, and therefore, larger bits of endometrial tissue could pass from the uterine cavity into the tubes than in the former. Illustration also published in 1918, in the legend of which I suggested that menstrual blood, at times, might escape through the tubes into the peritoneal cavity. Note the normal construction of the distal end of the tube at the origin of its fimbriae, also shown in the preceding specimen,

CASE 3.—Leiomyoma of the uterus. On exposing the pelvic organs at operation blood was observed escaping from both tubes. Endometrial tissue was present on the lateral surface of the left ovary which was adherent to the posterior surface of the uterus. A small patch of endometrial tissue was present on the posterior surface of the uterus mesial to the left ovary. The distal ends of both tubes were ligated and then the uterus, both tubes, and ovaries were removed. Bits of endometrial tissue were found embedded in blood in the lumen of the tubes, which were identical in their structure with fragments of the uterine mucosa present in blood obtained from the uterine cavity. The endometrial tissue on the sur-

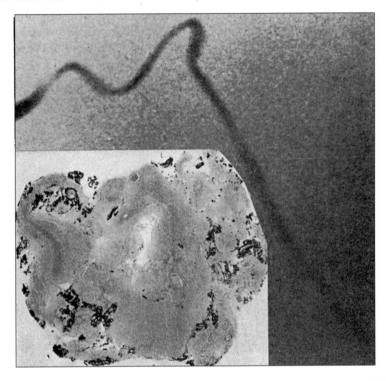

Fig. 42.—Photomicrograph (x 10) of a section of menstrual blood from the cavity of the uterus shown in the next illustration, placed beside an enlargement (x 10) of the very narrow thread-like interstitial portion of the tube shown in the roentgenogram of Fig. 40. The smaller bits of the uterine mucosa in this blood would easily pass through the lumen of the tube and the larger pieces would readily pass through a tube of greater caliber as the tube of the roentgenogram of Fig. 41. Blood escaping from the uterine cavity into the tubes during curettage and menstruation, at times, might carry with it bits of the uterine mucosa suspended in that blood (Fig. 46).

faces of the ovary and the uterus showed the same reaction to menstruation as did the mucosa lining the uterine cavity. I cannot exclude the possibility that blood, carrying with it endometrial tissue, had escaped into the abdominal ostia of the tubes from the menstruating endometrial tissue on the ovary and the uterus. From observations made at operation it appeared that the blood in the tube came from the uterine cavity. It was present in both tubes. The endometrial lesions on the surface of the left ovary were small and that aspect of the ovary was adherent to the uterus, thus lessening the chance of endometrial tissue escaping (see Figs. 43, 45, 46, 48, 49, and 50).

CASE 4.—Submucous leiomyoma of the uterus. On exposing the pelvic organs at operation blood was observed escaping from both tubes and apparently coming from the uterus. Peritoneal endometriosis was not present, nor was there any evidence of endometrial tissue on the surface of the ovaries. The fimbriated end of the left tube was ligated and the left tube and ovary and uterus were removed. A clump of epithelium-like cells, which I was unable to identify, was found in the lumen of the tube but no endometrial stroma. A mitotic figure was present in one of these cells (Fig. 57). I was unable to find any mitotic figures in epithelial cells in the blood obtained from the uterine cavity.

I fully realize that it is impossible definitely to state the origin of the blood in the lumen of the tubes in these eight cases. In all instances the blood was observed in the tubes of menstruating uteri prior to the opera-

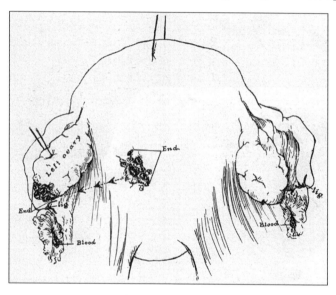

Fig. 43.—Myomatous uterus, tubes and ovaries drawn upwards (x ⅔). (Case 3 of this article.) The patient, forty-nine years old, married and having had children, was operated upon during menstruation. The left ovary (freed and lifted up) was adherent by its *lateral* and *under surfaces* to the posterior uterine wall, due to an endometriosis of the ovary (Fig. 48). A patch of endometrial tissue (Fig. 49) is present on the posterior uterine wall adjacent to the area to which the ovary had been adherent. Blood was observed coming from the abdominal ostia of both tubes. The distal ends of both tubes were first ligated in order to retain their contents, and then the uterus, tubes, and ovaries were removed. Did the blood in the tubes come from the uterine cavity or were the tubes disgorging blood obtained from the menstrual reaction of the misplaced endometrial tissue on the surface of the uterus and the lateral and under surface of the left ovary, the latter having been adherent to the uterus? Blood was present in *both tubes* and apparently was coming from the uterus and I believe that was its origin.

tive manipulation of that organ and if it came from the uterine cavity, as it apparently did, we know that it may carry with it bits of endometrial tissue. We should also expect that this endometrial tissue would be as capable of becoming implanted in suitable situations as that escaping into the venous circulation of the uterus and vagina and that escaping into the peritoneal cavity from ectopic endometrial foci in the pelvis.

THE LESIONS OF PERITONEAL ENDOMETRIOSIS OFTEN OCCUR IN SITUATIONS AND UNDER CONDITIONS INDICATING THEIR ORIGIN FROM MATERIAL ESCAPING INTO THE PERITONEAL CAVITY

One of the outstanding features of patients with peritoneal endometriosis is that the tubes are usually patent. In 293 cases of peritoneal lesions containing endometrium-like tissue encountered during the last five years both tubes appeared to be patent in 284, a unilateral hematosalpinx in three (in two of these blood was present in the opposite tube but the tube was patent), bilateral hematosalpinx in four, and bilateral pyosalpinx in two. Patent tubes apparently increase the incidence of peritoneal endometriosis and possibly the relatively large number of

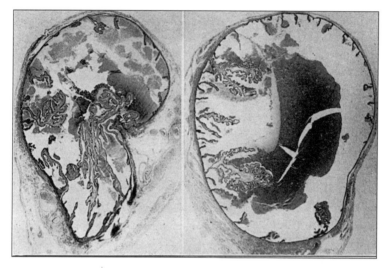

Fig. 44.—Photomicrograph (x 6) of a cross-section of the ampulla of a tube containing blood and bits of endometrial tissue (Fig. 46), carried with that blood from the uterine cavity during curettage. The abdominal operation had been preceded by a curettage of the uterus and repair of the pelvic floor. On exposing the pelvic contents, blood was observed dripping from the abdominal ostia of both tubes. I had planned to sterilize the patient. One tube was removed after ligating its distal end, so as to retain its contents. This tube was fixed in formalin. The opposite tube was cut at its uterine end and the stump buried. The bits of endometrial tissue (Fig. 46) floating about in blood in the lumen of the tube must have passed through its interstitial portion. Therefore, similar bits of endometrial tissue might be carried into the tube by menstrual blood escaping from the uterine cavity (Fig. 46).

Fig. 45.—Photomicrograph (x 6) of a cross-section of the ampulla of one of the tubes shown in Fig. 43. It contains blood and small bits of endometrial tissue, possibly carried with blood from the uterine cavity during menstruation, just as blood escapes from the uterine cavity into the tubes during curettage (Figs. 44 and 46). The ligated tubes, hardened in formalin, were cut into blocks and many sections were made from each block. Bits of endometrial tissue were found in sections from two different blocks. Unfortunately, the blocks removed from both tubes were run through the embedding solutions together and I was unable to determine whether the endometrial tissue was found only in one tube or in both. Blood was present, however, in both tubes.

patients with hematosalpinx (seven) may be of some significance. In the six cases with occlusion of both tubes, the peritoneal lesions might have been present prior to the closure of the fimbriated ends of the

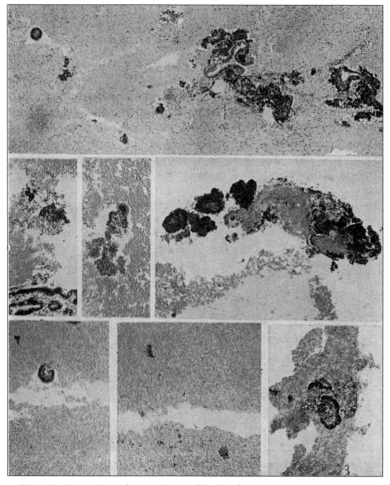

Fig. 46.—Seven photomicrographs (x 60), the lower three are from sections of the tube shown in Fig. 44 containing blood which had escaped from the uterine cavity during curettage. Bits of uterine mucosa are present in the blood and must have been carried with the latter through the interstitial portion of the tube.

The upper photomicrograph is of the section of the blood from the cavity of the menstruating uterus shown in Fig. 43. Blood apparently coming from the uterus was present in both tubes. Did the blood and endometrial tissue in these tubes come from the uterine cavity or from the menstruating ectopic endometrial tissue on the surface of the left ovary and adjacent surface of the uterus (Fig. 43, 48, 49, and 50)?

The middle three photomicrographs are from three different sections of the tube or tubes shown in Figs. 43 and 45. The first two photomicrographs show bits of endometrial tissue (epithelium and stroma) similar to those in the photomicrograph of the blood from the uterine cavity (above) and also those carried into the tubes during curettage (below). This suggests that they came from the uterine cavity but does not prove it. Both blood and endometrial tissue might escape into the tubes from the menstruating endometrial tissue on the surface of the ovary and the uterus (see Figs. 48, 49, and 50). The largest of the three middle photomicrographs shows a curved, elongated, "moulded" mass consisiting of bits of endometrial tissue and fibrin. Should the endometrial tissue in the photomicrogrph above it be forced into a narrow, curved tube, it would be moulded or fashioned into a mass like this. I believe that this moulded mass represents a cast of the lumen of a narrow portion of the tube and adds to the evidence already presented that the endometrial tissue in the tube or tubes was derived from the uterine cavity. The manipulation of the uterus during the operation may have forced endometrial tissue and blood from the uterine cavity into the tubes and dislodged this endometrial "plug." This is probably true. Blood was, however, observed escaping from the tubes before the uterus was handled.

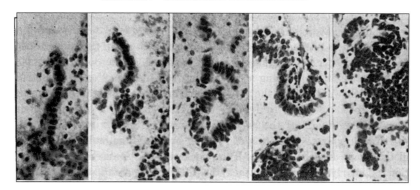

Fig. 47.—Five photomicrographs (x 250), the first two are of menstrual blood obtained from the vagina of two different patients. The third is from blood obtained from the uterus in curettage. The uterine epithelium in the first two appears just as healthy and just as much alive as that in the third. The fourth is from the menstrual blood of the uterine cavity (Case 3). The uterine epithelium stains as sharply as that in the third. The fifth is of a portion of the endometrial "cast" found in the tube of Case 3 and shown in Fig. 46. Epithelium, in the upper and lower ends of this photomicrograph, would seem to be alive. I have purposely photographed the healthiest appearing endometrial tissue that I could find in menstrual blood, the very kind I would choose to sow were I cultivating (implanting) this tissue.

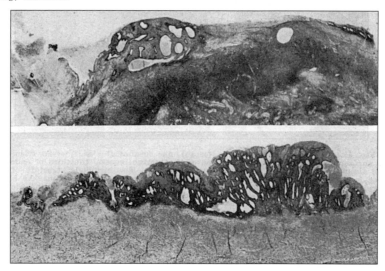

Figs. 48 and 49.—Two photomicrographs (x 10), one of the endometriosis on the surface of the left ovary and the other of the endometriosis on the surface of the uterus adjacent to the ovary. Both are of the same structure and of the same apparent age. They must have had either a common origin or one must have been secondary to the other. They are in a situation (Fig. 43) readily "soiled" by material escaping from the abdominal ostium, of the patent left tube.

tubes. It would seem that during the menstrual life of women some substance escapes from the tubes into the pelvis which plays an important rôle in the etiology of pelvic peritoneal endometriosis, including the development of endometrial tissue on the ovaries. This substance may be menstrual blood in some instances and tubal secretions in others.

In either case epithelium may be present. Endometrial tissue on the ovary nearly always occurs on the *lateral* and *under surfaces* of that organ. These surfaces are usually in contact with the side of the pelvis, the posterior layer of the broad ligament, or the posterior surface of the uterus, thus forming a crevice between the ovary and these structures which would favor the retention of any material escaping from the tubes into the pelvis. In freeing the ovary containing an endometrial hematoma, the wall of the hematoma is usually torn or reopened at the site of a previous perforation of the cyst or where the endometrial tissue in the ovary first developed. The tear in the cyst caused by the operation is nearly always on either the *lateral* or *under surface* of that structure.

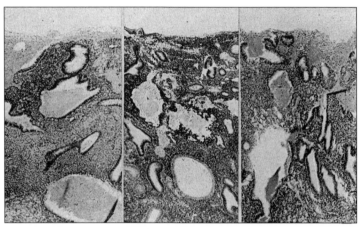

Fig. 50.—Three photomicrographs (x 40), the first of the endometrial tissue on the surface of the left ovary, the second of the uterine mucosa, the third of endometrial tissue on the surface of the uterus (Fig. 43). The histologic structure of all three is the same and they all show the same reaction to menstruation. As blood carrying with it bits of endometrial tissue escapes from the mucosa of the uterine cavity during menstruation, so might it likewise escape from these ectopic endometrial foci. Theoretically, it is possible that the blood in the tubes may have come from this source. It was, however, present in both tubes, was apparently coming from the uterus, and contained bits of endometrial tissue identical with those found in the blood of the uterine cavity. In addition, a moulded mass of endometrial tissue was found in this blood which conformed to a cast of the interstitial portion of the tube, through which it had apparently passed (Fig. 46).

Peritoneal endometriosis occurs most frequently in situations in the pelvis easily soiled by material escaping from the tubes and ovaries. It would seem that the tubes and ovaries are the chief distributing agents for the cause of pelvic peritoneal endometriosis. It is not peculiar to the pelvic peritoneum, as the appendix, cecum, small intestine and their mesenteries may be involved. The posture of mankind, whether standing, sitting, or lying down appears to be an important factor in determining the distribution of these lesions.

A comparative study of the lesions of peritoneal endometriosis with those of peritoneal carcinosis of implantation origin demonstrates that the peritoneal reaction is the same in both instances. Endometrial tissue and cancer may grow on the surface of the peritoneum. Both may become embedded in the peritoneum by the tissues of the latter growing over them. Both may be included in mesothelial lined pockets and may be caught in adhesions.

THE ETIOLOGY OF ENDOMETRIUM-LIKE TISSUE IN THE OVARY

The endometrial tissue in a direct or primary endometriosis of both uterine and tubal origin shows a variety of lesions, such as typical endometrium with glands and stroma identical with that of the müllerian mucosa from which it came, and also dilated glands or cyst-like cavities lined by epithelium with very little or no characteristic endometrial stroma about it.

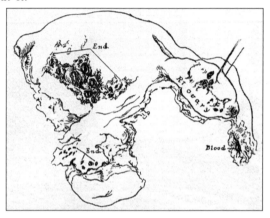

Fig. 51.—Posterior surface of the uterus, right tube and ovary (x ⅔), Case 1 of article. Uterus was retroflexed, and operation was performed on the second or third day of menstruation. Blood was observed escaping from both tubes on exposing the pelvic organs. Unfortunately, the distal end of the tube was not ligated and most of the blood in the tube was lost during the manipulation of the operation. Endometrial tissue was found in the tube (Fig. 53). Could the blood and the endometrial tissue in the tube have come from the ectopic endometrial tissue of the ovary and the posterior surface of the uterus? The endometrium-like tissue of the *lateral surface* of the ovary consisted of dilated glands filled with blood without any evidence of rupture. The endometriosis of the posterior uterine wall (Fig. 52) consisted of granulation tissue on its surface with deposits of endometrial tissue enmeshed in it and similar foci of endometrial tissue in the superficial portion of the uterine wall. Exposed endometrial tissue on the surface of the pelvic organs was not found. The endometriosis of the lateral surface of the ovary and the uterus are in situations readily soiled by material escaping from the tubes.

Marked changes in the mucosa lining the uterine cavity often occur. Of particular interest are those in the mucosa over a submucous leiomyoma. This mucosa becomes thin, the glands disappear, the stroma becomes less and less and in extreme cases the submucous leiomyoma is covered by a mucosa not unlike the mesothelial covering of a subserous leiomyoma. The endometrial epithelium in unfavorable conditions may be very similar to the peritoneal mesothelium and the surface epithelium of the ovary. Both the peritoneal mesothelium and the surface epithelium of the ovary, under the stimulation of any irritant, may become hypertrophied and resemble the epithelium of the uterine mucosa. We recognize the mucosal covering of a submucous leiomyoma to be of endometrial origin, even though it simulates the peritoneal mesothelium and the epithelial lining of a follicular cyst of the ovary. When we find patches of typical endometrial tissue in an ovarian cyst with a lining similar to the mucosal covering of a submucous leiomyoma, can it be truthfully said that the typical endometrial tissue represents a metaplasia of the epithelium of a follicular cyst of the ovary, just because the cyst is situated in the ovary and portions of its lining resemble that of a follicular cyst? Is it not more logical to claim that the entire cyst is lined by one kind of tissue and that endometrial, portions of which have failed to attain their full growth, and thus present a histologic picture identical with the linings of some of the atypical endometrial

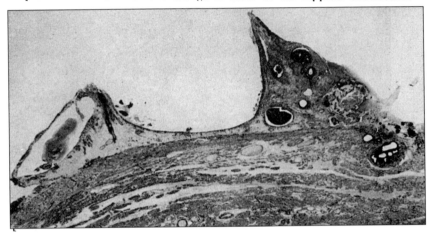

Fig. 52.—Photomicrograph (x 10) of a portion of the endometriosis of the posterior uterine wall. Granulation tissue, evidence of a reaction of the peritoneum to some irritant, has developed on the posterior surface of the uterus and has included in it endometrial tissue, just as cancer of implantation origin is included in the granulation tissue of peritoneal carcinosis. Endometrial "pockets" are also present in the superficial portion of the uterine wall. If this lesion is of implantation origin, it hardly could have come from the ovary. It is apparently an older lesion and could well be explained by the reaction of the peritoneum to material escaping from the tube; this material might contain uterine or tubal epithelium.

cavities of a direct endometriosis and the mucosal covering of submucous leiomyomas? See Figs. 59 and 60.

On account of the faculty of known endometrial epithelium to simulate peritoneal mesothelium and the surface epithelium of the ovary, it is often difficult to determine the origin of all misplaced endometrium-like tissue in the ovary.

Because a variety of epithelial structures develop in the ovary, it is natural to believe that müllerian tissue might also develop in that organ. Even if endometrial tissue arises on and in the ovary from the implantation of endometrial and tubal tissue on that organ, as I believe it does, this does not exclude the origin of similar tissue from other sources.

THE ETIOLOGY OF PERITONEAL ENDOMETRIOSIS

I have stated in this article that I have encountered 293 patients with these lesions in the last five years. The question arises: are all these instances of true peritoneal endometriosis? I cannot prove this. In

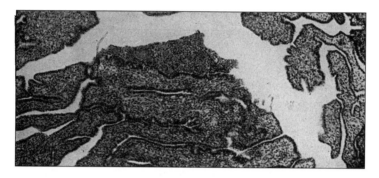

Fig. 53.—Photomicrograph (x 60) of a portion of the cross-section of the tube of Case 1. Endometrial tissue, consisting mostly of stroma infiltrated with blood and some epithelium, is adherent to the surface of the tubal mucosa. (The section unfortunately is thick.) This endometrial tissue resembled similar bits in the blood of the uterine cavity, from which the blood in the tubes was apparently coming.

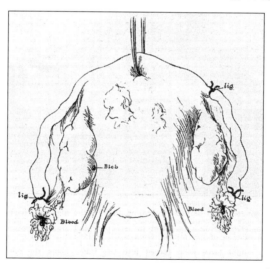

Fig. 54.—Uterus, tubes, and ovaries (x ⅓) of Case 2. The patient was menstruating at the time of the operation and blood could be seen coming from the abdominal ostia of both tubes. The distal end of the left tube and both the distal and proximal ends of the right tube were ligated before removing the uterus. The uterus, left tube and ovary, and the right tube were removed and hardened in formalin. Sections from both tubes showed blood and epithelial cells, a greater amount in the left tube as would be expected, because its proximal end, unfortunately, had not been ligated. Two small hemorrhagic blebs were found on the *under surface* of the left ovary, only one shown in the illustration. For the contents of the left tube and the structure of the larger bleb on the surface of the ovary, see Figs. 55 and 56.

many, typical endometrial tissue was found with a histologic structure identical with that of the mucosa of the uterus. In others, only atypical endometrial tissue was present, but similar to that often encountered in an endometriosis arising from the invasion of the uterine wall by its mucosa and by that of the tube. In still others, both typical and atypical endometrial tissue was found and one could trace the transition of one type of lesion into the other, just as one can follow a similar transition in the endometrial lesions of a direct endometriosis.

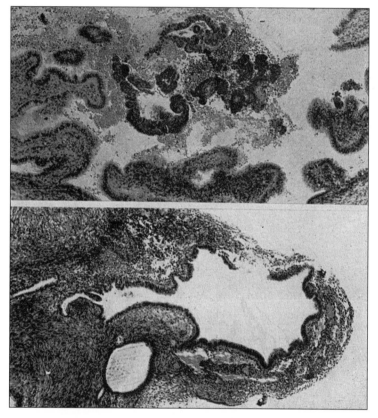

Figs. 55 and 56.—Two photomicrographs (x 60), the first of a portion of a cross-section of the left tube containing blood, strips of epithelium, a "gland" and fragments of *endometrial stroma* identical in structure and staining reaction with those present in the mucosa of the uterus, from which a larger amount of tissue had been cast off by menstruation. Compare with the ovarian lesion shown below. The endometrial tissue might have been forced into the tube during the operation, as the uterine end of the tube had not been ligated. Blood, however, was present in both tubes prior to the handling of the uterus.

The second photomicrograph (x 60) is of a section of the larger hemorrhagic bleb on the surface of the left ovary (Fig. 54). It is lined by epithelium of endometrial type with very *little stroma* and no *glands*. I was unable to find the loss of sufficient tissue to account for that in the tube, nor did the endometrium-like tissue of the ovary resemble that in the tube as closely as the mucosa lining the uterine cavity resembled it. It does not seem possible that the blood in the tubes (both) came from the small blebs on the left ovary (see Fig. 54).

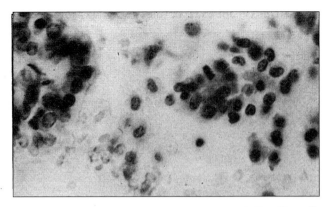

Fig. 57.—Photomicrograph (x 600) of a clump of epithelium-like cells in the lumen of the tube of a menstruating uterus (Case 4). Blood was observed escaping from the abdominal ostia of both tubes and apparently coming from the uterus. Peritoneal endometriosis was not present nor was there evidence of endometrial tissue in the ovaries. A clump of epithelium-like cells (to the right) is shown, surrounded by blood, in the lumen of the tubes. A mitotic figure is present in one of these cells. I am unable to state their origin. They certainly are not constituents of normal blood and they very closely resemble epithelium. Compare with the epithelium of the tubal mucosa to the left. Bits of uterine mucosa and clumps of epithelial cells were found in the blood obtained from the uterine cavity, but mitotic figures were not seen. If these are epithelial cells from the uterine or tubal mucosa they were alive at the time of the operation.

In four other cases blood was observed in the tubes of menstruating uteri at operation on patients without ectopic endometrial tissue in the pelvis, but the tubes were not removed. Films on slides were made of the blood obtained from the tubes by stripping them. Epithelium was found in these films and also cells which I was unable to identify. The trauma of stripping the tubes might dislodge tubal tissue and I have, therefore, discarded these. The blood in these cases apparently was coming from the uterine cavity and we know that, at times, it can carry with it bits of the uterine mucosa through the interstitial portion of the tubes, as shown by the bloody contents of tubes after curettage of the uterus.

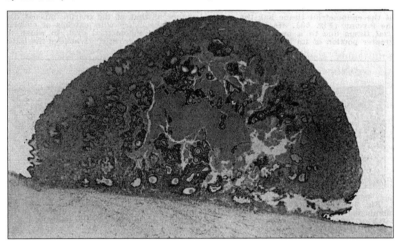

Fig. 58.—Photomicrograph (x 20) of a patch of "menstruating" uterine mucosa in the lining of the tube. Uterus, left tube and ovary were removed for uterine bleeding due to multiple leiomyomas; the patient was flowing at the time of the operation. The right tube and ovary were normal. A hematosalpinx was present on the left side adherent by its closed distal end to the ovary. Implantation-like lesions of endometrial tissue were present on the surface of the ovary adherent to the tube and in the wall of the tube. The blood in the tube evidently came from the endometrial tissue in the lining of the tube. The peritoneal endometriosis may have arisen from the same source, if the endometrial tissue was present in the tube prior to the closure of its fimbriated end. What is the origin of this patch of endometrial tissue? Is it misplaced endometrial tissue of congential origin, or a metaplasia of the tubal mucosa due to the influence of the ovarian hormone? Or even an implantation and subsequent growth of bit of uterine mucosa carried from the uterine cavity into the tube during menstruation or curettage? The patient had been curetted three years before.

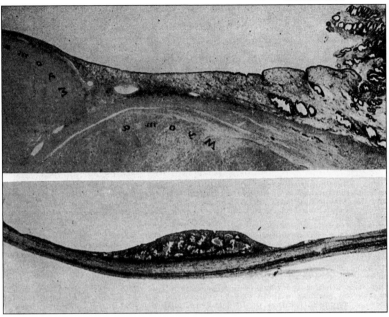

Fig. 59.—Two photomicrographs (x 10): the first of the uterine mucosa over a submucous leiomyoma and the second of the wall of an endometrial cyst of the ovary. The mucosa over the myoma is thin, there is very little stroma, the glands have disappeared and the surface epithelium is low. The patch of endometrial tissue in the lining of the ovarian cyst has the same histologic structure as that of the mucosa of the uterus removed with the cyst. The lining of the cyst on either side of the endometrial tissue has the same structure as that of the uterine mucosa over the myoma (Fig. 60). Is it a follicular cyst of the ovary with patches of endometrial tissue due to a metaplasia of its lining or an endometrial cyst, in which the greater portion of its lining had failed to reach its full growth? I believe the latter.

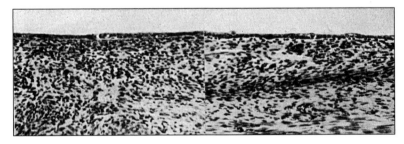

Fig. 60.—Two photomicrographs (x 130), the first of the uterine mucosa over the submucous myoma and the second of the lining of the ovarian cyst adjacent to the patch of typical endometrial tissue. Their histologic structure is the same.

The peritoneal mesothelium, when stimulated by any irritant, may assume an epithelium-like structure. Gland-like inclusions of the mesothelium may arise and also cavities lined by it. Should the irritant contain blood or cause bleeding, the conditions resulting from this might be incorrectly attributed to a menstrual reaction.

Even if peritoneal endometriosis arises from the implantation of endometrial and tubal tissue on the surface of the peritoneum, as I believe it does, this does not prove that all instances of endometrium-like tissue involving the peritoneum arise from this source.

SUMMARY

Menstrual blood escapes into the peritoneal cavity from (1) the rupture or perforation of endometrial cysts or cavities of the ovary and possibly of other pelvic structures; (2) menstruating endometrial tissue growing on the surface of the ovary and other pelvic structures; (3) the uterine cavity as a back flow through the tubes; (4) menstruating tubal mucosa.

Menstrual blood, irrespective of its source, at times, contains bits of endometrial tissue set free by menstruation.

Endometrial tissue disseminated by menstruation is sometimes alive and will continue to grow, if transferred to situations suited to its growth.

The peritoneum and surface of the ovary are suited to the growth of endometrial tissue.

The lesions of peritoneal endometriosis often occur in situations and under conditions indicating (at least suggesting) their origin from menstrual blood escaping from the above mentioned sources.

The local reaction of the peritoneum to the endometrial tissue in peritoneal endometriosis is similar to the local reaction of the peritoneum to cancer in peritoneal carcinosis of implantation origin.

CONCLUSIONS

These studies indicate that peritoneal endometriosis sometimes arises from the implantation of endometrial tissue disseminated by menstrual blood escaping into the peritoneal cavity.

Endometrial and tubal tissue disseminated by other means may do the same. This phase of the subject will be considered in a later paper.

REFERENCES

(1) *Sampson, J. A.:* Arch. Surg., 1921, iii, 245-323. (2) *Sampson, J. A.:* Am. Jour. Path., 1927, iii, 93-109. (3) *Meyer, R.:* Virchow's Arch. f. path. Anat., 1909, clcv, 487 (see 528). *Meyer, R.:* Ztsch. f. Geburtsh. u. Gynäk., 1900, xliii, 130 (see 159). *Kitai, I.:* Arch. f. Gynäk., 1925, cxxiv, 178 (see 202). (4) *Novak, E.:* AM. JOUR. OBST. AND GYNEC., 1926, xii, 501 and 503. (5) *Jacobson, V. C.:* Arch. Surg., 1922, v, 281-300; AM. JOUR. OBST. AND GYNEC., 1923, vi, 257-262; Arch. Path. and Lab. Med., 1926, i, 169-174. (6) *Novak, E.:* AM. JOUR. OBST. AND GYNEC., 1926, xii, 628. (7) *Sampson, J. A.:* Am. Jour. Obst., 1918, lxxxiii, 161-175. (8) *Davis, C. H.:* AM. JOUR. OBST. AND GYNEC., 1926, xii, 526, 527. (9) *Sampson, J. A.:* Surg., Gynec. and Obst., 1924, xxxviii, 287-311 (see Fig. 22).

180 WASHINGTON AVENUE.

Commentary on Classic Paper No.10

The evolution of our understanding of endometriosis is a fascinating chapter in gynecological pathology. This understanding will always be associated with the research of John A. Sampson, who, in 1921, gave this disease the name of 'peritoneal endometriosis' and also reflected on its pathogenesis 'due to menstrual dissemination of endometrial tissue into the peritoneal cavity'[1]. Sampson's research continued over several decades and careful reading gives the impression of a highly devoted clinician, gynecological surgeon and observer. All papers are without co-authors.

In 1921, Sampson presented a paper to the American Gynecological Society, on perforating hemorrhagic ovarian cysts, which he called chocolate cysts [2] (see figure below).

1. Sampson, J.A. (1927). Peritoneal endometriosis due to the menstrual dissemination of endometrial tissue into the peritoneal cavity. *Am. J. Obstet. Gynecol.*, **14**, 422

2. Sampson, J.A. (1921). Perforating hemorrhagic cysts (chocolate cyst) of the ovary: their importance and especially their relation to pelvic adenomas of endometrial type. *Arch. Surg.*, **3**, 245

Cross-section of the pelvis showing the condition found at operation. The ovarian cyst had ruptured and the perforation was sealed by the peritoneum on the side of the pelvis to which the ovary had become adherent. On freeing the ovary, its 'chocolate' contents escaped. Reproduced from Sampson (1921)[2] with permission. Copyright (1921) American Medical Association

3. Sampson, J.A. (1922).
The life history of ovarian
hematomas (hemorrhagic
cysts) of endometrial
(Müllerian) type.
Am. J. Obstet. Gynecol., **4**,
451

4. Sampson, J.A. (1924).
Benign and malignant
endometrial implants in the
peritoneal cavity and their
relation to certain ovarian
tumors.
Surg. Gynecol. Obstet., **38**,
287

5. Sampson, J.A. (1925).
Heterotopic or misplaced
endometrial tissue.
Am. J. Obstet. Gynecol.,
10, 649

6. Sampson, J.A. (1940).
The development of the
implantation theory for
the origin of peritoneal
endometriosis.
Am. J. Obstet. Gynecol.,
40, 549

7. von Recklinghausen, F.
(1896). *Die Adenomyome
und cystadenome der
Tubewandung.*
(Berlin: Hirschwald)

8. Meyer, R. (1919). Ueber
den Stand der Frage der
Adenomyositis und
Adenomyome im allge-
meinen und insbesondere
über Adenomyositis
seroepithelialis und
Adenomyometritis sarco-
matosa.
Zblt. Gynäkol., **36**, 745

In 1922, he presented additional data on the life history of ovarian hematomas[3] and two years later went on to distinguish between benign and malignant lesions[4].

In 1925, he used the terminology of 'misplaced endometrial tissue'[5] and in 1940, he reviewed the entire subject[6]. He concluded that endometriosis could be caused by the rupture of endometrial cysts of the ovary with implantation of such fragments onto the peritoneal pelvic surface, as well as by transtubal regurgitation of endometrial fragments during menstruation.

Uterine tumors, containing both smooth muscle and glandular elements, were described at the end of the nineteenth century, arousing considerable interest in the monograph by von Recklinghausen[7] in 1896, who proposed that these tumors were of 'Wolffian origin'.

In 1919, Robert Meyer[8], a gynecological pathologist, pointed out that adenomyositis (seroepitheliasis), adenomyoma and adenomyometritis sarcomatosa were in no sense malignant, but part of a healing process with pre-existing inflammation. He believed that the heterogeneity of serosal epithelium was the probable explanation for the existence of the extrauterine swellings. Today, theories about the pathogenesis of endometriosis still center around celomic metaplasia, implantation after retrograde menstruation, or a combination of both.

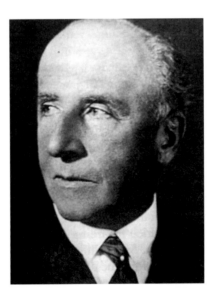

Robert Meyer (1864–1947)

At first sight, the concept of retrograde menstruation is not appealing because of the protective nature of the uterus and tubes which prevent the entry of anything but sperm. Nevertheless, there is now ample evidence that retrograde menstruation is a common event in women. In a study by Jouko Halme and colleagues, blood was found in the peritoneal fluid at laparoscopy in 90% of women with patent tubes during the perimenstrual part of their cycle. The authors concluded: *'The present observations indicate that retrograde menstruation through the fallopian tubes into the peritoneal cavity is a very common physiologic event in all menstruating women with patent tubes.'* [9]

The viability of the cast-off menstrual endometrium

In 1951, Keettel and Stein[10] reported the results of their investigations into the viability of cast-off endometrium obtained from menstrual fluid. The endometrium was cultured in a contraceptive diaphragm inserted in the vagina on the second day of menstrual bleeding and which was left in place from 8 to 12 hours. Cultures in Tyrode's solution were then examined at 24-hour intervals and refed with umbilical cord serum. They found that the cells in the outgrowths were either fibroblastic or epithelioid in appearance.

The search for endometrial cells in peritoneal fluid was carried out using cytology and cell culture, which disclosed mainly large intact glandular structures.

Willemsen and colleagues[11] reported the absence of adhering and proliferating glandular endometrial cells in any of 115 cultures from the peritoneal pouch in infertile women in the late proliferative phase of the cycle. After uterine–tubal irrigation, however, these glandular endometrial cells were found to be present in 67% of the cultures.

In another study which looked at an earlier phase of the menstrual cycle[12], endometrial epithelial cells could be identified in the majority of cultures (79%) from peritoneal fluid. In women with and without endometriosis, these cells also were capable of adhesion and proliferation.

Other routes by which endometrial cells are known to disseminate include the lymphatics[13], Bartholin's glands following excision[14] and utero–tubal flushing during tubal patency testing[11].

Studies in monkeys

Roger Scott, Richard W. Te Linde and L. R. Wharton[15], from Western Reserve University School of Medicine in Cleveland, Ohio, and the Johns Hopkins University, studied monkeys to tackle the problem of the histoge-

9. Halme, J., Hammond, M.G., Hulka, J.F., Raj, S.G. and Talbert, L.M. (1984). Retrograde menstruation in healthy women and in patients with endometriosis. *Obstet. Gynecol.*, **64**, 151

10. Keettel, W.C. and Stein, R.J.(1951). The viability of the cast-off menstrual endometrium. *Am. J. Obstet. Gynecol.*, **61**, 440

11. Willemsen, W.N.P., Mungyer, G., Smets, H., Rolland, R., Vemer, H. and Jap, P.H.K. (1985). Behavior of cultured glandular cells obtained by flushing of the uterine cavity. *Fertil. Steril.*, **44**, 92

12. Kruitwagen, R.F.P.M., Poels, L.G., Willemsen, W.N.P., de Ronde, I.J.Y., Jap, P.H.K. and Rolland, R. (1991). Endometrial epithelial cells in peritoneal fluid during the early follicular phase. *Fertil. Steril.*, **55**, 297

13. Halban, J. (1924). Hysteroadenosis metastatica. Die lympofene Genese der sogenannte Adenofibromatosis heterotopica. *Wien. Klin. Wochenschr.*, **37**, 1205

14. Scott, R.B. and Te Linde, R.W. (1954). Clinical external endometriosis. Probable viability of menstrually shed fragments of endometrium. *Obstet. Gynecol.*, **4**, 502

15. Scott, R.B., Te Linde, R.W. and Wharton, L.R. (1953). Further studies on experimental endometriosis. *Am. J. Obstet. Gynecol.*, **66**, 1082

16. Brosens, I.A., Koninckx, P.R. and Corveleyn, P.A. (1978). A study of plasma proges-terone, oestradiol-17β, prolactin and LH levels, and of the luteal phase appearance of the ovaries in patients with endometriosis and infertility. *Br. J. Obstet. Gynaecol.*, **85**, 246

17. Koninckx, P.R., Ide, P., Vandenbroucke, W. and Brosens, I.A.(1980). New aspects of the pathophysi-ology of endometriosis and associated infertility. *J. Reprod. Med.*, **24**, 257

18. Dmowski, W.P., Rao. R. and Scommegua, A. (1980). The luteinized unruptured follicle syndrome and endometriosis. *Fertil. Steril.*, **33**, 30

19. Dmowski, W.P., Steele, R.W. and Baker, G.F. (1981). Deficient cellular immunity in endometriosis. *Am. J. Obstet. Gynecol.*, **141**, 377

20. Steele, R.W., Dmowski, W.P. and Marmer, D.J. (1984). Immunologic aspects of human endometriosis. *Am. J. Obstet. Gynecol.*, **6**, 33

nesis of external endometriosis. Ten monkeys were altered surgically to permit intra-abdominal menstruation. Endometriosis developed in half of them. The authors concluded that endometriosis could develop by retro-grade menstruation, but they did not exclude lymphatic and vascular dis-semination. They found the metaplasia theory of celomic peritoneum to be the least likely.

Luteinized unruptured follicle syndrome

Brosens and colleagues[16] found the incidence of luteinized unruptured fol-licle (LUF) cycles in women with endometriosis to be 79% whereas in infertile controls with a male or tubal infertility factor, the incidence was only 6%. Because of the shorter onset of subsequent menstruation in patients with endometriosis, higher estradiol and lower progesterone lev-els, and less ovulation stigmata than in controls, luteinization *in situ* was proposed. The associated infertility could also be explained by anovula-tion.

The findings of Brosens and colleagues[16] together with those of Koninckx and co-workers[17], became known as the LUF syndrome. The existence of the LUF syndrome was, however, seriously questioned by Dmowski and associates[18] in 1980, but they did not deny that endocrine factors probably could play a role in the origin of LUF syndrome.

Deficient cellular immunity in endometriosis

Several alterations in the cellular and humoral immune system of women with endometriosis have been reported and in monkeys with spontaneous endometriosis, a decrease of the T-lymphocyte mediated response to autologous endometrial antigens has also been reported[19]. In women with endometriosis, these cellular mechanisms are known to be impaired, with the degree of impairment directly related to the severity of the endometrio-sis[20, 21].

The role of macrophages

A host response to implantation may involve macrophages as effector cells, active in the host defense mechanism. It is also known from the work of Muscato and colleagues[22] that peritoneal macrophages phagocytose menstrual detritus and sperm in the peritoneal cavity. Finally, phagocytes are known to be involved in inflammatory processes.

Halme and co-workers[23] investigated the possible role of peritoneal macrophages in the pathogenesis of endometriosis. They studied macrophages isolated from the peritoneal fluid of women with unex-plained infertility.

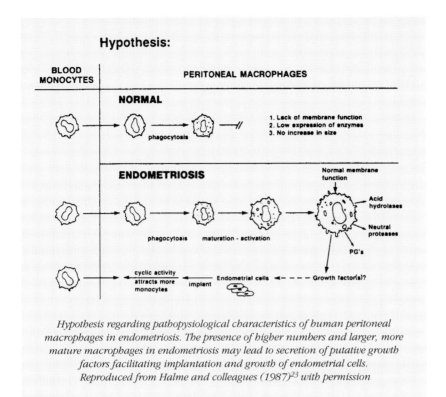

Hypothesis regarding pathophysiological characteristics of human peritoneal macrophages in endometriosis. The presence of higher numbers and larger, more mature macrophages in endometriosis may lead to secretion of putative growth factors facilitating implantation and growth of endometrial cells. Reproduced from Halme and colleagues (1987)[23] with permission

Flow cytometry was used to analyze the cell types, in addition to indirect immunofluorescence measurements.

The authors found a significantly increased number of peritoneal macrophages in women with endometriosis. Their hypothesis suggests that peritoneal macrophages may represent a population of monocyte-derived cells with a potential of secreting growth stimulating substances. The target cells for growth factors then could include endometrial cells that receive a stimulus to implantation and growth, eventually leading to endometriosis.

Even when normal ovulatory menstrual cycles and patent oviducts are present, endometriosis can be regarded as a chronic inflammatory process associated with infertility. In endometriosis patients, the number of macrophages of the peritoneal fluid is increased. Correlated with this finding is the fact that significantly elevated levels of interleukin-1 (IL-1) and the tumor necrosis factor (TNF), both products of activated macrophages, have been demonstrated in peritoneal fluid[24,25].

Cirkel and colleagues[26] performed an immunohistochemical study in endometriotic tissue using monoclonal antibodies for macrophage subtyping. They were able to demonstrate an immunological dynamic process within the lesion itself, in addition to that within the peritoneal fluid.

21. Dmowski, W.P. (1987). Visual assessment of peritoneal implants for staging endometriosis: do number and cumulative size of lesions reflect the severity of a systemic disease? *Fertil. Steril.*, **47**, 382

22. Muscato, J.J., Maney, A.F. and Weinberg, J.B. (1982). Sperm phagocytosis by human peritoneal macrophages: a possible cause of infertility in endometriosis. *Am. J. Obstet. Gynecol.*, **144**, 503

23. Halme, J., Becker, S. and Haskill, S. (1987). Altered maturation and function of peritoneal macrophages: possible role in pathogenesis of endometriosis. *Am. J. Obstet. Gynecol.*, **156**, 783

24. Fakih, H., Baggeh, B., Holtz, J., Tjang, K.Y., Lee, J.C. and Wilimson, H.O. (1987). Interleukin-1: a possible role in the infertility associated with endometriosis. *Fertil. Steril.*, **47**, 213

25. Eisermann, J., Fast, M., Pineda, J., Odem, R.R. and Collins, J.L. (1988). Tumor necrosis factor in peritoneal fluid of women undergoing laparoscopic surgery. *Fertil. Steril.*, **50**, 573

26. Cirkel, U., Ochs, H., Mues, B., Zwadlo, G., Sorg, C. and Schneider, H.P.G. (1993). Inflammatory reaction in endometriotic tissue: an immunohistochemical study. *Eur. J. Obstet. Gynecol. Reprod. Biol.*, **48**, 43

27. Barbieri, R.L., Niloff, J.M., Bast, R.C., Schaetzl, E., Kistner, R.W. and Knapp, R.C. (1986). Elevated serum concentrations of CA-125 in patients with advanced endometriosis. *Fertil. Steril.*, **45**, 630

28. Strathy, J.H., Molgaard, C.A., Coulam, C.B. and Melton, L.J. (1982). Endometriosis and infertility: a laparoscopic study of endometriosis among fertile and infertile women. *Fertil. Steril.*, **38**, 667

29. Kistner, R.W. (1975). Management of endometriosis in the infertile patient. *Fertil. Steril.*, **26**, 1151

The celomic epithelium

Barbieri and co-workers[27] demonstrated that patients with advanced endometriosis have significantly higher CA-125 levels in their serum than controls. CA-125 is an antigenic determinant, defined by the monoclonal antibody OC-125. Immunocytochemical studies, demonstrate that the antigen CA-125 is present in many tissues derived from embryonic celomic epithelium. Thus it seems possible that in advanced endometriosis, cell surface antigens are released into the systemic circulation.

The incidence and treatment of endometriosis

In 1982, Strathy and associates[28] demonstrated by laparoscopy, that endometriosis is more common in infertile than fertile women, with the risk of infertility estimated to be almost 20 times greater in patients with endometriosis.

When treating endometriosis there can be a number of goals:

- Treatment of symptoms such as dysmenorrhea, pelvic pain or dyspareunia

- Treatment of infertility

- Regression or elimination of endometriotic lesions

These goals may be approached by hormonal or surgical treatment, or both.

Hormonal therapy

The beneficial effect of pregnancy on endometriosis can be due to the typical hormonal status of pregnancy and the remarkable involutionary changes in the postpartum period, including lactation. Induction of a 'pseudopregnancy state' was probably the leading thought in the development of hormonal therapy with progestational agents as described by Kistner in 1975[29].

Sex steroids used in the treatment of endometriosis include progestins, estrogen and progestins, and androgen derivatives. All these steroids are capable of inhibiting ovulation, inducing decidualization and eventually causing atrophy of the endometrial tissue.

The progestins available include progesterone, dydrogesterone, 19-nor derivatives of testosterone (norethindrone, norethisterone, ethynodiol, norgestrel and lynestrenol), derivatives of testosterone (ethisterone and danazol) and derivatives of 17α-hydroxyprogesterone (medroxyprogesterone and megestrol).

Gonadotropin releasing hormone (GnRH) agonists are also effective in the treatment of endometriosis. Most synthetic GnRH agonists are characterized by a modification of the native decapeptide at position 6 or 9 or both, which creates a longer half-life.

The nor derivatives initially increase follicle stimulating hormone (FSH) and luteinizing hormone (LH) secretion from the pituitary gland until down-regulation of pituitary GnRH receptors occurs, leading to a decline in LH secretion. This creates a postmenopausal hypoestrogenic state, resulting in involution and atrophy of endometrial tissues.

A review of the literature on hormonal treatment demonstrates, in general, a relief of symptoms due to endometriosis and regression of lesions. In three studies that have reported the natural course of the disease within the placebo arms of the trials, the disease progressed in about half of the patients [30–32]. In the other half the disease was reported to either remain the same, improve or disappear.

It is worth noting the conclusion of Thomas[33], who stated that '*endometriosis should not be treated just because it is there*'.

This conclusion is further supported by evidence that treatment does not have a great impact on fertility rates (certainly not during treatment), plus the evidence that medical treatment works only temporarily, with the disease frequently recurring once stimulation by ovarian steroids returns[34].

Surgery

Surgical intervention is possible by laparoscopy (coagulation or laser treatment of lesions), the removal of pelvic masses, repair of tubal function, adhesiolysis or total hysterectomy.

As for hormonal therapy, the only clear recommendation for treatment is in symptomatic patients, bearing in mind – as with hormonal treatment – that the disease should be seen as a chronic one that can recur.

An effect of age

Redwine[35] studied 137 consecutive patients with endometriosis using laparoscopy, taking biopsies of lesions and using the presence of glands and stroma for the final diagnosis.

In Redwine's study, the dominant color of the lesions was noted carefully. These colors included clear, red, yellow, white, blue, gray, and black. The process of fibrosis gives rise to white or yellow colors, while hemorrhage results in many of the red-blue colors. When the colors of the lesions were arranged according to the age of the patients an evolution in appearance with advancing age is suggested. The table overleaf from Redwine's publi-

30. Thomas, E.J. and Cooke, I.D. (1987). The impact of gestrinone upon the course of asymptomatic endometriosis. *Br. Med. J.*, **294**, 272

31. Mahmood, T.A. and Templeton, A. (1990). The impact of the natural history of endometriosis. *Hum. Reprod.*, **5**, 965

32. Telimaa, S., Puolakka, J., Rönnberg, L. and Kauppila, A. (1987). Placebo controlled comparison of danazol and high-dose medroxyprogesterone acetate in the treatment of endometriosis. *Gynecol. Endocrinol.*, **1**, 13

33. Thomas, E.J. (1993). Endometriosis. *Br. Med. J.*, **306**, 158

34. Evers, J.L.H. (1987). The second-look laparoscopy for evaluation of the result of medical treatment of endometriosis should not be performed during ovarian suppression. *Fertil. Steril.*, **47**, 502

35. Redwine, D.B. (1987). Age-related evolution in color appearance of endometriosis. *Fertil. Steril.*, **48**, 1062

Evolution of Color Appearance
of Endometriosis with Age[*]

Color appearance	No. patients	Mean age in years ± SD	Age range in years
Clear papules only	6	21.5 ± 3.5	17–26
Clear papules plus other clear lesions	8	23.0 ± 4.0	17–28
Clear plus any others	14	23.4 ± 4.7	17–31
Red only	16	26.3 ± 5.4	16–38
Red plus any others	22	26.9 ± 5.7	17–43
All nonblack	55	27.9 ± 7.2	17–42
White plus any others	24	28.3 ± 6.9	17–43
Black plus any others	34	28.4 ± 5.8	17–43
White only	8	29.5 ± 5.9	20–39
Black only	48	31.9 ± 7.5	20–52

Total number of patients exceeds 137 because patients with more than one color appearance are listed in more than one appearance catagory. Color appearances 'gray', 'blue', and 'yellow' are not listed separately because of small numbers. They are included along with other colors where appropriate in the 'plus any other' color appearances. Reproduced from Redwine (1987)[35] with permission from the publisher, The American Fertility Society

36. Jansen, R.P.S. and Russell, P. (1986). Non-pigmented endometriosis: clinical, laparoscopic and pathologic definition. *Am. J. Obstet. Gynecol.*, **155**, 1154

cation demonstrates that young women start with clear papules and only at about 30 years of age do the colors appear to move through red to black. Non-pigmented endometriosis, as described by Jansen and Russell [36] therefore seems to be the first intra-abdominal lesion to appear.

Epilogue

Endometriosis is now defined as the growth of endometrium in an abnormal location, being internal when the endometrium is present in the uterine muscle and external when on the outside of the pelvic organs or the peritoneum.

Uterine tumors containing both smooth muscle and glandular elements were recognized and described as early as 1896 and at that time the glandular elements were thought to be of 'Müllerian' or 'Wolffian' origin.

Sampson, in his classic series of papers published between 1921 and 1940, made a fundamental contribution to our knowledge of endometriosis, by demonstrating that retrograde menstruation and implantation of endometrium into the peritoneal cavity provided the most likely explanation for the lesions seen at laparotomy. Research thereafter, finally established that retrograde menstruation occurs rather frequently and that the endometrial cells found in the peritoneal fluid are viable and capable of adherence and proliferation.

Implantation of these cells, and the formation of ectopic endometrial colonies and tumors, is, however, another enigma. It is here that other factors, such as heritable aspects, hormonal factors, inflammatory reactions (macrophages, interleukins, growth factors), immunological reactions and even oncological factors (CA-125), would appear to be involved.

Because the endometriotic lesions seem to be age related, appearing as colorless 'blisters' at a young age up to the white (fibrotic) and blue lesions at a later age, the most important hypothesis remains that endometriosis will be more likely to occur with increased exposure to menstruation. Women experience around 450 menstruations in their reproductive lifetime. With pregnancy, lactation and oral contraception, this may be reduced to between 30 and 50.

The effect of sex steroids and luteinizing hormone releasing hormone analogs on signs/symptoms of endometriosis and their effect on the endometriotic lesions seem to substantiate the hypothesis that continuous natural menstrual cycles are not so natural as was first thought.

Summary of references

1. Sampson, J.A. (1927). Peritoneal endometriosis due to the menstrual dissemination of endometrial tissue into the peritoneal cavity. *Am. J. Obstet. Gynecol.*, **14**, 422
2. Sampson, J.A. (1921). Perforating hemorrhagic cysts (chocolate cyst) of the ovary: their importance and especially their relation to pelvic adenomas of endometrial type. *Arch. Surg.*, **3**, 245
3. Sampson, J.A. (1922). The life history of ovarian hematomas (hemorrhagic cysts) of endometrial (Müllerian) type. *Am. J. Obstet. Gynecol.*, **4**, 451
4. Sampson, J.A. (1924). Benign and malignant endometrial implants in the peritoneal cavity and their relation to certain ovarian tumors. *Surg. Gynecol. Obstet.*, **38**, 287
5. Sampson, J.A. (1925). Heterotopic or misplaced endometrial tissue. *Am. J. Obstet. Gynecol.*, **10**, 649
6. Sampson, J.A. (1940). The development of the implantation theory for the origin of peritoneal endometriosis. *Am. J. Obstet. Gynecol.*, **40**, 549
7. von Recklinghausen, F. (1896). *Die Adenomyome und cystadenome der Tubewandung*. (Berlin: Hirschwald)
8. Meyer, R. (1919). Über den Stand der Frage der Adenomyositis und Adenomyome im allgemeinen und insbesondere über Adenomyositis seroepithelialis und Adenomyometritis sarcomatosa. *Zblt. Gynäkol.*, **36**, 745
9. Halme, J., Hammond, M.G., Hulka, J.F., Raj, S.G. and Talbert, L.M. (1984). Retrograde menstruation in healthy women and in patients with endometriosis. *Obstet. Gynecol.*, **64**, 151

10. Keettel, W.C. and Stein, R.J. (1951). The viability of the cast-off menstrual endometrium. *Am. J. Obstet. Gynecol.*, **61**, 440

11. Willemsen, W.N.P., Mungyer, G., Smets, H., Rolland, R., Vemer, H. and Jap, P. (1985). Behavior of cultured glandular cells obtained by flushing of the uterine cavity. *Fertil. Steril.*, **44**, 92

12. Kruitwagen, R.F.P.M., Poels, L.G., Willemsen, W.N.P., de Ronde, I.J.Y., Jap, P.H.K. and Rolland, R. (1991). Endometrial epithelial cells in peritoneal fluid during the early follicular phase. *Fertil. Steril.*, **55**, 297

13. Halban, J. (1924). Hysteroadenosis metastatica. Die lympofene Genese der sogenannte Adenofibromatosis heterotopica. *Wien. Klin. Wochenschr.*, **37**, 1205

14. Scott, R.B. and Te Linde, R.W. (1954). Clinical external endometriosis. Probable viability of menstrually shed fragments of endometrium. *Obstet. Gynecol.*, **4**, 502

15. Scott, R.B., Te Linde, R.W. and Wharton, L.R. (1953). Further studies on experimental endometriosis. *Am. J. Obstet. Gynecol.*, **66**, 1082

16. Brosens, I.A., Koninckx, P.R. and Corveleyn, P.A. (1978). A study of plasma progesterone, oestradiol-17β, prolactin and LH levels, and of the luteal phase appearance of the ovaries in patients with endometriosis and infertility. *Br. J. Obstet. Gynaecol.*, **85**, 246

17. Koninckx, P.R., Ide, P., Vandenbroucke, W. and Brosens, I.A.(1980). New aspects of the pathophysiology of endometriosis and associated infertility. *J. Reprod. Med.*, **24**, 257

18. Dmowski, W.P., Rao, R. and Scommegua, A. (1980). The luteinized unruptured follicle syndrome and endometriosis. *Fertil. Steril.*, **33**, 30

19. Dmowski, W.P., Steele, R.W. and Baker, G.F. (1981). Deficient cellular immunity in endometriosis. *Am. J. Obstet. Gynecol.*, **141**, 377

20. Steele, R.W., Dmowski, W.P. and Marmer, D.J. (1984). Immunologic aspects of human endometriosis. *Am. J. Obstet. Gynecol.*, **6**, 33

21. Dmowski, W.P. (1987). Visual assessment of peritoneal implants for staging endometriosis: do number and cumulative size of lesions reflect the severity of a systemic disease? *Fertil. Steril.*, **47**, 382

22. Muscato, J.J., Maney, A.F. and Weinberg, J.B. (1982). Sperm phagocytosis by human peritoneal macrophages: a possible cause of infertility in endometriosis. *Am. J. Obstet. Gynecol.*, **144**, 503

23. Halme, J., Becker, S. and Haskill, S. (1987). Altered maturation and function of peritoneal macrophages: possible role in pathogenesis of endometriosis. *Am. J. Obstet. Gynecol.*, **156**, 783

24. Fakih, H., Baggeh, B., Holtz, J., Tjang, K.Y., Lee, J.C. and Wilimson, H.O. (1987). Interleukin-1: a possible role in the infertility associated with endometriosis. *Fertil. Steril.*, **47**, 213

25. Eisermann, J., Fast, M., Pineda, J., Odem, R.R. and Collins, J.L. (1988). Tumor necrosis factor in peritoneal fluid of women undergoing laparoscopic surgery. *Fertil. Steril.*, **50**, 573

26. Cirkel, U., Ochs, H., Mues, B., Zwadlo, G., Sorg, C. and Schneider, H.P.G. (1993). Inflammatory reaction in endometriotic tissue: an immunohistochemical study. *Eur. J. Obstet. Gynecol. Reprod. Biol.*, **48**, 43

27. Barbieri, R.L., Niloff, J.M., Bast, R.C., Schaetzl, E., Kistner, R.W. and Knapp, R.C. (1986). Elevated serum concentrations of CA-125 in patients with advanced endometriosis. *Fertil. Steril.*, **45**, 630

28. Strathy, J.H., Molgaard, C.A., Coulam, C.B. and Melton, L.J. (1982). Endometriosis and infertility: a laparoscopic study of endometriosis among fertile and infertile women. *Fertil. Steril.*, **38**, 667

29. Kistner, R.W. (1975). Management of endometriosis in the infertile patient. *Fertil. Steril.*, **26**, 1151

30. Thomas, E.J. and Cooke, I.D. (1987). The impact of gestrinone upon the course of asymptomatic endometriosis. *Br. Med. J.*, **294**, 272

31. Mahmood, T.A. and Templeton, A. (1990). The impact of the natural history of endometriosis. *Hum. Reprod.*, **5**, 965

32. Telimaa, S., Puolakka, J., Rönnberg, L. and Kauppila, A. (1987). Placebo controlled comparison of danazol and high-dose medroxyprogesterone acetate in the treatment of endometriosis. *Gynecol. Endocrinol.*, **1**, 13

33. Thomas, E.J. (1993). Endometriosis. *Br. Med. J.*, **306**, 158

34. Evers, J.L.H. (1987). The second-look laparoscopy for evaluation of the result of medical treatment of endometriosis should not be performed during ovarian suppression. *Fertil. Steril.*, **47**, 502

35. Redwine, D.B. (1987). Age-related evolution in color appearance of endometriosis. *Fertil. Steril.*, **48**, 1062

36. Jansen, R.P.S. and Russell, P. (1986). Non-pigmented endometriosis: clinical, laparoscopic and pathologic definition. *Am. J. Obstet. Gynecol.*, **155**, 1154

ORAL CONTRACEPTIVES AND FERTILITY AWARENESS

Classic Paper No.11

The effects of progesterone and related compounds on ovulation and early development in the rabbit

GREGORY PINCUS AND MIN CHUEH CHANG

The Worcester Foundation for Experimental Biology, Shrewsbury, Massachusetts

1. Pincus, G. and Chang, M.C. (1953). The effects of progesterone and related compounds on ovulation and early development in the rabbit. *Acta Physiol. Latino-Americana.*, **3**, 177

The original work by Pincus and Chang on the effects of progesterone and related compounds on ovulation eventually had a great impact on women. The birth of the 'pill' led to the use of oral contraceptives in 63 million women throughout the world in 1988 alone, and it could be suggested that the pill did more for women than the United Nations. On the other hand, it became necessary to make changes to the dose of oral contraceptives as well as to the steroid structure in order to avoid side-effects. Education remains the key factor in fertility regulation and fertility awareness. To achieve 'reproductive health', all novel methods of hormonal contraception must be accompanied by education and political commitment.

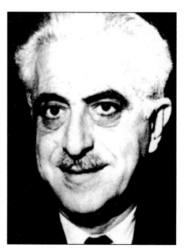

G. Pincus

THE EFFECTS OF PROGESTERONE AND RELATED COMPOUNDS ON OVULATION AND EARLY DEVELOPMENT IN THE RABBIT *

GREGORY PINCUS AND M. C. CHANG

(The Worcester Foundation for Experimental Biology. Shrewsbury, Massachusetts).

THAT PROGESTERONE is an effective inhibitor of ovulation was suggested by the difficulty of inducing ovulation in animals in which the ovaries contain active corpora lutea (Parkes, 1929). Direct demonstration of the ovulation-inhibiting effect in the rabbit was made by Makepeace *et al.* (1937), in the rat by Astwood and Fevold (1939), and in the sheep by Dutt and Casida (1948). Since progesterone also appears to inhibit fertilization in the rabbit (Boyarsky *et al.* 1947), we became interested in the further study of these phenomena and particularly if the ovulation-inhibiting effect and/or the fertilization-inhibition might be differentially affected by different substances. The mode of administration we have employed has failed to give any clear indication of an effect upon fertilization of the various compounds employed, but our data on ovulation inhibition are fairly clear cut, and seem worth recording.

METHODS AND MATERIALS

Mature rabbit does in estrus and of miscellaneous stocks were employed. The steroids employed in these studies were, with a few exceptions to be noted, administered in a single dose, and at appropriate intervals thereafter the does were mated to mature males. Twenty-four hours following the mating a laparotomy was performed and the occurrence of ovulation determined by the presence or absence of corpora lutea in the ovaries. If corpora lutea were found one fallopian tube was excised (and on ocasion the uterus on the same side), the incisions were sewn up, and the animal kept for further observation. The excised fallopian tube was flushed for ova which were then examined to determine if fertilization had taken place. Fertilized ova taken at this time are readily recognizable by the presence of cleavage and of sperm in the

---

* The investigations described in the paper were aided by grants from the Planned Parenthood Federation of America, Inc., the Ciba Co., Inc., and the Chemical Specialties Co., Inc.

TABLE I

Effects of a single subcutaneous injection of a macrocrystalline suspension of progesterone on the ovulation, transportation of spermatozoa and fertilization in the rabbit.

(The female rabbits were bred twice with fertile bucks at various days after injection, and examined 1 day after breeding).

Dose	Rabbit	Time of breeding: days after injection	Ovulation	Fertilization	N° of sperm in the tubes	N° of sperm in the uteri
	1	1	No	—	24 880	653 600
	11	1	No	—	0	1 976 700
	3	4	No	—	0	0
10 mg	4	8	Yes	4 of 16 ova	0	133 950
	13	8	No	—	2 667	1 836 00
	6	11	No	—	0	0
	9	14	Yes	7 of 9 ova	5 976	394 200
	14	14	Yes	9 of 9 ova	2 750	177 000
	2	1	No	—	4 140	8 300
	12	1	No	—	31 750	2 620 500
	8	4	No	—	0	0
30 mg	5	8	No	—	0	6 000
	7	11	No	—	0	142 240
	10	14	No	—	3 726	1 224 850
	15	18	No	—	0	12 834
	16	24	No	—	—	—

zona pellucida and/or the perivitteline space. In certain instances counts of sperm in the flushings from the tube and the uterus were also made. Nine to eleven days later, a second laparotomy was performed and the uterus on the unoperated side examined for implantations.

RESULTS

Before proceeding to a detailed account of our various experiments, we should state at once that in practically every instance in which ovulation occurred fertilization was observed if mating with fertile males was practised and implantation of fertilized eggs also took place. The ensuing

TABLE II

The effects on ovulation in rabbits of the intravaginal deposition of progesterone, 17α-hydroxyprogesterone and allopregnene-3β-ol-20-one. (The female rabbits were bred twice with bucks at various times after the deposition and examined 1 day after breeding).

Substance	Dosage mg	Nº rabbits	Time of breeding: hours after deposition	Nº ovulating
	30	1	24	0
	10	1	24	0
	1	2	24	0
Progesterone	1	2	5	0
	1	2	2	2
	0.5	1	24	1
	0.1	1	24	1
	2	4	24	0
17α-Hydroxy-progesterone	1	1	24	1
	0.5	1	24	1
Allopregnano-lone	5	2	24	1 (²)
	5 (¹)	2	24	2

(¹) Subcutaneous injection.
(²) Fertilization and implantation occurred.

account is therefore concerned with the influence of various substances on ovulation.

Our initial observations were concerned with the effects of progesterone injected subcutaneously as a macrocrystalline suspension. The data on the effects of 10 mg and 30 mg doses are presented in Table I. It is clear that the higher dosage effectively blocked the ovulation that normally follows copulation. In one instance ovulation occurred et eight days, and in two instances at fourteen days following the lower dose, suggesting somewhat reduced effectiveness of the lower dosage. Although great irregularities in sperm count were had, there is no obvious difference between the two dosages in relation to the frequency of appearance or number of sperm in either the fallopian tubes or the uterus.

In Table II we present data on the effects of the intravaginal deposition of various amounts of progesterone, 17-α-hydroxyprogesterone and allopregnanolone on ovulation. The data demonstrate: (a) That if mating is practised in less than five hours after the intravaginal administration of 1 mg of progesterone ovulation will occur; (b) that if mating

takes place at 24 hours after the deposition of 1 mg of progesterone the
block to ovulation is established as well at this dosage as at 10 and 30 mg
dosages; (c) that intravaginal dosages of 0.5 and 0.1 mg are not effective
at 24 hours following administration; (d) that 2 mg intravaginal dosages
of 17α-hydroxyprogesterone are effectively ovulation-inhibiting, but that
dosages of 1 mg or less are probably ineffective; and (e) that allopregnanolone is probably not effective as an inhibitor of ovulation by either
the intravaginal or subcutaneous route at a 5 mg dose level.

TABLE III

*Effect of oral administration of ethinyl testosterone on ovulation, fertilization and
implantation in the rabbit. (The animals were bred twice 1 day after feeding and
examined 1 day and 6-7 days after breeding).*

Dosage	Nº Rabbits	Nº Ovulating	Fertili- zation	Implan- tation
10 mg in a single feeding	8	1	? [1]	—
5 mg in a single feeding	13	8	Yes [2]	Yes [2]
2 mg in a single feeding	6	4	Yes [2]	Yes [2]
1.20 mg daily for 5 days	4	2	? [1]	—
1 mg daily for 5 days	4	2	?	No
0.75 mg daily for 5 days	2	2	?	—

[1] Bred to a sterile male.

[2] In females mated to fertile males.

Ethinyl testosterone (an oral progestin) was administered by mouth
in various courses as indicated in Table III. It will be noted: (a) That
seven out of eight rabbits given 10 mg in a single dose by mouth failed
to ovulate, whereas five out of thirteen failed at the 5 mg and two out
of six at the 2 mg levels; (b) that 1.25 mg and 1.0 mg fed daily for five
days were partially effective; and (c) that dubiously irregular effects on
fertilization and implantation occurred.

In Table IV we present data on the effects of the administration of
17-methyl progesterone in various experiments. The results suggest the
relative ineffectiveness of the oral route, but an effectiveness by subcutaneous or intravaginal injection comparable to that obtained with progesterone (*cf.* Table II) and with a duration of the effect at 5 mg comparable to that seen with progesterone (*cf.* Table I).

Intravenously into three rabbits one day after the subcutaneous
injection of 17-methyl progesterone, we injected a pituitary extract at a

TABLE IV

The effects of 17-methyl progesterone (dissolved in propylene glycol) on ovulation in the rabbit. Each rabbit was given the preparation in a single dose, and the determination of ovulation made 24 hours after mating.

Dosage mg	Nº of rabbits	Route of administration	Time of mating after administration, days	Nº ovulating
5	3	Subcutaneous	1	0
10	4	,,	1	0
5	2	Intravaginal	1	0
10	2	Oral	1	2
50	2	,,	1	1
5	2	Subcutaneous	2	0
5	3	,,	6	0
5	2	,,	7	1
5	2	,,	8	2

dosage level which was invariably ovulating in normal estrus females. Two of the three had ovulated when examined 24 hours later, suggesting that the methyl progesterone effect may involve a block to the release of pituitary gonadotrophin.

Using a standard tehnique of subcutaneous injection in 10 mg dose followed by mating in 24 hours, we have examined a series of pregnane and allopregnane derivatives as possible ovulation inhibitors. The data are presented in Table V. With the possible exception of pregnane-3,20 dione, no suggestion of ovulation inhibition at this dosage is had for any of the compounds tested.

DISCUSSION

The effectiveness of progesterone as an inhibitor of ovulation is reaffirmed by our data. Furthermore, certain active progestins, namely ethinyl testosterone and 17-methyl progesterone are also effective. Since 17-hydroxyprogesterone is also effective, it is suggested that substitutions at carbon 17 in the progesterone molecule do not notably interfere with the ovulation-inhibiting capacity. It is a matter of great interest that 17-methyl progesterone is roughly twice as active as progesterone in standard assay (Heusser *et al.*, 1950) whereas 17α-hydroxyprogesterone is inactive as a progestin (Pfiffner and North, 1940). A dissociation of progestational and ovulation-inhibiting effects is suggested. On the other hand, the ineffectiveness of 11α-hydroxyprogesterone at a dose notably effective for progesterone and 17-methyl progesterone suggests that substitutions at carbon 11 may interfere with ovulation-inhibiting capacity. It is notable (Byrnes *et al.*, 1953), that 11α-hydroxyprogesterone has less than one-half the activity of progesterone as a progestin, but in the

TABLE V

The effects on ovulation of various pregnane and allopregnane derivatives. Each compound, dissolved in propylene glycol, was administered in a single 10 mg. dose. Mating was practised 24 hours later, and examination for ovulation at 24 hours following mating.

Compound	Nº of females tested	Nº ovulating
Allopregnane-17α-ol-3, 20-dione	3	3
Allopregnane-3β, 17α, 21-triol	4	4
Allopregnane-21-ol-3, 20-dione	3	3
Pregnane-3, 20-dione	3*	1
Pregnane-3α, 20α-diol	3	2
Pregnane-3α, 20β-diol	3	3
Pregnane-3β, 20β-diol	3	3
Δ^4 ^{16}-Pregnadiene-3, 20-dione	3	3
11α-Hydroxyprogesterone	3	3

* 1 animal with small ovaries.

immature rat is only slightly less active as a pituitary gonadotrophin inhibitor. No reduction product of progesterone (with the possible exception of pregnane-3,20-dione) appears to have any significant ovulation-inhibiting capacity. Further studies of such compounds at varying dosages are, however, clearly necessary to rule out the possibility of any effect. We hope to report on such experiments as well as experiments with other types of progesterone relatives at a later date.

Some remark should be made about our failure to observe any effects on ovum fertilization. Boyarsky *et al.* (1947), found that pretreatment for ten days at 2 mg per day was necessary to block fertilization 95 %; the same dosage in a pretreatment for five days was completely ineffective. Also they had to ovulate the rabbits artificially with pituitary extract and artificially inseminate. It is clear that our experiments have been conducted under a different regime and that the fertilization-inhibiting treatment is inhibiting to ovulation induced by mating.

SUMMARY

The potency of progesterone as an inhibitor of ovulation in the rabbit has been reaffirmed. Its effectiveness when administered by subcutaneous or intravaginal routes is demonstrated. A single injection of 30 mg of progesterone may prevent ovulation for as long as 24 days.

Ethinyl testosterone administered orally is an effective inhibitor of ovulation in the rabbit, and the effect appears to be proportional to the dose over the range 2 to 10 mg in a single feeding. 17α-Hydroxyprogesterone administered intravaginally is an ovulation inhibitor. 17-Methyl progesterone is quite effective when administered intravaginally or subcutaneously, but is relatively ineffective when given by mouth. A series of ring-A reduced allo and normal reduction products of progesterone tested by subcutaneous injection at the 10 mg dose level appeared to be ineffective as ovulation inhibitors. 11α-Hydroxyprogesterone also is ineffective at this dosage.

ACKNOWLEDGEMENTS

We are indebted to Dr. I. V. Sollins of the Chemical Specialties Co. and to Dr. E. Oppenheimer of the Ciba Co. for supplies of compounds used in these studies. Miss Betty Hull offered valued technical assistence.

REFERENCES

ASTWOOD, E. B., FEVOLD, H. L.: *Amer. J. Physiol.*, 1939, *127*, 192.
BOYARSKY, L. H., BAYLIS, H., CASIDA, L. E., MEYER, R. K.: *Endocrinology*, 1947, *41*, 312.
BYRNES, W. W., STAFFORD, R. O., OLSON, K. J.: *Proc. Soc. Exper. Biol.*, N. Y., 1953, *82*, 243.
DUTT, R. H., CASIDA, L E.: *Endocrinology*, 1948, *43*, 208.
HEUSSER, H., ENGEL, C. R., HERZIG, P. T., PLATTNER, P. A.: *Helvetica chim. Acta*, 1950, *33*, 1229.
MAKEPEACE, A. W,. WEINSTEIN, G. L., FRIEDMAN, M. H.: *Amer. J. Physiol.*, 1937, *119*, 512.
PARKES, A. S.: *The Internal Secretions of the Ovary.* Longmans, Green, London, 1929.
PFIFFNER, J. J., NORTH, H. B.: *J. Biol. Chem.*, 1940, *132*, 459.

This paper has been reproduced by kind permission of
Acta Physiologica Pharmacologica et Therapeutica Latinoamericana.

Commentary on Classic Paper No.11

In 1929, Parkes[2] observed that the induction of ovulation is difficult in animals in which the ovaries contain active corpora lutea, and, from this observation, he suggested that progesterone should be an effective inhibitor of ovulation. The potential use of steroids for contraception, however, was hampered by the fact that they were not active when administered orally. This hurdle was finally overcome in 1938, when it was discovered that the addition of an ethinyl group at the 17 position made estradiol orally active[3]. This led to the introduction of sex steroids that were active when taken orally.

Ethinylestradiol

In 1953, Pincus and Chang[1] published their classic paper which developed from the original work of Parkes[2]. For their studies they used mature rabbits and, by laparotomy, checked the effects of various doses of progesterone, 17α-hydroxyprogesterone and ethinyltestosterone on the ovulatory process. They also studied the effects of intravaginal administration. The results of their work established the potency of progesterone as an inhibitor of ovulation and paved the way for the development of oral contraception.

After 1944, a host of new progestational agents became available, of which norethindrone[4] and norethynodrel[5] have had wide clinical application. The discovery of ethinyl substitution at the 17 position and oral activity led to the preparation of ethisterone, an orally active derivative of testosterone. In 1951, it was demonstrated that removal of the 19 carbon from ethisterone changed the effect from that of an androgen to a progestational agent. The progestational derivatives of testosterone were named 19 nortestosterone (nor = no radical).

Ethisterone

1. Pincus, G. and Chang, M.C. (1953). The effects of progesterone and related compounds on ovulation and early development in the rabbit. *Acta Physiol. Latino-Americana*, **3**, 177

2. Parkes, A.S. (1929). *The Internal Secretions of the Ovary.* (London: Longmans, Green)

3. Inhoffen, H.H. and Hohlweg, W. (1938). New female glandular derivates active per os: 17-ethinyl-estradiol and pregnenein-3-one-17-06. *Naturwissenschaften*, **26**, 96

4. Djerassi, C., Miracontes, G., Rosenkranz, G. and Sondheimer, F. (1954). Synthesis of 19-nor-17-ethinyl-testosterone and 19-nor-17-methyltestosterone. *J. Am. Chem. Soc.*, **76**, 4092

5. Pincus, G., Chang, M.C., Hafez, E.S.E., Zarrow, M.X. and Merrill, A. (1956). Effects of certain 19-nor-steroids on reproductive processes in animals. *Science*, **124**, 890

In Pincus and Chang's original paper, they commented that *'The mode of administration we have employed has failed to give any clear indication of an effect upon fertilization of the various compounds employed, but our data on ovulation inhibition are fairly clear cut, and seem worth recording.'* When this classic paper is viewed in the context of the development of oral contraception, we can see just how true their original comment has proved to be.

The history of oral contraceptives

6. Roberts, R.M. (1989). *Serendipity: Accidental Discoveries in Science.* pp. 128–30. (New York: John Wiley and Sons)

The history of steroid use for contraception starts with Russell E. Marker, a chemist who never received his PhD[6]. From 1927 to 1935, Marker worked at the Rockefeller Institute in New York on configuration and optical rotation as methods for identifying compounds. When he moved to Pennsylvania State University in 1935, he trained in steroid chemistry and became interested in solving the problem of cheap production of progesterone. At that time ovaries of 2500 pregnant pigs were needed to produce 1 mg of progesterone! Marker discovered that a species of Trillium (the Mexican yam), collected as Beth's root in North Carolina, and popular at that time for the relief of menstrual pains, contained a plant steroid, diosgenin.

In 1942, he visited Mexico and collected roots of the Mexican yam and back home worked out the degradation of diosgenin to progesterone. At that time, pharmaceutical companies were not interested in his finding! Returning to Mexico in 1943, he prepared several pounds of progesterone and joined Hormone Laboratories in Mexico City and then, with two partners, formed a company called Syntex.

In 1947, Marker sold his share of the company and Syntex recruited George Rosenkranz to manufacture progesterone commercially. In 1949, it was discovered that cortisone relieved arthritis. Dr Carl Djerassi then joined Syntex to work on the synthesis of cortisone, taking the same Mexican yam plant steroid, diosgenin, as the starting point.

The Syntex chemists again turned their attention to the sex steroids and discovered that the removal of the 19 carbon from progesterone increased the progestational activity of the molecule. Ethisterone was now available and in 1951 norethindrone was synthesized.

It can be seen from this sequence of events that, although the origin of the 'pill' was not purely a serendipitous event, serendipity certainly represented one part of the story. Gregory Pincus went on to test these sex steroids in women in Puerto Rico and the pill was born.

Development of the pill: side-effects, lower doses and structural changes

After more than a decade of research, the US Food and Drug Administration approved the first combined oral contraceptive on 9th May, 1960. This oral contraceptive, Enovid-10®, contained 9.85 mg of the progestogen norethynodrel and 150 µg of the estrogen mestranol. By 1970, around 8–10 million women in the US and a similar number in other developed countries were using the pill. Due to the efforts of family planning programs in the developing world, an estimated 20–30 million women were using oral contraceptives in these countries by the early 1970s. In the 1980s, the pill became even more popular. In developed countries, use of an oral contraceptive reached 24 million married women, or 14% of married women of reproductive age. In the developing countries, over 38 million married women used the pill which is about 6% of married women of reproductive age. According to a Population Report (November, 1988), 63 million women throughout the world were using an oral contraceptive in 1988[7].

Thrombosis and estrogen dose reduction

In 1961, a general practitioner described the occurrence of pulmonary embolism in a women taking Enovid-10[8]. Several other reports of thromboembolic events in women taking oral contraceptives followed, and this focused attention on a possible relationship between oral contraceptives and thrombosis. Investigations into this phenomenon began, including cohort studies like the Royal College of General Practitioners' study, published in 1967[9]. In the late 1960s, epidemiological studies[10,11] showed that the high-dose oral contraceptives used at that time increased the risk of thromboembolic diseases and that the risk was related to the estrogen dose. Consequently, the Committee on Safety of Medicines recommended in 1969 that oral contraceptives with an estrogen content higher than 50 µg should not be used routinely. The first of the low-dose pills, which contained 30 µg ethinylestradiol and a new progestogen, levonorgestrel, was introduced in 1973, and the first 20 µg ethinylestradiol oral contraceptive, with the progestogen desogestrel, appeared in 1988. With the continuous estrogen dose reductions, the incidence of thromboembolic diseases in pill users steadily decreased[12,13] and today, the risk is only marginally higher than in non-users.

Levonorgestrel

7. Population Reports, November 1988, The Johns Hopkins University, Series A, no.7, p.1

8. Jordan, W.M. (1961). Pulmonary embolism. *Lancet*, **2**, 1146

9. Royal College of General Practitioners (1967). Oral contraception and thromboembolic disease. *J. R. Coll. Gen. Pract.*, **13**, 267

10. Vessey, M.P. and Doll, R. (1968). Investigation of relation between use of oral contraceptives and thromboembolic disease. *Br. Med. J.*, **2**, 199

11. Sartwell, P.E., Masi, A.T., Arthes, F.G., Greene, G.R. and Smith, H.E. (1969). Thromboembolism and oral contraceptives: an epidemiologic case-control study. *Am. J. Epidemiol.*, **90**, 365

12. Bottiger, L.E., Boman, G. and Westerholm, B. (1980). Oral contraceptives and thromboembolic disease: effects of lowering oestrogen content. *Lancet*, **1**, 1097

13. Lidegaard, O. (1993). Oral contraception and risk of a cerebral thromboembolic attack: results of a case-control study. *Br. Med. J.*, **306**, 956

Cardiovascular disease and new progestogens

14. Mann, J.I., Vessey, M.P. and Doll, R. (1975). Myocardial infarction in young women with special reference to oral contraceptive practice. *Br. Med. J.*, **2**, 445

15. Jick, H., Dinan, B. and Rothman, K.J. (1978). Oral contraceptives and non-fatal myocardial infarction. *J. Am. Med. Assoc.*, **239**, 1403

16. Gordon, T., Castelli, W.P., Hjortland, M., Kannel, W.B. and Dawber, T. (1977). High density lipoprotein as a protective factor against coronary heart disease. *Am. J. Med.*, **62**, 707

17. Op ten Berg, M.T. (1991). Desogestrel: using a selective progestogen in a combined oral contraceptive. *Adv. Contracept.*, **7**, 241

In 1977, the Royal College of General Practitioners' study found an association between risk of cardiovascular disease and the progestogen in the pill, while several other epidemiological studies showed a higher incidence of cardiovascular disease in women using oral contraceptives[14,15]. Around the same time, population studies, such as the Framingham study, showed that men and women with low serum levels of high-density lipoprotein (HDL)-cholesterol had a higher risk of ischemic heart disease than those with higher levels[16]. In 1978, the Walnut Creek study from the US reported a connection between the pill and lipid metabolism. As a result of all this, the focus in developing new oral contraceptives shifted from the estrogen to the progestogen component of the pill.

The progestogens used in oral contraceptives in the 1970s all had substantial androgenic activity which resulted in adverse effects on lipid metabolism and, therefore, progestogens could be improved by minimizing their intrinsic androgenicity. In 1981, the first new progestogen with low androgenicity, desogestrel, was introduced and this was followed by gestodene and norgestimate.

Gestodene   Norgestimate

The hormonal characteristics of the different progestogens can be studied properly by means of receptor binding studies. The binding affinity to the progesterone receptor is a good standard for its progestational activity, as is binding to the androgenic receptor for its androgenicity. The most relevant information that can be obtained from receptor binding studies is the selectivity index (see figure below), which is the ratio of the binding affinity to the progesterone receptor over that to the androgen receptor.

This index has been shown to correlate well with the metabolic impact of a progestogen on lipid metabolism. The new progestogens are far more selective than the older ones, with 3-keto-desogestrel (the active metabolite of desogestrel) the most selective available[17]. A large number of prospective longitudinal and cross-sectional studies confirm that these pills

Desogestrel

containing progestogens lack negative effects on lipid parameters and are, in some cases, even beneficial[17,18].

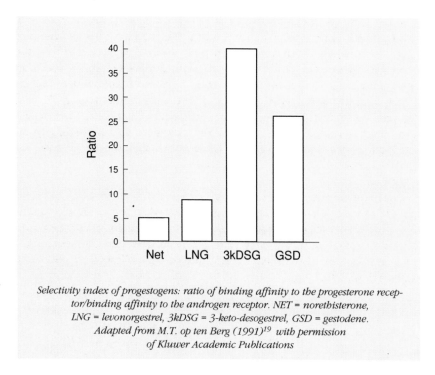

Selectivity index of progestogens: ratio of binding affinity to the progesterone receptor/binding affinity to the androgen receptor. NET = norethisterone, LNG = levonorgestrel, 3kDSG = 3-keto-desogestrel, GSD = gestodene. Adapted from M.T. op ten Berg (1991)[19] with permission of Kluwer Academic Publications

Cancer studies

A large number of studies have been undertaken to investigate the pill's potential effects on female reproductive cancers. In particular, much attention has been focused on the relationship between the pill and breast cancer. In 1983, a world pill scare developed when Pike and his colleagues suggested a positive association between the use of the pill before the age of 25 and risk of breast cancer[19]. However, in 1986, Paul and colleagues reported an inverse association between these factors[20]. Although at this moment there is consensus in the literature that the use of combined oral contraceptives does not increase the overall risk of breast cancer, there remain some doubts about the effects of early use (before the age of 25)[21].

The first epidemiological study, in which a protective effect of the pill in relation to ovarian cancer was suggested, was reported in 1977 by Newhouse and colleagues[22]. All subsequent studies confirmed this protective effect after 3 or more years of oral contraceptive use, with a risk reduction of 40%. A reduction of 50% after 4 years and 60–80% after 7 or more years of use has also been suggested[21]. A similar duration-related protective effect against endometrial cancer occurs with combined oral contraceptives. After 2 years of use, the risk is reduced by about 40% and by about 60% after 4 or more years of use[21]. The protection against ovarian and endometrial cancer persists in ex-users of the pill for at least 10 years.

18. Godsland, I.F., Crook, D., Simpson, R., Proudler, T., Felton, C., Lees, B., Anyaoku, V., Devenport, M. and Wynn, V. (1990). The effects of different formulations of oral contraceptive agents on lipid and carbohydrate metabolism. *N. Engl. J. Med.*, **323**, 1375

19. Pike, M.C., Henderson, B.E., Krailo, M.D., Duke, A. and Roy, S. (1983). Breast cancer in young women and use of oral contraceptives: possible modifying effect of formulation and age at use. *Lancet*, **2**, 926

20. Paul, C., Skegg, D.C.G., Spears, G.F.S. and Kaldor, J.M. (1986). Oral contraceptives and breast cancer: a national study. *Br. Med. J.*, **293**, 723

21. Schlesselmen, J.J. (1989). Cancer of the breast and reproductive tract in relation to use of oral contraceptives. *Contraception*, **40**, 1

22. Newhouse, M.L., Pearson, R.M., Fullerton, J.M., Boesen, E.A.M. and Shannon, H.S. (1977). A case-control study of carcinoma of the ovary. *Br. J. Prev. Soc. Med.*, **31**, 148

Studies of cervical dysplasia and carcinoma of the cervix *in situ* have suggested an elevated risk after 2 or more years of use, but the results of these studies are difficult to interpret, due to confounding variables such as sexual history, regular screening for cervical cancer in oral contraceptive users and lack of barrier methods (which protect against sexually transmitted disease)[21].

The pill has been shown clearly to have a protective long-lasting effect on ovarian and endometrial cancer. Studies on cervical cancer are difficult to interpret and it will take the results of on-going epidemiological studies with low-dose oral contraceptives possibly finally to resolve the remaining questions about the association between the pill and breast cancer.

Beneficial effects

23. Vessey, M.P. (1990). The Jephcott Lecture. An overview of the benefits and risks of combined oral contraceptives. In Mann, R.D. (ed.) *Oral Contraceptives and Breast Cancer*, pp.121–32. (Carnforth: Parthenon Publishing Group)

Apart from its high contraceptive reliability, the pill has a number of established benefits[23]. Combined oral contraceptives protect against menstrual problems such as menorrhagia and dysmenorrhea. The risk of heavy, prolonged, frequent, irregular and painful periods is reduced. This also implies a protective effect against the development of iron deficiency anemia. Benign breast lumps occur to a lesser extent in women currently using the pill. This effect increases with duration of use and is probably brought about by the progestogen component of the pill.

There is some evidence that combined oral contraceptives reduce the risk and severity of pelvic inflammatory disease in general, although the risk of infection of the cervix by Chlamydia seems to be enhanced.

Because the main mode of action of the pill is to arrest follicular development and inhibit ovulation, women using oral contraceptives are at a greatly reduced risk of corpus luteum cysts and follicular cysts of the ovary.

As mentioned previously, the pill reduces the risk of ovarian and endometrial cancer by about 50%, a protection which lasts for several years once a woman has stopped using the pill.

Benefits of the pill which have not, as yet, been clearly confirmed, but which are expected to be confirmed in the future, include protection against thyroid disease, rheumatoid arthritis, peptic ulcer and fibromyomata of the uterus.

A well-established benefit of the pill is that it allows menstruation to be delayed, and recent evidence suggests that newer oral contraceptives improve acne.

Benefits and risks

Vessey used a simple approach to weigh up the benefits and risks of combined oral contraceptives[23]. In the table below, morbidity (in terms of hospital admissions) experienced by women aged 25–39 years using a combined oral contraceptive is compared with that of women using condoms. The non-obstetric events are based on hospital admission rates, whereas the obstetric data are derived directly from the Oxford-Family Planning Association study, taking the failure rate for combined oral contraceptive users as 5/1000 per year and for condom users as 50/1000 per year.

Morbidity (in terms of hospital admissions) experienced by women aged 25–39 years using either combined oral contraceptives or relying on the condom to try and prevent pregnancy for 1 year.

	Number of hospital admissions in 1 year among 100 000 women relying on:	
Reasons for hospital admission	*Combined oral contraceptives*	*Condom*
Beneficial effects of combined oral contraceptives		
menstrual problems	375	500
anemia	22	30
benign breast disease	115	230
pelvic inflammatory disease*	60	60
functional ovarian cysts	15	60
ovarian cancer	5	10
endometrial cancer	2	4
Harmful effects of combined oral contraceptives		
acute myocardial infarction	10	5
thrombotic stroke	50	10
hemorrhagic stroke	7	5
venous thromboembolism	100	20
hepatocellular adenoma	2	0
hepatocellular carcinoma	0	0
Accidental pregnancy†		
term birth	300	3040
spontaneous abortion	63	640
extrauterine pregnancy	3	20
induced abortion	134	1300

* These rates are equal because both combined oral contraceptives and a condom offer protection against pelvic inflammatory diesease. † The failure rate for combined oral contraceptives has been taken to be 5/1000 per year and for the condom to be 50/1000 per year

Adapted from M.P. Vessey (1990)[23] with permission

It must be kept in mind that the cardiovascular risks with the use of modern low-dose oral contraceptives may be considerably lower than indicated. Besides, the protective effect against ovarian and endometrial cancer persists in ex-users and is of greater importance beyond the childbearing years than during these years. The overall effect on morbidity is clearly in favor of the oral contraceptive.

The benefits of oral contraceptive use (and probably even more so for the low-dose oral contraceptives) appear to outweigh the risks. One of the consequences of benefit/risk equations for oral contraceptives is that there is currently no age limit for pill use in non-smoking women.

Contragestion

24. Beaulieu, E.E. and
Segal, S.J. (1985). *The
Antiprogestin Steroid
RU 486 and Human
Fertility Control*. (New
York: Plenum Press)

An interesting development in the regulation of fertility is the use of a progesterone antagonist (RU 486)[24] as an alternative addendum to post-conception regimens. Its structure resembles that of norethindrone, with a longer 17α side-chain, to increase affinity to the receptor and an 11β phenyl group which acts as the antagonist.

RU 486 interrupts the menstrual cycle, whether fertilization and implantation have occurred or not. Clinical studies report that 600 mg given once interrupts more than 90% of early pregnancies for up to 41 days of amenorrhea. The term 'contragestion' was introduced to distinguish this anti-progesterone action from a way of avoiding conception.

Lactation and contraception

Lactational amenorrhea is an important mechanism for 'natural' fertility regulation, especially in developing countries. The mechanisms by which ovulation is suppressed are, however, incompletely understood, but the frequency and duration of suckling, i.e. the mechanical stimulation of the nipple, appears to be crucial. A prompt and large release of prolactin is known to be associated with suckling.

25. Yen, S.S.C. (1986).
Prolactin in human repro-
duction. In Yen, S.S.C.
and Jaffe, R.R. (eds.)
*Reproductive
Endocrinology*, 2nd edn.,
pp. 237–63.
(Philadelphia: W.B.
Saunders Co.)

Once supplementary feeding of the newborn begins and suckling time decreases, prolactin concentration also decreases and ovarian activity recommences, leading to ovulatory cycles after 5 weeks. Prolactin, oxytocin, but especially β-endorphins seem to be involved in the mechanisms of lactational amenorrhea. It would seem likely that new trends for contraception may emerge based on lactational amenorrhea[25], especially from work with neurohormones.

Breast feeding is associated with prolonged hyperprolactinemia, normal levels of luteinizing hormone (LH) and follicle stimulating hormone (FSH), and low levels of estradiol and progesterone. In long-term lactational amenorrhea, the actual duration of amenorrhea is associated with the degree of hyperprolactinemia, which in turn is related to the suckling frequency.

The antifertility effects of lactation have been recognized for many years and still are the normal method of contraception in developing countries. The efficacy of lactational amenorrhea as an effective inhibitor of ovulation is questioned, however, because 5–10% of women become pregnant during the suckling period. Breast feeding can have an optimal contraceptive effect for 6 months, but that after this period it becomes less effective. At this time, menstruation or spotting are not predictive of subsequent ovulation.

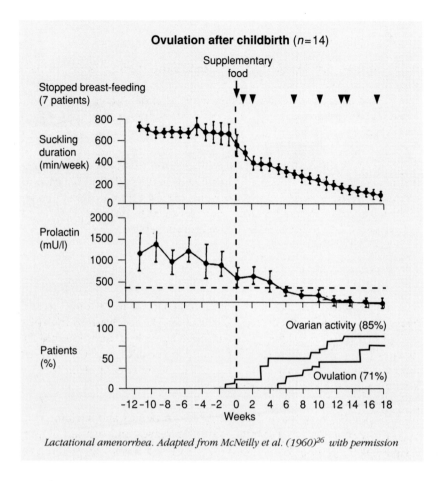

Ovulation after childbirth (*n*=14)

Lactational amenorrhea. Adapted from McNeilly et al. (1960)[26] with permission

Natural family planning

Herman Knaus (1892–1970) worked at the Department of Obstetrics and Gynecology in Graz, Austria. During his studies at the University of Cambridge in England, Knaus was involved in research to understand the physiology of the uterus. In experiments with rabbits, he found that the pituitary gland lost its contractile property on the uterus after ovulation. He attributed this phenomenon to the action of the corpus luteum.

Knaus extended his studies to women, using a uterosalpingograph mercury manometer and kymograph. In women with regular cycles, he found that there was always a uterine reaction to pituitrin, in the first 14 days of the menstrual cycle. After day 16, however, not only did the pattern of uterine activity change but also the reaction to pituitrin was virtually absent. He related these findings to the time of ovulation, being 2 days before the loss of sensitivity of the uterus to pituitrin.

From these studies, Knaus concluded that the fertile period in the menstrual cycle was between day 11 and day 17. Infertile periods were, therefore, the first 10 days of the cycle and after the 18th day[27,28].

26. McNeilly, A.S., Howie, P.W. and, Houston, M.J. (1980). Relationship of feeding patterns, prolactin and resumption of ovulation postpartum. In Zatuchni, G., Labbu, M.H. and Sciarra, J.J. (eds.) *Research Frontiers in Fertility Regulation.* pp. 102–116. (Philadelphia: Harper and Row)

27. Knaus, H. (1929). Ueber den Zeitpunkt der Konzeptionsfahigkeit des Weibes im Intermenstruum. *München Med. Wochensch.,* 76, 1157

28. Knaus, H. (1929). Eine neue Methode zur Bestimmung des Ovulationstermines. *Zblt. Gynäkol.,* 35, 2193

29. Ogino, K. (1930).
Ovulationstermin und
Konzeptionstermin.
Zbit. Gynäkol., **54**, 469

30. Schröder, R. (1913).
Ueber die zeitlichen
Beziehungen der Ovulation
und Menstruation.
Verh. Dtsch. Ges. Gynäk.,
15, 251

31. Billings, J.J. (1964).
The Ovulation Method.
(Melbourne, Australia:
Advocate Press)

32. Djerassi, C. (1990).
Fertility awareness: jet-age
rhythm method?
Science, 248, 1061

While Knaus was working in Europe, Kyusaku Ogino (1882–1975), the 'chef de clinique' of the Department of Gynecology in Niigata, was carrying out similar studies in Japan. He had already published his research in Japanese and in 1930 commented on the work of Knaus[29].

Ogino categorized the observations which he made during laparotomy in women and the histological examination of corpora lutea and endometrium. In his approach to determining the point of ovulation, Ogino used an original methodology. He determined the ovulation period in days preceding the next menstruation, basing this on the work of Schröder[30] who concluded that ovulation preceded menstruation. In later years, the methods of Ogino and Knaus became known as the symptothermic method of natural family planning[31], going back to the observation of temperature changes within the menstrual cycle made originally in 1904, by van de Velde (see Commentary No. 8).

Fertility awareness

In 1990, Djerassi[32] called for a new look at the role of natural family planning. To be effective, this method requires daily measurements of basal body temperature, together with assessments of vaginal discharge or cervical mucus qualities. Together, these allow ovulation to be predicted. The poor reliability of these methods means, however, that sexual abstinence is prolonged, even up to 17 days per cycle!

Djerassi believed that improvements to natural family planning would be possible if certain biochemical measurements could be made, where a change of more than 50% would indicate fertility. One such marker is the rise in levels of estrogens which increase steadily in different women over a period of 48–168 hours. Saliva or urine can be used for testing. Another marker might be the increasing level of progesterone soon after ovulation, accompanied by a second rise in estrogens. Both indicate that the danger of conception has passed. Finally, research into the changing immuno-chemistry of the cervical mucus could prove a promising approach to fertility regulation.

Epilogue

The history of the development of steroids as oral contraceptives represents a fascinating story and one in which the pioneering work of Pincus and Chang played an important part. The way in which today's oral contraceptive has evolved is based on fundamental research into the factors that regulate the menstrual cycle.

A new approach towards contraceptive practice, including lactational amenorrhea and natural family planning, might be of value, increasing our awareness of fertility. Such interest invites more research on the prediction of ovulation. Also, as judged by the number of abortions still carried out, education still has a major role to play in helping women to avoid pregnancy.

Nevertheless, today an almost complete armamentarium of methods is available for women and doctors to use in order to avoid unwanted pregnancies.

Summary of references

1. Pincus, G. and Chang, M.C. (1953). The effects of progesterone and related compounds on ovulation and early development in the rabbit. *Acta Physiol. Latino-Americana,* **3**, 177
2. Parkes, A.S. (1929). *The Internal Secretions of the Ovary.* (London: Longmans, Green)
3. Inhoffen, H.H. and Hohlweg, W. (1938). New female glandular derivates active per os: 17-ethinyl-estradiol and pregnenein-3-one-17-06. *Naturwissenschaften,* **26**, 96
4. Djerassi, C., Miracontes, G., Rosenkranz, G. and Sondheimer, F. (1954). Synthesis of 19-nor-17-ethinyl-testosterone and 19-nor-17-methyltestosterone. *J. Am. Chem. Soc.,* **76**, 4092
5. Pincus, G., Chang, M.C., Hafez, E.S.E., Zarrow, M.X. and Merrill, A. (1956). Effects of certain 19-nor-steroids on reproductive processes in animals. *Science,* **124**, 890
6. Roberts, R.M. (1989). *Serendipity: Accidental Discoveries in Science,* pp. 128–30. (New York: John Wiley and Sons)
7. Population Reports, November 1988, The Johns Hopkins University, Series A, no.7, p.1
8. Jordan, W.M. (1961). Pulmonary embolism. *Lancet,* **2**, 1146
9. Royal College of General Practitioners (1967). Oral contraception and thromboembolic disease. *J. R. Coll. Gen. Pract.,* **13**, 267
10. Vessey, M.P. and Doll, R. (1968). Investigation of relation between use of oral contraceptives and thromboembolic disease. *Br. Med. J.,* **2**, 199
11. Sartwell, P.E., Masi, A.T., Arthes, F.G., Greene, G.R. and Smith, H.E. (1969). Thromboembolism and oral contraceptives: an epidemiologic case-control study. *Am. J. Epidemiol.,* **90**, 365
12. Bottiger, L.E., Boman, G. and Westerholm, B. (1980). Oral contraceptives and thromboembolic disease: effects of lowering oestrogen content. *Lancet,* **1**, 1097
13. Lidegaard, O. (1993). Oral contraception and risk of a cerebral thromboembolic attack: results of a case-control study. *Br. Med. J.,* **306**, 956
14. Mann. J.I., Vessey, M.P., Thorogood, M. and Doll, R. (1975). Myocardial infarction in young women with special reference to oral contraceptive practice. *Br. Med. J.,* **2**, 445
15. Jick, H., Dinan, B, and Rothman, K.J. (1978). Oral contraceptives and non-fatal myocardial infarction. *J. Am. Med. Assoc.,* **239**, 1403

16. Gordon, T., Castelli, W.P., Hjortland, M., Kannel, W.B. and Dawber, T. (1977). High density lipoprotein as a protective factor against coronary heart disease. *Am. J. Med.*, **62**, 707

17. Op ten Berg, M.T. (1991). Desogestrel: using a selective progestogen in a combined oral contraceptive. *Adv. Contracept.*, **7**, 241

18. Godsland, I.F., Crook, D., Simpson, R., Proudler, T., Felton, C., Lees, B., Anyaoku, V., Devenport, M. and Wynn, V. (1990). The effects of different formulations of oral contraceptive agents on lipid and carbohydrate metabolism. *N. Engl. J. Med.*, **323**, 1375

19. Pike, M.C., Henderson, B. E., Krailo, M.D. Duke, A. and Roy, S. (1983). Breast cancer in young women and use of oral contraceptives: possible modifying effect of formulation and age at use. *Lancet,* **2**, 926

20. Paul, C., Skegg, D.C.G., Spears, G.F.S. and Kaldor, J.M. (1986). Oral contraceptives and breast cancer: a national study. *Br. Med. J.*, **293**, 723

21. Schlesselman, J.J. (1989). Cancer of the breast and reproductive tract in relation to use of oral contraceptives. *Contraception,* **40**, 1

22. Newhouse, M.L., Pearson, R.M., Fullerton, J.M., Boesen, E.A.M. and Shannon, H.S. (1977). A case-control study of carcinoma of the ovary. *Br. J. Prev. Soc. Med.*, **31**, 148

23. Vessey, M.P. (1990). The Jephcott Lecture. An overview of the benefits and risks of combined oral contraceptives. In Mann, R.D. (ed.) *Oral Contraceptives and Breast Cancer*, pp.121–32. (Carnforth: Parthenon Publishing Group)

24. Beaulieu, E.E. and Segal, S.J. (1985). *The Antiprogestin Steroid RU 486 and Human Fertility Control.* (New York: Plenum Press)

25. Yen, S.S.C. (1986). Prolactin in human reproduction. In Yen, S.S.C. and Jaffe, R.R. (eds.) *Reproductive Endocrinology,* 2nd edn., pp 237–63. (Philadelphia: W.B. Saunders & Co)

26. McNeilly, A.S., Howie, P.W. and, Houston M.J. (1980). Relationship of feeding patterns, prolactin and resumption of ovulation postpartum. In Zatuchni, G., Labbu, M.H. and Sciarra, J.J. (eds.) *Research Frontiers in Fertility Regulation,* pp. 102–116. (Philadelphia: Harper and Row)

27. Knaus, H. (1929). Ueber den Zeitpunkt der Konzeptionsfähigkeit des Weibes im Intermenstruum. *München. Med. Wochensch.*, **76**, 1157

28. Knaus, H. (1929). Eine neue Methode zur Bestimmung des Ovulationstermines. *Zblt. Gynäkol.*, **53**, 2193

29. Ogino, K. (1930). Ovulationstermin und Konzeptionstermin. *Zblt.Gynäkol.*, **54**, 469

30. Schröder, R. (1913). Ueber die zeitlichen Beziehungen der Ovulation und Menstruation. *Verh. Dtsch. Ges. Gynäk.*, **15**, 251

31. Billings, J.J.(1964). *The Ovulation Method.* (Melbourne, Australia: Advocate Press)

32. Djerassi, C. (1990). Fertility awareness: jet-age rhythm method? *Science,* **248**, 1061

THE PERIMENOPAUSE

Classic
Paper
No.12

Treatment of perimenopausal complaints
with dried ovarian extract

LUDWIG FRAENKEL

1. Fraenkel, L. (1903). Die
Funktion des Corpus
Luteum.
Arch. Gynäkol., **68**, 438

Fraenkel's paper has been selected because it represents one of the earliest attempts by a clinician to treat the physical complaints associated with the menopause with ovarian extracts. Fraenkel was one of the first clinicians to not only recognize the symptoms of the perimenopause, but to investigate forms of treatment. In the perimenopause, which is characterized by shorter or longer interval lengths of the menstrual cycle, marked changes occur in hormonal balance. Most significant are the reduced levels of estrogen, increased levels of gonadotropins, the extraglandular conversion of androstenedione to estrone, and ovarian androgen production. Many of the complaints associated with the menopause, such as hot flushes and genital atrophy, are estrogen-dependent, but estrogen supplementation, which was initially thought to be of benefit for every woman, has led, on some occasions, to unwanted effects.

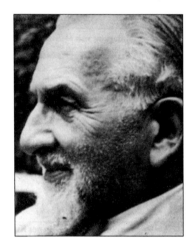

Die Function des Corpus luteum.

Von

L. Fraenkel.

Only Section III of the paper is reproduced here

III. Haupttheil.
Therapeutische Nutzanwendungen.

Ein Gesetz, dessen Richtigkeit mit Präcision erwiesen worden ist, und welches dazu eine grössere Anzahl physiologischer und pathologischer Vorgänge im Geschlechtsleben der Frau zu erklären geeignet ist, muss schliesslich auf seine Verwendbarkeit im praktischen Leben zum Nutzen der Kranken geprüft werden. Bezüglich hier zu erzielender Resultate ist eine gewisse Skepsis durchaus am Platze, weil lange nicht alle theoretisch richtig construirten Nutzanwendungen im praktischen Leben Stich halten; würden also Versuche dieser Art erfolglos seinen, so dürfte uns das in keiner Weise an der Richtigkeit des von uns ermittelten Gesetzes über die Function des Corpus luteum stutzig machen. Das Räderwerk der menschlichen Maschine ist zu complicirt, als dass ein theoretisch noch so folgerichtig construirtes Eingreifen auch sofort die erwartete Wirkung haben muss. Nicht immer folgt die Praxis der Theorie nach, wie sie ihr allerdings häufig genug vorauseilt.

Dennoch bin ich in der Lage, eine praktisch wichtige Schlussfolgerung aus meiner Arbeit ziehen zu können, und ein neues Heilpräparat vorzulegen, welches den theoretisch gestellten Anforderungen vollständig entsprach. Bekanntlich wurde vor ungefähr 6 Jahren nahezu gleichzeitig von Mainzer (82) aus der Landau'schen (83) und von Mond (84) aus der Kieler Klinik ein neues Präparat empfohlen, das Oophorin oder Ovariin, welches das Trockenextract der ganzen Eierstöcke von Kühen, Kälbern, Schafen oder Schweinen darstellt. Es war das zu der Zeit, als die Organpräparate sehr beliebt waren, und man sich gerade der in ihrer Function noch unbekannten Drüsen mit supponirter innerer Secretion, wie der Thyreoidea, Nebenniere, Milz, Thymus u. s. w. bediente, um Wirkungen zu erzielen. (Von diesen hat bekanntlich das Thyreoidin die auffallendste und beste Wirkung gezeigt, die indessen nicht frei von üblen Nebenwirkungen ist.)

Nun wusste man von den Eierstöcken, dass sie nicht nur eine Wirkung auf den Zustand des Uterus und das Zustandekommen der Menstruation ausüben, sondern auch das Allgemeinbefinden in einem gewissen Gleichgewicht erhalten; man wusste, dass durch plötzlichen Ausfall der Eierstocksfunction bei der geschlechtsreifen Frau, besonders durch die Castration, nicht nur eine mit Amenorrhoe einhergehende Uterusatrophie, sondern auch eine Anzahl Allgemeinsymptome hervorgerufen werden, die man als „Ausfallserscheinungen" bezeichnete. Darunter versteht man neben gewissen psychischen Alterationen hauptsächlich Anfälle von überlaufender Hitze, Wallungen zum Kopf mit Ohrensausen und intensiver Rötung des ganzen Gesichtes, Kopfschmerzen, Schwindelanfälle, Herzklopfen, Schweissausbrüche, Zittern in den Gliedern und andere lästige Symptome, ferner gewisse für die Menstruation vicariirend eintretende Blutungen, wie Nasenbluten u. s. w. Folgerichtig, weil durch Ausfall der Eierstocksfunction hervorgerufen, glaubten die erwähnten Autoren, dass Eierstockssubstanz, innerlich verabreicht, den Schaden wieder gut machen könnte; sie liessen also die Eierstöcke von Thieren zu Tabletten verarbeiten und den an Ausfallserscheinungen leidenden Kranken verabreichen. Der Erfolg war ein zum Theil eclatanter. Seitdem hat sich in der Litteratur (85—95) eine grössere Zahl von Arbeiten angehäuft, in welchen über die Wirkung des Mittels die widersprechendsten Erfahrungen mitgetheilt werden; einige sahen günstige, mehrere unzuverlässige, manche gar keine Wirkung; einen schädlichen Einfluss hat kein Autor dem Oophorin oder Ovariin nachsagen können. Alles das kann auch ich nur bestätigen. Neben vielen Fällen, wo jeder Erfolg ausblieb, sah ich einige sich deutlich dadurch bessern. Nicht nur bei Ausfallserscheinungen nach Castration, sondern auch bei Beschwerden der natürlichen Climax, ferner bei Dysmenorrhoe und Amenorrhoe wurde das Mittel versucht, meist ohne in die Augen springenden Erfolg, doch sind auch einige Frauen anscheinend dadurch mehr oder minder gebessert worden.[1] Nachdem wir wissen, dass das Corpus luteum der einzig in Betracht kommende

---

1) Besonders erinnere ich mich eines Falles von mehrmonatlicher Amenorrhoe bei einer jungen Frau (Polikl. Journ.-No. 226). Hier wurden viele andere Mittel: Aloë, Sabina, Ferrum, Eumenol, heisse Bäder und Injectionen, Faradisation etc., erfolglos versucht. Sofort nachdem Oophorin gegeben war, trat die Menstruation ein und blieb längere Zeit, auch nach Aussetzen des Mittels regelmässig. Ein späteres Recidiv konnte wiederum nur durch Oophorin beseitigt werden.

Theil des Eierstocks ist, welcher der Ernährung des
Uterus und dem Zustandekommen der Menstruation
vorsteht, wird uns der schwankende Erfolg bei Oopho-
rinverabreichung klar: Nicht die ganze Eierstocksub-
stanz ist wahrscheinlich das nützliche Agens, sondern
ihr Gehalt an gelbem Körper, und von der Menge dieser
Substanz, die naturgemäss stark differirt, hängt der
Erfolg ab.

Diese Vermuthung forderte dazu auf, die gelben Körper isolirt
zu Organpräparaten zu verarbeiten. Bei der Kuh ist dies nicht
schwer, weil der meist in Einzahl vorhandene gelbe Körper über
wallnussgross wird und mehr als $^2/_3$ des Eierstocks für sich in
Anspruch nimmt; man kann ihn leicht, theils stumpf, theils mit
Scheere und Pincette herauspräpariren, im Trockenofen des Wassers
berauben, dann pulverisiren und mit irgend einem Vehikel zu
Tabletten comprimiren; an jedem Orte, wo ein Schlachthaus sich
befindet, wird man stets eine grössere Menge derartiger frischer
Präparate finden, weil ca. jeder vierte Eierstock einen gelben
Körper enthält. Solche Tabletten habe ich, weil ich die Wirkung
nicht kannte und Anfangs keine grossen Hoffnungen damit
verband, unterschiedslos bei verschiedenen vermuthlich primär-
ovariellen Erkrankungen verordnet, besonders bei Amenorrhoe zwecks
Herbeiführung der Menstruation und bei Dysmenorrhoe zur Milde-
rung der Schmerzen. Im Allgemeinen ohne Erfolg; einige Frauen
gaben einen solchen bei Dysmennorhoe an, den ich jedoch zum
Theil auf Suggestion oder auf den Zufall beziehe. Erst später
hatte ich Gelegenheit das Präparat bei Ausfallserscheinungen zu verordnen und war erstaunt über die Wirkung,
die in keinem einzigen Falle im Stiche liess. Ich notirte
vor Benutzung des Mittels genau die Beschwerden, speciell die
Zahl der Anfälle am Tage nnd besonders in der Nacht, weil
die Kranken durch die Anfälle in ihrer Nachtruhe gestört werden
und erwachen. Ich sagte den Frauen, dass das verordnete Mittel
neu und in der Wirkung noch unerprobt sei, und bat sie, sorgfältige
Notizen und Angaben zu machen und nicht etwa aus Gefälligkeit
die eventuelle Wirkung zu übertreiben. Ich gab 3 mal täglich 0,3
der getrockneten Corpus luteum-Substanz, die ich von
nun ab der Kürze wegen als „Luteïn" bezeichne; ich habe
daraufhin nie die geringste üble Wirkung gesehen, dagegen sank
alsbald die Zahl und Intensität der Anfälle am Tage stark herab,

und in der Nacht wurden die Kranken durch die Wallungen entweder nur einmal oder gar nicht aus dem Schlafe geweckt. Setzte ich das Mittel aus, so hörte häufig entweder bald oder nach einiger Zeit die Wirkung auf. Es handelt sich also um kein Heil-, sondern um ein symptomatisches Mittel. Man muss die Kranken während der kritischen Zeit mit Luteïn füttern, um dauernden Erfolg zu erzielen. Das ist jedoch kein Nachtheil, weil das Leiden sich selten über viele Jahre erstreckt, das Luteïn unschädlich ist, 2—3 Tabletten täglich genügen und ihr Preis[1]) nicht über den eines feineren Genussmittels hinausgeht. Die Frauen waren mit dem Erfolg so sehr zufrieden, dass selbst minder wohlhabende es sich von Zeit zu Zeit verschreiben liessen. Die Kranken machten häufig recht prägnante Angaben; so erklärt z. B. eine Patientin (No. 9), dass die kaum zu ertragenden Kopfschmerzen, die sie bisher alle vier Wochen an Stelle der Menstruation gehabt habe, jedes Mal nach Genuss von 1—2 Tabletten sofort verschwinden, fügte jedoch spontan hinzu, dass sie bei Kopfschmerzen ausser dieser Zeit durch das Mittel nicht die geringste Erleichterung verspüre. Bei folgenden Fällen von Ausfallserscheinungen habe ich Luteïntabletten verordnet.

1. Alwine K., Pkl. Journ. No. 987. 6. 1. 1902. Pat., 27 Jahre alt, vor 2½ Jahren wegen „Geschwulstbildung" castrirt, klagt seitdem über heftige Wallungen zum Kopf, Angstgefühl, Zittern und Herzklopfen. (Eine derartige überlaufende intensive Gesichtsröthung von über einer Minute Dauer wird von mir beobachtet.) Dieselben kommen alle 45 Minuten und sind so heftig, dass Pat. Nachts jedesmal erwacht. — Pat. hat viele Mittel erfolglos versucht, darunter auch Oophorin. Es wird Luteïn 0,3 dreimal täglich eine Tablette verordnet. Die Wirkung ist eine augenblickliche. Die Wallungen kommen seltener, sind viel schwächer, dauern kürzer (1—2 Secunden) und treten ohne Herzklopfen auf. Der Schlaf ist von da ab ungestört, sehr tief und gut bis 7 Uhr Morgens. — Nach Aussetzen des Mittels treten die Anfälle wieder häufiger, intensiver und auch des Nachts auf. Nach Anwendung von Luteïn II (s. u.) nicht die geringste Besserung, neuerliche Verabreichung von Luteïn I auf Bitte der Patientin führt wieder bedeutende Besserung herbei, schliesslich kommen nur noch Abends einige Anfälle, der Schlaf ist ausgezeichnet und ungestört. Die doppelte Dosis Luteïn lässt keinen Unterschied in der Wirkung erkennen. Vom 21. April ab keine Tabletten mehr. Am 5. Mai meldet Pat., dass sie sich vollkommen wohl fühle, keine Anfälle mehr habe und dass der Schlaf vorzüglich sei.

---

1) Die Apotheke Hygieia in Breslau, Tauentzienstrasse 33, giebt 100 Tabletten analog dem Oophorin für 4,50 Mk. ab.

2. Mathilde T., Prv.-Journ. 1901 No. 214, 24 Jahre alt, wird am 11. Juli 1901 wegen Pyosalpinx duplex von mir castrirt. 17. Januar 1902 erscheint Pat. wieder mit der Klage über Ausfallserscheinungen. — Luteïn 0,3 dreimal täglich eine Tablette. — Bei der nächsten Consultation am 25. 4. 1902 giebt sie an, dass es ihr besser gehe und dass sie deswegen seit vier Wochen die Tabletten nicht mehr zu nehmen brauche.

3. Marie J. Pkl. Journ. No. 1059, 30 Jahre, am 20 Februar 1900 doppelseitige Ovariotomie in unserer Klinik, kommt am 18. Februar 1902 mit Magenbeschwerden und giebt ausserdem auf Befragen an, dass sie täglich 4—6 Anfälle von überlaufender Hitze, Herzklopfen und Schweissausbruch habe, jedesmal ein paar Minuten lang; Nachts desgleichen, wobei sie etwa viermal erwacht. Es wird Luteïn 0,3 dreimal täglich eine Tablette verordnet. Am 12. 3. 1902 erscheint sie wieder und giebt an, dass sie nur mehr täglich 2 Anfälle ohne Schweissausbruch habe, Nachts wacht sie nur noch einmal auf. Verordnung von dreimal täglich zwei Tabletten. 22. 10. 1902. Pat. hat keine Tabletten mehr und seitdem wieder mehr Anfälle.

4. Pauline Sch. Pkl. Journ. No. 1088, 30 Jahre alt, Consultation am 6. 3. 02: Pat. hat viermal geboren, zuletzt vor zwei Jahren, stillte das letzte Kind 5/4 Jahre, seitdem klagt sie über Amenorrhoe und alle vier Wochen an Stelle der Menstruation über Fluor und Schmerzen. Dreimal täglich 0,3 Luteïn. Am 17. 3. giebt Pat. an, dass diesmal deutliche Besserung der Beschwerden zu bemerken gewesen sei.

5. Anna P. Pkl. Journ. No. 592, 27 Jahre alt, am 17. 7. 1901 vaginale Radicaloperation durch mich wegen doppelseitiger Adnextumoren. Von da ab volles Wohlbefinden, nur alle vier Wochen heftige Kopfschmerzen und Aufregungszustände. Phenacetin erweist sich erfolglos. Luteïn 0,3 dreimal täglich eine Tablette. Von da ab jedesmal nach einer Tablette sofortige Besserung bis zum vollständigen Wegbleiben der Symptome. Bei Weglassen der Tabletten neuere Verschlechterung. Die Tabletten werden daher weiter mit vollem Erfolge genommen. Gelegentliche Kopfschmerzen ausser der regelmässigen Zeit werden durch Luteïn nicht beeinflusst. Am 1. 11. 1902 erscheint Pat. wieder mit genau den gleichen Angaben und von da ab wiederholt und lässt sich das Mittel mehrfach neu verordnen.

6. Elisabeth W. Prv.-Journ. No. 144, 1902, 24 Jahre alt, kommt am 7.4.02 zur Consultation. Ein Partus vor neun Monaten, das Kind wurde nicht gestillt; Menstruation seitdem sehr schwach, regelmässig, vierwöchentlich. Pat. klagt über Blutandrang zum Kopf, überlaufende Hitze und Herzbeschwerden bei der Menstruation. Es besteht horizontale Retroversion, welche in Narkose behoben wird. Pessartherapie. Gegen die obengenannten Beschwerden wird später Luteïn verordnet, worauf dieselben vollkommen aufhören. Am 4. 11. 02 giebt Pat. an, dass sie von neuem vor der Menstruation Blutandrang zum Kopf, überlaufende Hitze und Herzbeklemmungen habe. — Auf neue Luteïnverordnung sofortige Wirkung.

7. Anna L. Pkl. Journ. No. 340, 46 Jahre alt. Pat. steht vom 30. 1. 1901 ab in Behandlung mit heftigen Blutungen in Folge climacterischer Endometritis und Retroflexio uteri. Auf Curettement und wiederholte Liquor ferri-Pinselung steht die Blutung nicht, daher wird am 2. 4. 1901 der Uterus in Narkose reponirt und die Höhle 20 Sec.

lang mit 120 ⁰ heissem Dampf kauterisirt. Von da ab steht die Blutung vollständig, die Menstruation tritt nicht mehr ein.   Am 8. 4. werden
der Pat. wegen Ausfallserscheinungen (Herzklopfen, Gesichtshyperämien)
Luteïntabletten in der üblichen Dosis verordnet; daraufhin verschwinden die Ausfallserscheinungen vollständig; bei der
letzten Consultation am 10. 9. 1902 besteht volles Wohlbefinden.

8. Emma K. Pkl. Journ. No. 1264. 30 Jahre alt. Wegen Sal-
pingo-Ooph. dpl. chronica (5 Jahre lang erfolglos von uns behandelt)
vaginale Radicaloperation am 18. 9. 02. Nach 14 Tagen mit glatter
Heilung entlassen. Pat. klagt am 21. 10. über viel Kopfschmerz und
mehrmals täglich überlaufende Hitze. Luteïn 0,3 dreimal täglich.
28. 10. Kopfschmerz nicht mehr so stechend. Anfälle von überlaufender
Hitze viel seltener und schwächer.

9. Marie P. Pkl. Journ. No. 440, 55 Jahre alt, Climax seit mehreren
Jahren. Am 1. 5. 1902 klagt Pat. über Wallungen und überlaufende Hitze
alle Viertelstunden. Luteïnverordnung. 17. 8. 1902 bedeutende
Besserung der Wallungen, die jetzt nur noch 2—3mal im Tage
auftreten.

10. Fanny B. Pkl. Journ. No. 1224, 52 Jahre alt, Climax seit sechs
Jahren. Faustgrosses, subseröses Myom in zwei Knollen. Klagen über
Schweissausbruch, überlaufende Hitze und Herzklopfen. Am 12. 5.
Luteïnverordnung. Pat. ist bisher nicht mehr erschienen.

11. Marie L. Pkl. Journ. No. 812, 46 Jahre alt, 8 Entbindungen,
zuletzt vor 7 Jahren. Pat. stillte nicht; Menstruation stets regulär, drei-
wöchentlich, letzte Menstruation vor 3 Monaten. Am 27. 5. 1902 erscheint Pat. und klagt über „Brausen" im Unterleib, Uebelkeiten und
Kopfschmerzen in Anfällen, durch die sie Nachts 2—3mal erweckt wird.
Verordnung von Luteïntabletten. Am 3. 6. 1902 sind die Kopfschmerzen verschwunden, das „Brausen" ist etwas gebessert.
Pat. schläft besser und wacht Nachts nur einmal auf. Luteïn-
gebrauch fortzusetzen. Am 3. 7. bedeutende Besserung, un-
gestörter, sehr guter Schlaf, sämmtliche oben erwähnte
Beschwerden haben aufgehört. Am 8. 7.: Seit 4—5 Tagen
hat Frau L. den Gebrauch der Tabletten ausgesetzt und
seitdem haben sich die Beschwerden ein wenig wieder ein-
gestellt.

12. Franziska H. Pkl. Journ. No. 1288, 40 Jahre alt, vor 7 Jahren
anderwärts beide Eierstöcke entfernt, seitdem Amenorrhoe. Pat. klagt
am 14. 6. 1902 über Hitze und Herzklopfen. Uterus atrophisch. Luteïntabletten. Am 26. 6. etwas Besserung. Auf Ersuchen erscheint Pat.
am 18. 10. wieder und erklärt, dass die Anfälle selten (Tags ca. 3mal,
Nachts gar nicht) und so schwach seien, dass sie dadurch nicht wesentlich sich gestört sehe.

13. Dorothea D. Prv.-Journ. No. 249, 50 Jahre alt, 30 Jahre ver-
heirathet, 0p. Climax seit 12 Jahren; am 25. 7. 1902 klagt sie über
überlaufende Hitze, ca. 3—4mal Tags und 1—2mal Nachts. Luteïntabletten. Pat. ist bisher nicht wieder erschienen.

14. Helene K. Pkl. Journ. 1309, 40 Jahre alt, 1892 Castration
anderwärts. Am 25. 6. 1902 erscheint Pat. mit Klagen über typische
Ausfallserscheinungen. Seit der Operation besteht Amenorrhoe. — Es
findet sich Castrationsatrophie des Uterus und Adipositas universalis.
Verordnung dreimal täglich eine Luteïntablette 0,3. Am 4. 7. erheb-

liche Besserung bezüglich der Ausfallserscheinungen; die
Anfälle von überlaufender Hitze vorher fast alle Stunden,
desgleichen Nachts, jetzt höchstens einmal täglich, Nachts
gar nicht.

15. Helene v. S. Prv.-Journ. No. 335, 1902, 41 Jahre alt. Am
9. 7. 1902 wegen Myom bei schwerer Myocarditis Castration. Prima
intentio. Am 25. 10. klagt Pat. über häufige Schweissausbrüche seit
der Operation. Luteïntabletten 0,3 dreimal täglich eine Tablette. Am
3. 11. die Schweissausbrüche sofort gebessert und nach Gebrauch von 50 Tabletten ganz beseitigt. — Neuerdings, seit Aussetzen des Mittels, wieder etwas eingetreten.

Ausser diesen, wie man sieht, durchweg soweit festgestellt
[13 von 15][1]) erfolgreichen Fällen, habe ich bei weiteren 36 Frauen
mit verschiedenartigen, andern gynäkologischen Beschwerden Luteïn
verordnet, mit sehr wechselndem Erfolge; nicht den geringsten er-
zielte ich gegen Lactationsatrophie und andere Formen von
Atrophie und Amenorrhoe. Ich glaube, dass die Wirkung sich
auf die sog. Ausfallserscheinungen im wesentlichen be-
schränken wird. Da diese Symptome ungemein quälen und
bisher oft nicht wesentlich gebessert werden konnten (bis sie sich
von selbst bisweilen erst nach langer Zeit verloren), so können wir
auch mit diesem Resultat zufrieden sein. Zu mancher sonst
indicirten Radicaloperation werden wir uns jetzt leichter ent-
schliessen, als früher, wo wir glauben mussten, den Teufel durch
den Belzebub zu vertreiben.

Möglicherweise lässt sich durch Vergrösserung der Dosis oder
Herstellung des Präparates von andern Thieren oder auf andere
Weise, z. B. durch Extrahiren mit Wasser oder Kochsalzlösung[2]),
oder Einverleibung auf anderem Wege die Wirkung noch steigern.

---

1) Anmerkung bei der Correctur: Inzwischen habe ich das Mittel
in folgendem weiteren Falle angewendet. 16. Beate Sch. Polikl. Journ.-
No. 1490. 46 J. alt. Am 30. 10. 02 vag. Hysterectomie wegen kindskopfgrossen
intraligam. Myom mit Morcellement. — Glatter Verlauf. Am 6. 12. 02 giebt
Pat. an, dass sie zur Zeit, wo sonst die Menstruation eintrat, überlaufende
Hitze und Schwindelanfälle von 10 Min. Dauer alle $1/_2$—2 Stunden verspüre.
Auf Luteïn sofortige Besserung, nur 2—3 Anfälle täglich von ganz
kurzer Dauer. — 4 Wochen später geringe Hitzewallungen, die
auf Luteïntabletten sofort verschwanden.

2) Bei Glycerinextracten müsste man Vorsicht walten lassen. Neumann
und Vas (96) haben in einer sorgfältigen, experimentellen Arbeit nachgewiesen,
dass Verabreichung der Ovarialsubstanz an castrirte oder normale Hündinnen,
selbst in sehr grossen Dosen, unschädlich ist, dagegen mit Glycerin herge-
stellte Extracte starken Eiweisszerfall hervorrufen.

Erfahrungen hierüber habe ich nicht. Am besten wäre es, das Präparat vom menschlichen Corpus luteum herzustellen, wenn nicht ethische und andere Schwierigkeiten im Wege ständen. Wir nahmen die Substanz des gelben Körpers von Kühen, die nicht tragend waren und haben dieselbe mit dem Apotheker zunächst als „Luteïn I" vereinbart. Auch von dem Corpus luteum graviditatis der Kuh habe ich Tabletten herstellen lassen (Luteïn II), davon jedoch erklärlicher Weise keine Wirkung bei Ausfallserscheinungen gesehn. Eher könnte man sich von diesem Präparat Wirkungen bei gewissen Graviditätsbeschwerden versprechen, doch kann ich darüber noch keine zuverlässigen Angaben machen.

Ich verwende das Präparat „Luteïn I" gegen Ausfallserscheinungen mit nur gutem Erfolge seit über einem Jahr und glaube nach einigem Zögern (man kann mit neuen Präparaten nicht vorsichtig genug sein) mit meinen Resultaten an die Oeffentlichkeit treten zu sollen. Ich weiss wohl, wie zahlreich die Schwierigkeiten sind, die sich der objectiven Beurtheilung eines neuen Heilpräparates entgegenstellen, und wie gross die Abneigung der Praktiker ist, auf jede Empfehlung hin in eine Prüfung einzugehen, weil sie durch üble Erfahrung allesammt misstrauisch gemacht sind. Dennoch glaube ich nunmehr, mich zu einer Empfehlung des Luteïn herbeilassen zu dürfen und thue es zunächst nur in diesem streng wissenschaftlichen Organ, um das Urtheil der engeren Fachgenossen[1]) abzuwarten, ehe ich das Luteïn einem grösseren Aerztepublicum empfehle. Der einzelne kann zu leicht bezüglich der Wirkung eines Mittes bei einer immerhin beschränkten Anzahl von Kranken sich täuschen, und anfänglich gute Erfolge können sich später in schlechte umwandeln; ich stelle daher ohne jede Präsumtion anheim, das Mittel zu versuchen und kann das um so eher, weil es

1. sicher unschädlich,
2. auf rationeller, theoretischer Basis aufgebaut ist,
3. weil andere, zuverlässige Mittel gegen Ausfallserscheinungen fehlen.

Wie oben gesagt, hängt keineswegs die Richtigkeit meines Corpus luteum-Gesetzes von dem Erfolg des Mittels ab, denn Theorie und Praxis müssen sich nicht decken. Jedenfalls ist es

---

1) Mehrere Kliniker haben sich bereits Tabletten senden lassen. Bis jetzt habe ich nur günstiges gehört.

erfreulich, wenn, wie hier, ein neues physiologisches Gesetz sogleich zu therapeutischen Erfolgen verwerthbar ist.

Der gelbe Körper, eine Drüse, die in den Blutkreislauf Substanzen absondert, welche dem Uterus der geschlechtsreifen Frau das für diesen nöthige Ernährungsplus zuführen, lässt sich zu einer Substanz verarbeiten, welche den der Ovarialfunction beraubten Frauen innerlich verabreicht, die lästigen Ausfallserscheinungen zu mildern geeignet ist.

Wir können die Menstruation durch Ausschalten der Corpora lutea zwar isolirt unterdrücken und den Uterus zur Atrophie bringen, wir können aber nicht umgekehrt durch innerliche Verabreichung von Luteïn, die Atrophie heilen, die Menstruation hervorrufen. Wohl aber können wir gewisse, zweifellos an die fehlende Function des Corpus luteum gebundene Symptome durch Verabreichung einer derartigen Substanz beseitigen. (Wir haben hier ein Analogon zu unseren Experimenten am Kaninchen, die in der Transplantation der Corpora lutea beim graviden Thier bestanden. Niemals konnten wir dadurch die Fruchtkammern, deren Lebensfaden durch Wegnahme der gelben Körper unterbunden war, retten; wenn aber das Luteïngewebe nach einigen Tagen anderwärts eingeheilt war, wurde der Rückgang der Schwangerschaft ganz deutlich und erheblich verzögert. Ebenso konnten wir durch das Luteïn niemals die Menstruation hervorrufen, welche durch Fehlen eines gelben Körpers unausgelöst blieb; die dadurch entstehenden subjectiven Symptome hingegen konnten wir mildern oder coupiren.) —

Dieses ist die Hauptnutzanwendung, welche wir für die Therapie aus unserem Gesetz gezogen haben.

Commentary on Classic Paper No.12

Climacterium and postmenopause are periods in which women can have serious complaints and the symptoms can be traced back to the loss of ovarian function, i.e. to a decrease in estrogen production. These complaints, which can be summarized as flushes, transpiration and atrophy of the vaginal wall, are often also accompanied by symptomatology of the central nervous system including depression, fatigue and general malaise.

The first clinician to recognize this symptomatology in women and to attempt to develop a form of treatment that would bring symptomatic relief was Fraenkel. In 1903, Fraenkel[1] published the results of his experiments, carried out in animals, especially rabbits, into the function of the corpus luteum and its hormonal activity. In this publication (Section III: Hauptteil), he also reported on climacteric complaints in castrated or aged women, which he relieved by giving them dry extracts of corpora lutea of cows, sheep or pigs (three times daily).

1. Fraenkel, L. (1903). Die Funktion des Corpus Luteum. *Arch. Gynäkol.*, **68**, 438

Timing of the perimenopause

The studies of Treloar and colleagues[2] have provided a greater understanding of when the climacteric menopausal and perimenopausal periods occur and the variability that occurs. In their study, they collected information on intraperson variation in menstrual interval over a period of 22 754 calendar years. Treloar and colleagues were interested in the mathematical/statistical analysis of the interval length of the human menstrual cycle.

2. Treloar, A.E., Boynton, R.E., Behn, B.G. and Brown, B.W. (1967). Variation of the human menstrual cycle through reproductive life. *Int. J. Fertil.*, **12**, 77

Knowing the centiles of these intervals, it is clear that approximately 8 years before the last vaginal bleeding (i.e. menopause) the interval centiles begin to become wider than between 20–40 years of chronological age. This transitional period is known as the climacteric period, while postmenopause starts after the last vaginal bleeding. During the transitional phase, unusually long and short cycles are often present.

Throughout life, there is a continuous depletion of primary ovarian follicles that begins during fetal life and continues until the menopause. In perimenopausal women, histological examination of the ovaries shows a reduced number of primary follicles with few Graafian follicles or corpora lutea[3].

3. Costoff, A. (1974). In Greenblatt, R.B., Mahesh, V.B. and Mc Donough, P.S. (eds.) *The Menopausal Syndrome.* (New York: Medcom Press)

After menopause, there are no follicles left in the ovary[4]. Vaginal bleeding can occur at the end of an inadequate luteal phase or after a peak of estradiol without ovulation or adequate corpus luteum formation.

4. Gosden, R.G. (1987). Follicular status at menopause. *Hum. Reprod.*, **2**, 617

Hormonal changes associated with the perimenopause

Endocrine transition

5. Albright, F. (1936). Studies on ovarian dysfunction. III. The menopause. *Endocrinology*, **20**, 24

Increased secretion of pituitary gonadotropins and decreased secretion of estrogens have been recognized as characteristics of the menopause[5].

6. Sherman, B.M., West, J.H. and Korenman, S.G. (1976). The menopausal transition: analysis of LH, FSH, estradiol and progesterone concentrations during menstrual cycles of older women. *J. Clin. Endocrinol. Metab.*, **42**, 629

Sherman and colleagues[6] investigated levels of luteinizing hormone (LH), follicle stimulating hormone (FSH), estradiol and progesterone during menstrual cycles in older women. They found that, during the perimenopausal period, estradiol levels were lower and FSH levels increased. FSH levels were found to increase 10–20-fold, whilst levels of LH showed a threefold increase, reaching a maximum 3 years after menopause.

The concentrations of FSH were elevated strikingly in the early follicular phase and fell as estradiol increased during follicular maturation. The LH concentrations during these cycles were indistinguishable from those observed in younger women. These elevated concentrations of FSH may be indicative of a reduced number of functional, residual ovarian follicles.

7. Longcope, C. (1971). Metabolic clearance and blood production rates of estrogens in postmenopausal women. *Am. J. Obstet. Gynecol.*, **11**, 778

Sherman and colleagues concluded: *'Cycles of variable length during the menopausal transition may be due either to irregular maturation of residual follicles with diminished responsiveness to gonadotropin stimulation, or to anovulatory vaginal bleeding that may follow estrogen withdrawal without evidence of corpus luteum function. The observation of elevated FSH concentrations and normal LH levels in perimenopausal women emphasizes the complexity of the hypothalamic–pituitary–ovarian regulatory system and suggests that LH and FSH are modulated independently at the level of the pituitary.'*

8. Ross, G.T., Cargille, C.M., Lipsett, M.B., Rayford, P.L., Marshall, J.R., Strott, C.A. and Rodbard, D. (1970). Pituitary and gonadal hormones in women during spontaneous and induced ovulatory cycles. *Rec. Prog. Horm. Res.*, **26**, 162

The lower estradiol secretion during both the follicular and luteal phases in perimenopausal women must reflect diminished capacity of residual follicles to secrete estradiol, since the clearance rate of estradiol in pre- and postmenopausal women is similar[7]. The divergent FSH and LH levels might also initiate the maturation of one or more follicles in the subsequent cycle[8].

9. Yen, S.S.C. and Tsai, C.C. (1971). The effect of ovariectomy on gonadotrophin release. *J. Clin. Invest.*, **50**, 1149

In cases of premenopausal oophorectomy, a more rapid increase in FSH than LH has also been demonstrated[9].

Extraglandular estrogen

Pentti K. Siiteri and Paul C. MacDonald[10] focused on the possibility of extraglandular formation of estrogens. They postulated that estrogen might arise in women either by glandular secretion of adrenals and ovaries or be produced by extraglandular aromatization of circulating C19 precursors.

By injecting tracer doses of estrone and androstenedione intravenously by continuous infusion and measuring plasma and urinary concentrations, they were able to calculate the extent of conversion of plasma androstenedione to estrone, the production rate of androstenedione, the production of estrone from androstenedione, total estrone production, and plasma production of estrone derived from androstenedione (see figure below).

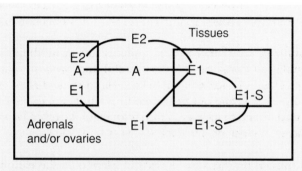

Possible sources of estrone (E1) and estradiol (E2) in postmenopausal women. E1-S = estrone sulfate and A = androstenedione. Adapted from Siiteri and MacDonald (1973)[10] with permission

In these studies, Siiteri and MacDonald demonstrated that in premenopausal women the extraglandular formation of estrone from androstenedione results in a relatively constant basal level of estrogen (40 µg estrone/day) upon which the fluctuating secretion of estradiol by the developing follicles or corpus luteum is superimposed.

In postmenopausal women the average conversion of plasma androstenedione to estrone was about 2.7% as compared to 1.3% in premenopausal women. The major source of estrogen in the postmenopausal female was derived from the peripheral formation of estrone from plasma androstenedione and not from ovarian or adrenal secretion. They also found that, in cases of postmenopausal bleeding, the extent of conversion of androstenedione to estrone or estrone sulfate was approximately twice (5.1%) that obtained from studies performed in non-bleeding patients.

The extent of conversion of androstenedione to estrone was found to correlate with body weight in postmenopausal women (correlation coefficient = 0.74). Although estrone is a weaker estrogen than estradiol, both hormones can bind to the cytoplasmic receptor and prolonged exposure to either estrone or estradiol may lead ultimately to abnormal endometrial proliferation and neoplasia.

10. Siiteri, P.K. and MacDonald, P.C. (1973). Role of extraglandular estrogens in human endocrinology. In Greep, R.O. and Astwood, E.B. (eds.) *Handbook of Physiology*, Section 7, Vol II, Part 1, p.615. (New York: Oxford University Press)

11. Longcope, C., Pratt, J.H., Schneider, S.H. and Finberg, S.E. (1978). Aromatization of androgens by muscle and adipose tissue *in vivo*. *J. Clin. Endocrinol. Metab.*, **46**, 14

The observation of extragonadal aromatization was also documented by Longcope and colleagues[11] who used isotope studies in the forearm. The muscle accounted for 25–30% of the total extragonadal aromatization of androgens to estrogens in men, and adipose tissue for 10–15% . This fractional rate of extragonadal aromatization is greater in men than in women. This finding could explain the fact that heavier, overweight women experience less climacteric (hypoestrogenic) complaints than underweight women.

Ovarian testosterone production

12. Judd, H.L., Judd, G.E., Lucas, W.E. and Yen, S.S.C. (1974). Endocrine function of the post-menopausal ovary: concentration of androgens and estrogens in ovarian and peripheral vein blood. *J. Clin. Endocrinol. Metab.*, **39**, 1020

In 1974, Judd and co-workers[12] published the results of their study into endocrine function of the postmenopausal ovary. At the time of total hysterectomy and bilateral salpingo-oophorectomy, blood samples were taken from each ovarian vein and from the antecubital vein.

The mean ovarian testosterone level was found to be 15-fold higher than the peripheral concentration. This suggests that the ovarian secretion of testosterone contributes significantly to the peripheral circulating hormone.

The mean ovarian level for androstenedione was four- to fivefold higher than peripheral levels; however, the magnitude of the difference for estradiol and estrone was small and would only account for minimal ovarian estrogen secretion. These findings are consistent with the demonstration of peripheral conversion of androstenedione to estrone.

13. Mattingly, R.F. and Huang, W.Y. (1969). Steroidogenesis of the menopausal and post-menopausal ovary. *Am. J. Obstet. Gynecol.*, **103**, 679

Using specific histochemical enzyme techniques, Mattingly and Huang[13] have shown that ovarian androgen production takes place in the hilus and stroma theca cells. From this study, one is reminded that the postmenopausal human ovary is not an inactive organ, probably due to the drive of the elevated gonadotropins.

The preponderance of circulating estradiol in postmenopausal women is derived from the peripheral conversion of estrone, which in turn is the product of the peripheral aromatization of circulating androgens.

Perimenopausal complaints

14. Tilt, E.J. (1870). *The Change of Life in Health and Disease*, 3rd edn. (London: J. Churchill)

In 1870, 135 conditions were ascribed to the 'change of life' ranging from aortic pulsation, hysterical flatulence, blind piles and boils in the seat through to pseudonarcotism, temporary deafness, melancholia and hot flushes[14]. Today, the main symptoms associated with the menopause about which patients complain are hot flushes and atrophy of the urogenital tract.

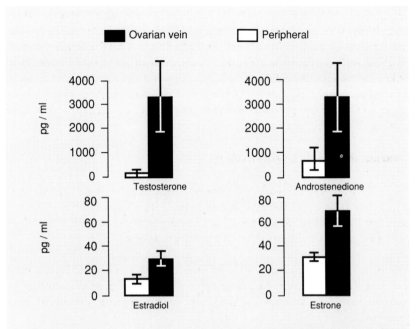

The mean ± SE serum testosterone, androstenedione, estradiol, and estrone levels in peripheral and ovarian veins in ten postmenopausal women. Endocrine function of the postmenopausal ovary: concentration of androgens and estrogens in ovarian and peripheral blood. Adapted from Judd and colleagues (1974)[12] with permission. Copyright, The Endocrine Society

Hot flushes

Hot flushes are characteristically climacteric or postmenopausal complaints and are felt by women as a dermovascular reaction. An association between ovarian failure (estrogen withdrawal) and flushes has long been postulated. In 1941, Reynolds[15] investigated this reaction and noted a rapid rise of skin temperature lasting for 10–15 minutes which was noticed by the patient in the rising temperature phase only. A change in finger volume was also noted. Collet[16] observed not only a rise in skin temperature but also an increase in basal metabolic rate and respiratory rate.

In a study by Molnar[17], changes in temperature were noted on the surfaces of fingers and cheeks, with an increase of 0.7°C during flushes. At the same time, a corresponding decrease in temperature in the vagina and rectum of 0.6°C was recorded. The onset of the flush was observed to be accompanied by tachycardia and sweating. Nesheim and Seatre have demonstrated that the flush is associated with an increase in the velocity of blood flow in radial, temporal and lateral thoracic arteries[18].

15. Reynolds, S.R.M. (1941). Dermovascular action of estrogen, the ovarian follicular hormone. J. Invest. Dermatol., **4**, 7

16. Collet, M.E. (1948). Basal metabolism at the menopause. J. Appl. Physiol., **1**, 629

17. Molnar, G.W. (1975). Body temperatures during menopausal hot flushes. J. Appl. Physiol., **38**, 499

18. Nesheim, B.J. and Seatre, T. (1982). Changes in skin blood flow and body temperatures during climacteric hot flushes. Maturitas, **4**, 49

19. Tataryn, I.V., Meldrum, D.R., Lu, K. H., Frumar, A.M. and Judd, H.L. (1979). LH, FSH and skin temperature during the menopausal hot flash. *J. Clin. Endocrinol. Metab.*, **49**, 152

20. Casper, R.F., Yen, S.S.C. and Wilkes, M.M. (1979). Menopausal flush episodes: link with pulsatile luteinizing hormone secretion. *Science*, **205**, 823

21. Studd, J., Chakravardi, S. and Oram, D. (1977). The climacteric. *Clin. Obstet. Gynaecol.*, **4**, 3

22. Paul, S.M. and Axelrod, J. (1977). Catechol estrogen – presence in brain and endocrine tissue. *Science*, **197**, 657

23. Davies, I.J., Naftolin, F., Ryan, K.J., Fishman, J. and Siu, J. (1975). The affinity of catecholestrogen for estrogen receptors in the pituitary and anterior hypothalamus of the rat. *Endocrinology*, **97**, 554

24. Adashi, E.Y., Rakoff, J., Divers, W., Fishman, J. and Yen, S.S.C. (1979). The effect of acutely administered 2-hydroxyestrone on the release of gonadotropins and prolactin before and after estrogen priming in hypogonadal women. *Life Sci.*, **25**, 2051

Hormonal changes during hot flushes indicate that these are associated with a pulsatile increase of LH[19,20] (see figure below). No changes have been found in plasma catecholamines or prolactin[20]. Because hot flushes can also occur after hypophysectomy, the hot flush must be mediated by centers above the pituitary.

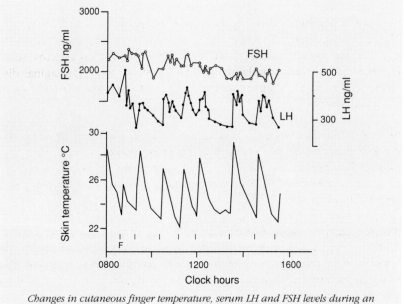

Changes in cutaneous finger temperature, serum LH and FSH levels during an 8-hour study in a postmenopausal patient. The vertical bars indicate subjective hot flushes. Adapted from Tataryn and colleagues (1979)[19] with permission

The autonomic nervous system seems to play a predominant role because there is a similarity between the symptoms of pheochromocytoma and menopausal flushes[21]. An attractive hypothesis that forms a link with estrogens and catecholamines is the possible relationship between 2-hydroxylated estrogens and catecholamines. These 2-hydroxylated estrogens have two hydroxyl groups on the benzene ring thus forming a catechol ring. Because of this arrangement, the 2-hydroxylated estrogens act as catecholestrogens.

A concentration of catecholestrogens ten times higher than the parent estrogen has been found in the pituitary and hypothalamus by Paul and Axelrod[22], which interacts with estrogen receptors[23]. Infusion of catecholestrogens in hypogonadal women pretreated with estrogen resulted in an initial rise in serum LH followed by a suppression of gonadotropins[24]. Thus, a link was established between catecholestrogens and gonadotropins.

Norepinephrine plays an important role as a neurotransmitter, in the release of gonadotropin releasing hormone (GnRH) and central thermoregulation[25]. Although the pathophysiology of perimenopausal hot flushes is not fully understood, the mechanisms involved point to an alteration of the central autonomic nervous system.

It seems likely that, due to an estrogen decline, catecholestrogens decrease. Conversion to norepinephrine leads to increased GnRH secretion, with an accompanying downward setting of the central thermostat, activating heat-loss mechanisms with impaired vasomotor control.

Atrophy of the urogenital tract

During the perimenopause, hypoestrogenicity results in vaginal changes. The vaginal epithelium becomes thinner, rugae and fornices become less marked and vaginal secretion becomes less than in the reproductive state. Common associated complaints include irritation, burning, vaginal discharge and even bleeding which can lead also to dyspareunia and loss of sexual interest[26].

In 44% of postmenopausal Scandinavian women aged approximately 60 years of age, dryness of the vagina and urinary problems were considered to be indications for estrogen therapy. Estrogen replacement restored the glycogen deposition in the vaginal epithelium restoring vaginal acidity and bacterial flora[27].

Atrophic changes can also affect the epithelium of the bladder and urethra resulting in pollakiuria, dysuria, urge incontinence and infections of the lower urinary tract. A study by Tapp and Cardozo[28] demonstrated that estrogen therapy can influence fibroblast activity, thus improving urethral and urogenital collagen content and urethral functions. Estrogen receptors are present both in vaginal and urethral epithelium and respond to the exogenous administration of estrogens.

Osteoporosis

In 1941, Fuller Albright and colleagues[29] pointed out the existence of postmenopausal osteoporosis and described its clinical features. They concluded that *'calcium deficiencies of the skeleton due to metabolic disorders are divided into those due to increased resorption of bone and those due to decreased formation of bone'*. Albright noted a constant tendency of osteoporosis (too little formation of bone) to occur in women after the menopause and a beneficial effect of estrogen therapy on the retention of calcium in this condition.

Osteoporosis is a disease characterized by low bone mass and microarchitectural deterioration of bone tissue leading to enhanced bone fragility and a consequent increase in fracture risk. Osteoporotic fractures affect mainly the spine, the distal radius and the proximal femur. It is estimated that, in the USA, osteoporosis affects more than 20 million individuals with 1.5 million fractures/year, including 250000 hip fractures. Of these, 90% are postmenopausal women.

Several studies have demonstrated that estrogen therapy prevents osteoporosis and, thereby, fractures. In one long-term prospective study of 1000

25. Cox, B. and Lomax, P. (1977). Pharmacologic control of temperature regulation. *Annu. Rev. Pharmacol. Toxicol.*, **17**, 341

26. Semmens, J.P., Tsai, C.C., Semmens, E.C. and Loadholt, C.B. (1985). Effects of estrogen therapy on vaginal physiology during menopause. *Obstet. Gynecol.*, **66**, 15

27. Privette, M., Cade, R., Peterson, J. and Mars, D. (1988). Prevention of recurrent urinary tract infections in postmenopausal women. *Nephron*, **50**, 24

28. Tapp, A.J.S. and Cardozo, L. (1986). The postmenopausal bladder. *Br. J. Hosp. Med.*, **35**, 20

29. Albright, F., Smith, P.H. and Richardson, A.M. (1941). Postmenopausal osteoporosis. *J. Am. Med. Assoc.*, **116**, 2465

30. Burch, J.C., Byrd, B.V.
and Vaughn, W.K. (1978).
Results of estrogen
treatment in one thousand
hysterectomised women
for 14.318 years.
*Annu. Rev. Pharmacol.
Toxicol.*, **18**, 164

31. Nachtigall, L.E.,
Nachtigall, R.H.,
Nachtigall, R.D. and
Beckman, E. (1979).
Estrogen replacement
therapy. 1. A 1-year
prospective study in the
relation to osteoporosis.
Obstet. Gynecol., **53**, 277

32. Eriksen, E.F., Colvard,
D.S., Berg, N.J., Graham,
M.L., Mann, K.G.,
Spelsberg, ThC. and
Riggs, B.L. (1988).
Evidence of estrogen
receptors in normal human
osteoblast-like cells.
Science, **241**, 84

33. Jilka, R.L., Hangoc, G.,
Girasole, Passeri, G.,
Williams, D.C., Abrams,
J.S., Boyce, B.,
Broxmeyer, H. and
Manolagas, S.C. (1992).
Increased osteoclasts
development after estro-
gen loss: medication by
interleukin-6.
Science, **257**, 88

34. Lindsay, R., McKay
Hart, D. and Kraszewski,
A. (1980). Prospective
double-blind trial of synthetic steroid (Org OD 14)
for preventing post-
menopausal osteoporosis.
Br. Med. J., **280**, 1207

hysterectomized women treated with estrogens for 15 years, wrist fractures were reduced by 70% from the expected rate[30].

The recommendations of the National Institutes of Health Consensus Development Conference on osteoporosis stated that estrogen therapy is the best prevention of osteoporosis. They also recommended that calcium supplementation should begin 10 years before menopause at a dose of 1000 mg daily and that exercise should be taken, as this can help to prevent osteoporosis.

The combination of estrogen–progestin therapy also increases bone formation. In a 10-year double-blind study, significant differences were observed with the placebo group on bone density, when therapy started less than 3 years after menopause[31].

It is now known that different factors control bone mass, including genetics, lifestyle, nutrition and medication. Loss of estrogen in the postmenopausal state leads to excessive osteoclast activity.

There is now evidence that estrogen receptors are present in osteoblasts[32] giving a scientific basis for the effect of estrogens on bone mass. It is thought possible that there is a direct effect of estrogen on these cells and this may explain the fact that estrogen is the major hormone responsible for the maintenance of bone mass.

The effects of estrogen may be mediated also by changes in the concentration of systemic and local factors. Possibilities include calcitonin, growth factors, prostaglandins, tumor necrosis factors, insulin-like growth factors and interleukin[33].

A new approach towards the prevention of postmenopausal osteoporosis was published by Lindsay and colleagues[34] in 1980. They proposed the administration of a steroid, Org OD 14 or Livial®, that has weak progestational, estrogenic and central effects. This steroid has a positive significant effect on bone mineral content without causing endometrial stimulation.

However, reports on prevention and treatment of osteoporosis tend to be in favor of estrogen treatment, but also consider the relevance of factors such as diet, calcium supplements, exercise, calcitonin and biphosphonates.

Estrogen therapy

In 1963, Wilson and Wilson[35] claimed estrogen therapy to be essential '*from puberty to the grave*'. This rather exaggerated statement promoted estrogens as a panacea for all postmenopausal problems and illnesses and became known in the USA as the 'Wilson-treatment'. Even the problems of ageing would be solved: 'feminine forever'.

In 1938, long before the studies of Wilson and Wilson, Bishop[36], with a more scientific approach, had advocated replacement therapy when castration in young women was performed.

Estrogens can be administered orally, intramuscularly or by subcutaneous implantation. A novel way of administering estrogens was introduced by Schenkel[37] in 1981. He developed percutaneous administration of estradiol which gives the advantage that the first pass through the liver could be circumvented, so avoiding possible liver damage.

Many reports have been published to demonstrate the benefits of treatment of perimenopausal symptomatology with estrogens and this form of treatment can be cost-effective. Weinstein[38] reported that estrogen treatment is highly cost-effective in women who had a hysterectomy and in women who were at risk of osteoporosis. In symptomatic women who did not have a hysterectomy and who were at average risk for osteoporosis, the cost-effectiveness of treatment was dependent on the importance attached to the attenuation of symptoms.

Cancer risk

In 1946, Fremont-Smith and colleagues[39] raised the suspicion, in a case-report, that estrogen stimulation may be a key factor in the development of endometrial cancer.

Jensen and co-workers[40] studied 105 cases of endometrial carcinoma and, although no controls were used, the authors found that menopause commenced late, often preceded by periods of metrorrhagia and less frequently accompanied by hot flushes. Often, treatment with estrogens was recorded.

Carcinoma of the breast will strike approximately one woman in ten. The incidence of breast cancer increases steadily and steeply in relation to age and is the leading cause of death in women (see figure below).

Studies of both endometrial and breast cancer in estrogen users have suggested a modest association with estrogen therapy. The association between estrogens and carcinoma of the breast was, however, less than with endometrial carcinoma[41].

Studies on the addition of progestin in estrogen therapy show inconsistent results. Progestogens decrease estrogen receptors in endometrial cells and induce estradiol dehydrogenase and isocitrate activity, which is the mechanism whereby cells metabolize estrogens. Breast cells are not cyclically shed by progesterone and an eventual protective mechanism (if any) awaits further studies at the cellular level. Combined estrogen–progestin

35. Wilson, R.A. and Wilson, ThA. (1963). The fate of the non-treated postmenopausal woman: a plea for the maintenance of adequate estrogen from puberty to the grave. J. Am. Geriatr. Soc., 11, 347

36. Bishop, P.M.F. (1938). A clinical experiment in oestrin therapy. Br. Med. J., 1, 939

37. Schenkel, L. (1981). A new method of controlled percutaneous oestradiol administration. Rev. Fr. Endocr. Clin., 22, 269

38. Weinstein, M.C. (1980). Estrogen use in postmenopausal women – costs, risks and benefits. N. Engl. J. Med., 303, 308

39. Fremont-Smith, M., Meigs, J.V., Graham, R.M. and Gilbert, H.H. (1946). Cancer of endometrium and prolonged estrogen therapy. J. Am. Med. Assoc., 131, 805

40. Jensen, E., Denmark, V. and Ostergaard, E. (1954). Clinical studies concerning the relationship of estrogens to the development of cancer of the corpus uteri. Am. J. Obstet. Gynecol., 67, 1094

41. Gambrell, R.D. Jr. (1986). The menopause. Invest. Radiol., 21, 369

42. Geusens, P., Dequeker, J., Gielen, J. and Schot, L.P.C. (1991). Non-linear increase in vertebral density induced by a synthetic steroid (Org OD14) in women with established osteoporosis. *Maturitas,* **13**, 155

43. Grady, D., Cummings, S.R., Petitti, D., Rubin, S.M. and Audet, A.M. (1992). Hormone therapy to prevent disease and prolong life in post-menopausal women. *Ann. Intern. Med.,* **117**, 106

therapy has, however, been shown to reduce the risk of endometrial hyperplasia and cancer. For the future, it seems wise to direct research directly to those steroids that act specifically on bone metabolism. The development of Livial®, which has an effect on cortical and trabecular bone, represents a start in that direction[42].

A review of the benefits and risks of hormone therapy in postmenopausal women by Grady and colleagues[43] concluded that estrogen therapy decreases the risk of coronary heart disease and of hip fracture. Long-term estrogen therapy, if unopposed by progestogen, increased the risk for endometrial cancer and might be associated with a small increase in risk for breast cancer.

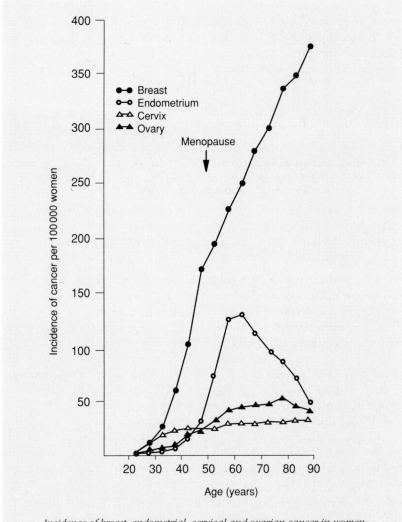

Incidence of breast, endometrial, cervical and ovarian cancer in women according to age. Adapted from Gambrell (1986)[41] with permission

Prevention of osteoporosis

From both a clinical and cost–benefit point of view, it is certainly worthwhile to prevent osteoporosis where possible, because of the increased incidence of fractures of the spine, wrist and hip and the associated risk of mortality that hip fractures, in particular, carry in old age.

In a cross-over study by Christiansen and co-workers[44] which compared the effects of estrogen–progestogen therapy with a placebo, the bone mineral content was found to increase during the 3 years of combination hormone therapy but continued to decline in the placebo-treated group.

44. Christiansen, C., Riis, B.J. and Rodbro, P. (1981). Prediction of rapid bone loss in post-menopausal women. *Lancet*, **1**, 459

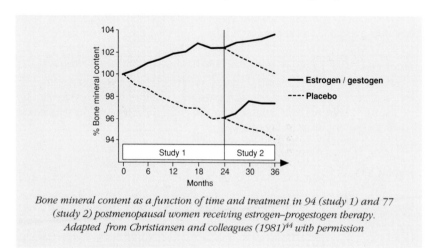

Bone mineral content as a function of time and treatment in 94 (study 1) and 77 (study 2) postmenopausal women receiving estrogen–progestogen therapy. Adapted from Christiansen and colleagues (1981)[44] with permission

Prevention of cardiovascular disease

The most well-known study on the risk of cardiovascular disease and the menopause is the 'Framingham study'. This prospective study, under the guidance of the National Institutes of Health, Bethesda, Maryland, has offered a thorough standardized cardiovascular examination biennially since 1948, with a satisfactory follow-up.

Of the 2873 women in the original Framingham cohort, 1972 were identified as having a natural menopause and 752 a surgical menopause by the tenth examination. The incidence of cardiovascular disease in postmenopausal women was observed to be higher than in premenopausal women. This higher risk could not be accounted for by other known risk factors.

A later report from the same Framingham population found an increased risk for coronary heart disease, especially among estrogen users. However, in a survey of over one hundred thousand nurses, a 70% reduction of cardiovascular disease was found among users of estrogens[45]. A 10-year follow-up from the study concluded that the overall relative risk of coronary disease in women taking estrogens was 0.56 and that there was less benefit in women taken more than 1.25 mg of estrogen daily[46].

45. Stampfer, M.J., Willett, W.C., Colditz, G.A., Rosner, B., Speizer, F.E. and Hennekens, C.H. (1985). A prospective study of postmenopausal estrogen therapy and coronary heart disease. *N. Engl. J. Med.*, **313**, 1044

46. Stampfer, M.J., Colditz, G.A., Willett, W.C., Manson, J.E., Rosner, B., Speizer, F.E. and Hennekens, C.H. (1991). Postmenopausal estrogen therapy and cardiovascular disease: ten year follow-up from the Nurses' Health Study. *N. Engl. J. Med.*, **325**, 756

47. Stampfer, M.J. and Colditz, G. A. (1991). Estrogen replacement therapy and coronary heart disease: a quantitative assessment of the epidemiologic evidence. *Prev. Med.*, **20**, 47

48. The Coronary Drug Project Research Group (1970). The coronary drug project: initial findings leading to modifications of its research protocol. *J. Am. Med. Assoc.*, **214**, 1303

49. Nabulsi, A. A., Folsom, A. R., White, A., Patsch, W., Weiss, G., Wu, K.K. and Szklo, M. (1993) Association of hormone replacement therapy with various risk factors in post-menopausal women. *N. Engl. J. Med.*, **328**, 1069

More than 20 studies have been conducted to assess the effects of estrogen therapy on coronary heart disease. The prospective studies revealed a protective effect of estrogen replacement therapy; however, controversy exists as to the benefit of estrogen therapy for preventive reasons[47]. Men given 5mg of conjugated estrogens daily experienced a twofold increase in the number of non-fatal myocardial infarctions, a threefold increase in the number of pulmonary emboli and one and a half times the number of deaths as did the placebo group[48].

Much emphasis has been given in the literature to the observation that estrogens decrease the serum level of low-density lipoprotein (LDL) cholesterol and increase the level of high density lipoprotein (HDL) cholesterol. Total and LDL-cholesterol levels are lower in premenopausal women but after menopause they rise rapidly.

The relationship between cholesterol levels and death from cardiovascular disease seems to be strong and the recent study of Nabulsi and colleagues[49] suggests that the effect of estrogens on lipoprotein levels may be beneficial. However, the mechanism of estrogen protection for cardiovascular disease remains, as yet, unclear.

Epilogue

Menopause can be a major event in a woman's life and marks the last vaginal bleeding, thus indicating the end of reproductive capacity. Some years before menopause the interval length of the menstrual cycle starts varying, announcing the premenopausal or climacteric state. The work of Ludwig Fraenkel in the early 1900s marked the beginning of the research into this clinical area and contributed significantly to our knowledge of the menopause and its management.

The endocrine transition through menopause is characterized by increasing FSH levels, a sign of oocyte depletion. Also LH levels increase up to about one-third of those of FSH. Ovarian hormonal activity, however, does not stop after menopause; most notably, androstenedione is produced which forms a source (together with the adrenal) for peripheral aromatization in adipose and muscle tissue to estrone. The extent of this conversion is correlated with body weight.

In the perimenopause, women may experience complaints, most notably estrogen-dependent flushes producing a rise in skin temperature. Flushes are preceded by LH release and catecholestrogens seem to be involved with the autonomic dysregulation in the brain that can occur in the perimenopausal state. Hypoestrogenicity can lead also to atrophic changes in the urogenital system, leading to complaints of dyspareunia, vaginal discharge or urinary problems, as well as problems due to osteoporosis.

Current research is focused on the management of osteoporosis and an understanding of this aspect of the menopause continues to increase. Future research must also measure the cost–benefit ratios of hormone replacement, as well as quality of life.

Summary of references

1. Fraenkel, L. (1903). Die Funktion des Corpus Luteum. *Arch. Gynäkol.,* **68**, 438
2. Treloar, A.E., Boynton, R.E., Behn, B.G. and Brown, B.W. (1967). Variation of the human menstrual cycle through reproductive life. *Int. J. Fertil.,* **12**, 77
3.' Costoff, A. (1974). In Greenblatt, R.B., Mahesh, V.B. and Mc Donough, P.S. (eds.) *The Menopausal Syndrome.* (New York: Medcom Press)
4. Gosden, R.G. (1987). Follicular status at menopause. *Hum. Reprod.,* **2**, 617
5. Albright, F. (1936). Studies on ovarian dysfunction. III. The menopause. *Endocrinology,* **20**, 24
6. Sherman, B.M., West, J.H. and Korenman, S.G. (1976). The menopausal transition analysis of LH, FSH, estradiol and progesterone concentration during menstrual cycles of older women. *J. Clin. Endocrinol. Metab.,* **42**, 629
7. Longcope, C. (1971). Metabolic clearance and blood production rates of estrogens in postmenopausal women. *Am. J. Obstet. Gynecol.,* **11**, 778
8. Ross, G.T., Cargille, C.M., Lipsett, M.B., Rayford, P.L., Marshall, J.R., Strott, C.A. and Rodbard, D. (1970). Pituitary and gonadal hormones in women during spontaneous and induced ovulatory cycles. *Rec. Prog. Horm. Res.,* **26**, 162
9. Yen, S.S.C. and Tsai, C.C. (1971). The effect of ovariectomy on gonadotrophin release. *J. Clin. Invest.,* **50**, 1149
10. Siiteri, P.K. and MacDonald, P.C. (1973). Role of extraglandular estrogens in human endocrinology. In Greep, R.O. and Astwood, E.B. (eds.) *Handbook of Physiology,* Section 7, Vol II, Part 1, p.615. (New York: Oxford University Press)
11. Longcope, C., Pratt, J.H., Schneider, S.H. and Finberg, S.E. (1978). Aromatization of androgens by muscle and adipose tissue *in vivo. J. Clin. Endocrinol. Metab.,* **46**, 146
12. Judd, H.L., Judd, G.E., Lucas, W.E. and Yen, S.S.C. (1974). Endocrine function of the postmenopausal ovary: concentration of androgens and estrogens in ovarian and peripheral vein blood. *J. Clin. Endocrinol. Metab.,* **39**, 1020
13. Mattingly, R.F. and Huang, W.Y. (1969). Steroidogenesis of the menopausal and postmenopausal ovary. *Am. J. Obstet. Gynecol.,* **103**, 679
14. Tilt, E.J. (1870). *The Change of Life in Health and Disease,* 3rd edn. (London: J. Churchill)

15. Reynolds, S.R.M. (1941). Dermovascular action of estrogen, the ovarian follicular hormone. *J. Invest. Dermatol.*, **4**, 7

16. Collet, M.E. (1948). Basal metabolism at the menopause. *J. Appl. Physiol.*, **1**, 629

17. Molnar, G.W. (1975). Body temperatures during menopausal hot flushes. *J. Appl. Physiol.*, **38**, 499

18. Nesheim, B.J. and Seatre, T. (1982). Changes in skin blood flow and body temperatures during climacteric hot flushes. *Maturitas*, **4**, 49

19. Tataryn, I.V., Meldrum, D.R., Lu, K. H., Frumar, A. M. and Judd, H.L. (1979). LH, FSH and skin temperature during the menopausal hot flash. *J. Clin. Endocrinol. Metab.*, **49**, 152

20. Casper, R.F., Yen, S.S.C. and Wilkes, M.M. (1979). Menopausal flush episodes: link with pulsatile luteinizing hormone secretion. *Science.*, **205**, 823

21. Studd, J., Chakravardi, S. and Oram, D. (1977). The climacteric. *Clin. Obstet. Gynaecol.*, **4**, 3

22. Paul, S.M. and Axelrod, J. (1977). Catechol estrogen–presence in brain and endocrine tissue. *Science*, **197**, 657

23. Davies, I.J., Naftolin, F., Ryan, K.J., Fishman, J. and Siu, J. (1975). The affinity of catecholestrogen for estrogen receptors in the pituitary and anterior hypothalamus of the rat. *Endocrinology*, **97**, 554

24. Adashi, E.Y., Rakoff, J., Divers, W., Fishman, J. and Yen, S.S.C. (1979). The effect of acutely administered 2-hydroxyestrone on the release of gonadotropins and prolactin before and after estrogen priming in hypogonadal women. *Life Sci.*, **25**, 2051

25. Cox, B. and Lomax, P. (1977). Pharmacologic control of temperature regulation. *Annu. Rev. Pharmacol. Toxicol.*, **17**, 341

26. Semmens, J.P., Tsai, C.C., Semmens, E.C. and Loadholt, C.B. (1985). Effects of estrogen therapy on vaginal physiology during menopause. *Obstet. Gynecol.*, **66**, 15

27. Privette, M., Cade, R., Peterson, J. and Mars, D. (1988). Prevention of recurrent urinary tract infections in postmenopausal women. *Nephron*, **50**, 24

28. Tapp, A.J.S. and Cardozo, L. (1986). The postmenopausal bladder. *Br. J. Hosp. Med.*, **35**, 20

29. Albright, F., Smith, P.H. and Richardson, A.M. (1941). Postmenopausal osteoporosis. *J. Am. Med. Assoc.*, **116**, 2465

30. Burch, J.C., Byrd, B.V. and Vaughn, W.K. (1978). Results of estrogen treatment in one thousand hysterectomised women for 14.318 years. *Annu. Rev. Pharmacol. Toxicol.*, **18**, 164

31. Nachtigall, L.E., Nachtigall, R.H., Nachtigall, R.D. and Beckman, E. (1979). Estrogen replacement therapy. 1. A 1-year prospective study in the relation to osteoporosis. *Obstet. Gynecol.*, **53**, 277

32. Eriksen, E.F., Colvard, D.S., Berg, N.J., Graham, M.L., Mann, K.G., Spelsberg, ThC. and Riggs, B.L. (1988). Evidence of estrogen receptors in normal human osteoblast-like cells. *Science*, **241**, 84

33. Jilka, R.L., Hangoc, G., Girasole, Passeri, G., Williams, D.C., Abrams, J.S., Boyce, B., Broxmeyer, H. and Manolagas, S.C. (1992). Increased osteoclasts development after estrogen loss: medication by interleukin-6. *Science*, **257**, 88

34. Lindsay, R., McKay Hart, D. and Kraszewski, A. (1980). Prospective double-blind trial of synthetic steroid (Org OD 14) for preventing post-menopausal osteoporosis. *Br. Med. J.,* **280**, 1207

35. Wilson, R.A. and Wilson, ThA. (1963). The fate of the non-treated post-menopausal woman: a plea for the maintenance of adequate estrogen from puberty to the grave. *J. Am. Geriatr. Soc.,* **11**, 347

36. Bishop, P.M.F. (1938). A clinical experiment in oestrin therapy. *Br. Med. J.,* **1**, 939

37. Schenkel, L. (1981). A new method of controlled percutaneous oestradiol administration. *Rev. Fr. Endocr. Clin.,* **22**, 269

38. Weinstein, M.C. (1980). Estrogen use in postmenopausal women – costs, risks and benefits. *N. Engl. J. Med.,* **303**, 308

39. Fremont-Smith, M., Meigs, J.V., Graham, R.M. and Gilbert, H.H. (1946). Cancer of endometrium and prolonged estrogen therapy. *J. Am. Med. Assoc.,* **131**, 805

40. Jensen, E., Denmark, V. and Ostergaard, E. (1954). Clinical studies concerning the relationship of estrogens to the development of cancer of the corpus uteri. *Am. J. Obstet. Gynecol.,* **67**, 1094

41. Gambrell, R.D. Jr. (1986). The menopause. *Invest. Radiol.,* **21**, 369

42. Geusens, P., Dequeker, J., Gielen, J. and Schot, L.P.C. (1991). Non-linear increase in vertebral density induced by a synthetic steroid (Org OD 14) in women with established osteoporosis. *Maturitas,* **13**, 155

43. Grady, D., Cummings, S.R., Petitti, D., Rubin, S.M. and Audet, A.M. (1992). Hormone therapy to prevent disease and prolong life in post menopausal women. *Ann. Intern. Med.,* **117**, 106

44. Christiansen, C., Riis, B.J. and Rodbro, P. (1981). Prediction of rapid bone loss in postmenopausal women. *Lancet,* **1**, 459

45. Stampfer, M.J., Willett, W.C., Colditz, G.A., Rosner, B., Speizer, F.E. and Hennekens, C.H. (1985). A prospective study of postmenopausal estrogen therapy and coronary heart disease. *N. Engl. J. Med.,* **313**, 1044

46. Stampfer, M.J., Colditz, G.A., Willett, W.C., Manson, J.E., Rosner, B., Speizer, F.E. and Hennekens, C.H. (1991). Postmenopausal estrogen therapy and cardiovascular disease: ten year follow-up from the Nurses' Health Study. *N. Engl. J. Med.,* **325**, 756

47. Stampfer, M.J. and Colditz, G. A. (1991). Estrogen replacement therapy and coronary heart disease: a quantitative assessment of the epidemio-logic evidence. *Prev. Med.,* **20**, 47

48. The Coronary Drug Project Research Group (1970). The coronary drug project: initial findings leading to modifications of its research protocol. *J. Am. Med. Assoc.,* **214**, 1303

49. Nabulsi, A. A., Folsom, A. R., White, A., Patsch, W., Weiss, G., Wu, K.K. and Szklo, M. (1993). Association of hormone replacement therapy with various risk factors in postmenopausal women. *N. Engl. J. Med.,* **328**, 1069

Index of authors

Numbers in italics refer to figures.

Index of commentaries

Numbers in italics refer to figures.

WZ 40 Esk